Psychocutaneous Diseases

Gianni Angelini • Domenico Bonamonte
Anna Belloni Fortina • Iria Neri • Luca Stingeni
Editors

Psychocutaneous Diseases

A Clinical Dermatological Approach

Springer

Editors
Gianni Angelini
Professor of Dermatology
University "Aldo Moro"
Bari, Italy

Anna Belloni Fortina
Professor of Dermatology and Venereology,
Department of Women's and Child's Health
University of Padua
Padova, Italy

Luca Stingeni
Department of Medicine and Surgery
University of Perugia
Perugia, Italy

Domenico Bonamonte
Unit of Dermatology, Department
of Precision and Regenerative Medicine
and Ionian Area
A.O.U.C. Policlinico of Bari – University
"Aldo Moro"
Bari, Italy

Iria Neri
Dermatology Unit
Policlinic S.Orsola-Malpighi
Bologna, Italy

ISBN 978-3-031-70295-2 ISBN 978-3-031-70296-9 (eBook)
https://doi.org/10.1007/978-3-031-70296-9

This Springer imprint is published by the registered company Springer Nature Switzerland AG
The registered company address is: Gewerbestrasse 11, 6330 Cham, Switzerland

Preface

Psychocutaneous disorders represent one of the most challenging problems in clinical medicine. Recent studies have shown that 35–40% of dermatological patients have psychiatric/psychological comorbidities that impact the outcome of their skin disease.

The skin and central nervous system arise from the same embryonal tissue, the ectoderm, which is the reason for the continual two-way interaction between the skin and the psyche. Adopting a highly simplified model, the diseases that involve skin and psyche can be grouped as follows: "somatopsychic" disorders (when the body is primarily involved, and mental disturbances are a consequence of the psychical damage) and "psychosomatic" disorders (when psychological or psychiatric disorders lie at the origin of the problem, while the somatic disturbances are the secondary effect).

Undoubtedly, psychocutaneous diseases are in the great majority of cases correlated to mental disorders, and so they are generally included among psychiatric disorders. This is also because the treatment primarily targets the mental rather than the dermatological problem. Despite these valid reasons, in this work we have preferred to adopt a classification that highlights the dermatological aspect of the problem, starting from the various skin pictures that can, in turn, be induced by or else induce psychiatric or psychological disturbances.

The management of patients with psychocutaneous disorders is quite challenging: a joint liaison between psychiatry and dermatology (that has led to the origin of psychodermatology), however, has proven very helpful to patients.

The purpose of this work, resulting in decades of field experience and of the joint efforts of both dermatologists and psychiatrists, is to clarify the terminology of these disorders and, above all, to analyze their clinical characteristics in detail, the first and pivotal sign of suspicion and diagnosis. The topic is completed by the addition of chapters by psychiatric specialists, in order to address pathogenetic problems and therapeutic guidelines, as well as contributions that integrate the approach with medico-legal expertise. It is hoped that this manual will offer a helpful tool for dermatologists, psychologists, psychiatrists and forensic doctors, will provide a handy update on this complex medical area, and in particular, an in-depth analysis of the clinical aspects of this important field of psychodermatology.

Bari, Italy Gianni Angelini
Bari, Italy Domenico Bonamonte
Padova, Italy Anna Belloni Fortina
Bologna, Italy Iria Neri
Perugia, Italy Luca Stingeni

Acknowledgments

This book has been produced, thanks to the valuable contributions of colleagues, infantile neuropsychiatrists, and forensic doctors, to whom we extend our sincerest gratitude.

We would like to thank the publishers Springer-Verlag (Berlin) and Edizioni Minerva Medica (Turin, Italy), editor of the Italian Journal of Dermatology and Venereology, John Wiley & Sons A/S, editor of the journal Contact Dermatitis, and Lippincott Williams & Wilkins, editor of the journal Medicine (Baltimore), for kindly authorizing the reproduction of various figures.

Finally, we are grateful to Springer-Verlag for their assiduous commitment to producing this volume.

Gianni Angelini, M.D.
Domenico Bonamonte, M.D., Ph.D.
Anna Belloni Fortina, M.D.
Iria Neri, M.D.
Luca Stingeni, M.D.

Contents

Contributors

Gianni Angelini Dermatology, University of Bari "Aldo Moro", Bari, Italy

Anna Belloni Fortina Pediatric Dermatology Regional Center, Department of Medicine (DIMED) and Department of Women's and Children's Health (SDB), University of Padua, Padua, Italy

Marcello Benevento Department of Interdisciplinary Medicine, University of Bari "Aldo Moro", Bari, Italy

Domenico Bonamonte Department of Precision and Regenerative Medicine and Ionian Area, University of Bari "Aldo Moro", Bari, Italy

Luigi Buongiorno Department of Interdisciplinary Medicine, University of Bari "Aldo Moro", Bari, Italy

Francesca Caroppo Department of Woman and Child Health and Department of Medicine, University of Padua, Padua, Italy

Elisa Cecchini Department of Medicine and Surgery, Dermatology Section, University of Perugia, Perugia, Italy

Marco Adriano Chessa Department of Experimental, Diagnostic and Specialty Medicine, University of Bologna, Bologna, Italy

Davide Ferorelli Department of Interdisciplinary Medicine, University of Bari "Aldo Moro", Bari, Italy

Alessandra Gabellone Department of Translational Biomedicine and Neuroscience, University of Bari "Aldo Moro", Bari, Italy

Katharina Hansel Department of Medicine and Surgery, Dermatology Section, University of Perugia, Perugia, Italy

Gabriele Mandarelli Department of Interdisciplinary Medicine, University of Bari "Aldo Moro", Bari, Italy

Aurora De Marco Department of Precision and Regenerative Medicine and Ionian Area, University of Bari "Aldo Moro", Bari, Italy

Lucia Margari Department of Precision and Regenerative Medicine and Ionian Area, University of Bari "Aldo Moro", Bari, Italy

Lucia Marzulli Department of Translational Biomedicine and Neuroscience, University of Bari "Aldo Moro", Bari, Italy

Emilia Matera Department of Precision and Regenerative Medicine and Ionian Area, University of Bari "Aldo Moro", Bari, Italy

Iria Neri Dermatology Unit, Department of Experimental, Diagnostic and Specialty Medicine, University of Bologna, Bologna, Italy

Dermatology Unit, IRCCS Azienda Ospedaliero-Universitaria di Bologna, Bologna, Italy

Maria Giuseppina Petruzzelli Department of Translational Biomedicine and Neuroscience, University of Bari "Aldo Moro", Bari, Italy

Biagio Solarino Department of Interdisciplinary Medicine, University of Bari "Aldo Moro", Bari, Italy

Luca Stingeni Department of Medicine and Surgery, Dermatology Section, University of Perugia, Perugia, Italy

Annalucia Virdi Department of Experimental, Diagnostic and Specialty Medicine, University of Bologna, Bologna, Italy

Chapter 1
Psychodermatology: When Psyche and Skin Interact

Lucia Margari, Alessandra Gabellone, Lucia Marzulli, Emilia Matera, and Maria Giuseppina Petruzzelli

1.1 Definition

Psychodermatology is a rapidly growing medical specialty that results from the merging of two medical specialties: psychiatry and dermatology (Fig. 1.1). Psychodermatology studies the biological basis and clinical expression of the bidirectional interaction between skin and psyche [1].

There is no single, globally accepted definition of psychodermatology. Synonyms for psychodermatology include "mind and skin medicine," "skin and mind medicine," "sensory neuronal dermatology," "psycho-somatic dermatology," "psychosomatic medicine," "cutaneo-somatic dermatology," and "cutaneo-somatic medicine" [2].

L. Margari (✉) · E. Matera
Department of Precision and Regenerative Medicine and Ionian Area (DiMePRe-J), University of Bari "Aldo Moro", Bari, Italy
e-mail: lucia.margari@uniba.it; emilia.matera@uniba.it

A. Gabellone · L. Marzulli · M. G. Petruzzelli
Department of Translational Biomedicine and Neuroscience (DiBraiN), University of Bari "Aldo Moro", Bari, Italy
e-mail: alessandra.gabellone@uniba.it; lucia.marzulli@uniba.it; maria.petruzzelli@uniba.it

G. Angelini et al. (eds.), *Psychocutaneous Diseases*,
https://doi.org/10.1007/978-3-031-70296-9_1

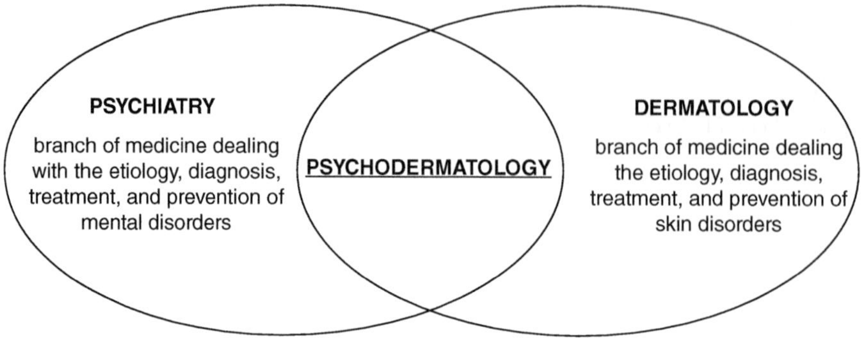

Fig. 1.1 Psychodermatology: a branch of medicine resulting from the merging of psychiatry and dermatology

1.2 History of Psychodermatology

Psychodermatology has gained momentum and interest among medical disciplines in recent years, even though its origins go back a long way, as philosophers and physicians described the first psychodermatological cases in ancient times [3, 4]. The first case described in history seems to date back to the eighteenth century B.C. and concerns a Persian prince who developed a skin condition (compatible with what we now call "psoriasis") due to the stress he felt about his imminent succession to the royal throne [5]. In the fourth century B.C., Hippocrates described cases of people who had pulled out their hair due to stress, describing a clinical picture that corresponds to what we know today as "trichotillomania" [6]. In the same century, Aristotle recognized the role of the inseparability of the mind and the skin, considering them as two complementary and inseparable entities [3]. Anecdotal cases are also reported in sacred texts. Descriptions of trichotillomania were mentioned in the Bible [3, 7], and the ancient Buddhist texts transmit the story of a woman whom Buddha taught to control her anger to improve her skin disease [8]. More recently, in the eighteenth century, the dermatologist Robert Willan described a patient who was convinced he had skin parasites that were causing him harm (describing the condition we would now call "delusional parasitosis") [3]. Interest in this disorder continued in the following centuries. In the twentieth century, the neurologist Karl Axel Ekbom studied the difference between insect phobia and delusional parasitosis, which was later definitively defined in 1946 with this terminology [3]. In recent centuries, the close connection between skin and mind has been increasingly explored. In his book, the dermatologist William James Erasmus Wilson described some the so-called skin neurosis" (such as alopecia areata, hyperhidrosis, pruritus, and delirious infestation) and investigated the relationship between these manifestations and depressive and anxious states [3, 9]. In 1933, the dermatologist John Thornton Ingram stated that the skin is an extension of the mind and that, consequently, an assessment of the external condition of the skin should be performed to obtain a complete evaluation of a person's personality [10].

1.3 Fields of Interest of Psychodermatology

Psychodermatology deals with:

1. primary dermatological disorders with secondary psychiatric implications (e.g., atopic eczema, psoriasis, vitiligo, alopecia areata, albinism);
2. primary psychiatric disorders with secondary dermatological manifestations (e.g., obsessive-compulsive disorder including skin picking disorder and trichotillomania; somatic symptom disorders including factitious disorder with artifact dermatitis; non-suicidal self-injury; self-injury associated with autism spectrum disorder, intellectual disability, psychosis with delirium of parasitosis);
3. secondary dermatological disorders associated with treatments for psychiatric disorders (e.g., lithium may be associated with psoriasis or acne; fluoxetine, lithium, valproic acid may be associated with alopecia);
4. psychiatric disorders associated with treatments for dermatological disorders (e.g., isotretinoin and methotrexate may be associated with mood disorders; minocycline may be associated with depersonalization; dapsone and hydroxychloroquine may be associated with psychosis) [2, 11].

1.4 Current Subspecialties in Psychodermatology

To date, psychodermatology has gained such interest that the following subspecialties are recognized within it [12]:

- *pediatric psychodermatology*, which is specifically concerned with the assessment and comprehensive treatment of psychodermatologic manifestations in children and adolescents [13];
- *geriatric psychodermatology*, which addresses psychodermatologic pathologies in the elderly population and also examines the psychological impact of advancing age on the quality of life of geriatric patients [14];
- *trichopsychodermatology*, which addresses the etiopathogenetic, psychological, and social aspects of both hair loss and excessive hair growth, as well as the impact of these conditions on the quality of life of those affected [15];
- *psychodermato-oncology*, which focuses on the psychological impact of skin cancer and the role of stress in the development of skin cancer. It is worth noting that skin cancer is the only type of cancer that is immediately visible externally (as a cancerous lesion or as disfigurement resulting from previous surgery to remove it). This, together with the feeling of guilt for not having prevented it and the fear of death, can cause anxiety and depression in these particularly vulnerable individuals [16];
- *cosmetic psychodermatology*, a new science that aims to evaluate the psychological aspects, expectations, and previous experiences of patients who increasingly undergo cosmetic procedures [17];

- *tropical psychodermatology*, which deals with tropical skin diseases (infectious or non-infectious), the psychological and social aspects associated with them, and the resulting impact on the quality of life of those affected [18];
- *sports psychodermatology*, which deals specifically with skin diseases in athletes (such as infections, aberrant growths, and trauma) and the resulting psychological and social implications [19];
- *environmental psychodermatology*, which studies the interaction between skin, environment, and stress factors (biological, physical, and chemical) and evaluates their impact on the quality of life of affected patients [20].

1.5 Pathophysiology

The connection between skin and psyche is bidirectional and complex. In summary, as shown in Fig. 1.2, chronic exogenous stressors, such as psychological ones, may play a role in the development of primary psychiatric disorders that may also have secondary dermatologic manifestations. Similarly, chronic physical stress can lead to primary dermatologic disorders with secondary psychiatric effects. Like exogenous stress, endogenous stress conditions (e.g., hormonal changes or autoimmune disorders) can also affect the development and duration of psychodermatological disorders, potentially affecting both the skin and nervous system. Regardless of the pathogenic noxa, the manifestations that affect one organ end up having repercussions on the other, creating a vicious circle that inextricably links psyche and skin.

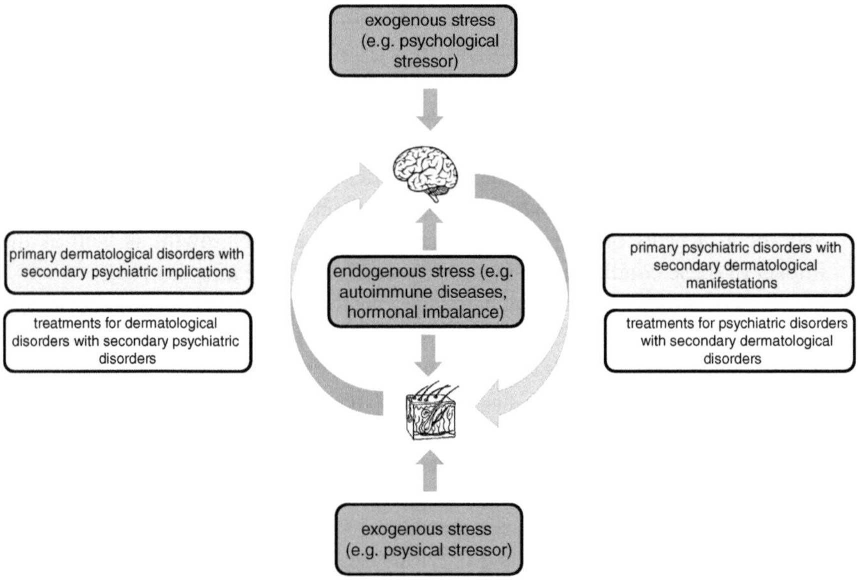

Fig. 1.2 The bidirectional connection between skin and psyche and the fields of interest of psychodermatology

For example, a patient can get dermatosis due to a stressful event and at the same time be stressed due to dermatosis.

The relationship between skin and brain begins in the embryonic period, as both organs arise from the same germ layer, the embryonic ectoderm. The ectodermis differentiates to form the epidermis (including the skin appendages) and the nervous system (brain, spine, and peripheral nerves, including the free nerve endings in the skin) [21]. The brain and skin not only share a common origin, but also a development influenced by the same hormones and neurotransmitters. The interaction between these two organs continues throughout life and is so complex that it is often difficult to distinguish in which of the two organs a problem first occurs that inevitably affects the other [22]. Various studies have been and are being conducted to determine the cause-and-effect relationship and to identify the pathophysiology of psychodermatological disorders. Over the past 30 years, research has shown that stress plays an important role in the development and exacerbation of these problems [23, 24]. This hypothesis seems to have been confirmed during the recent Covid 19 pandemic, a highly stressful event that saw an increase in alopecia, psoriasis, and urticaria [25–28]. Psychological and physical stress is physiologically associated with the activation of two main axes: the hormonal pathway, called the hypothalamic-pituitary-adrenal (HPA) axis [24, 29] and the nervous pathway, which is therefore more immediate, called the sympathetic-adrenal-medullary axis (SAM) [30] (see Fig. 1.3).

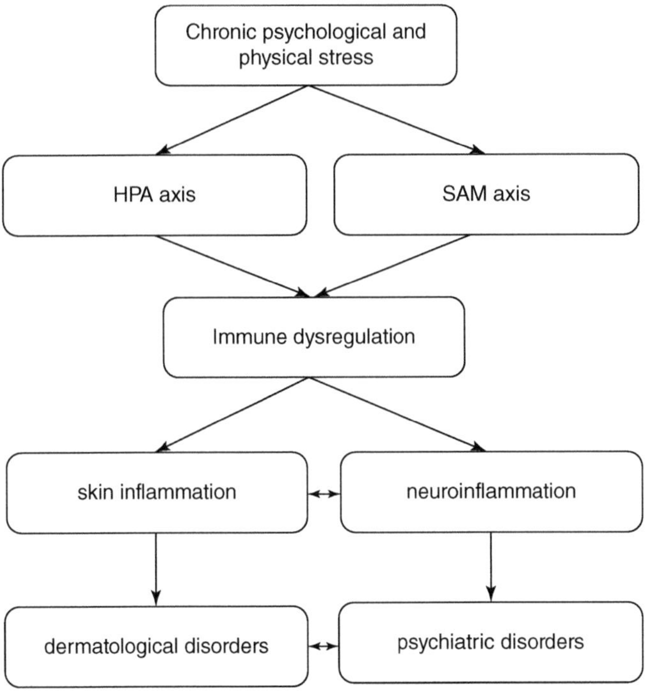

Fig. 1.3 Pathogenesis of dermatological and psychiatric disorders due to chronic stress. HPA hypothalamic-pituitary-adrenal, SAM sympathetic-adrenal-medullary

1.5.1 The HPA Axis

The HPA axis includes central and peripheral cutaneous components.

Under stress conditions, at the level of the central HPA axis, neurons in the hypothalamus secrete corticotropin-releasing hormone (CRH) into the hypothalamic-hypophyseal portal circulation. CRH is transported to the anterior pituitary where it stimulates the secretion of adrenocorticotropic hormone (ACTH), also called adrenocorticotropin or corticotropin. Through the bloodstream, ACTH in turn reaches the adrenal cortex and stimulates the production of glucocorticoids (GCs), including cortisol [31]. Cortisol, also known as stress hormones, when transiently released, supports the homeostasis of the organism in the face of a threat by stimulating catabolic pathways (and acting on the metabolism of proteins, lipids, and carbohydrates), promoting glycogenesis, increasing immune activity, stimulating the production of catecholamines, and increasing cardiovascular tone to support any physical exertion. In addition, cortisol inhibits the release of its precursors through a negative feedback mechanism (it acts on the pituitary gland by inhibiting further release of ACTH, and on the hypothalamus by inhibiting further release of CRH). After cessation of the acute stress event, there is rapid depletion of the hormones, whereas the increase in the duration and magnitude of the release of cortisol and catecholamines in chronic stress leads to desensitization of the receptors and consequent dysfunction of the HPA axis. This dysfunction also affects the immune system, mainly in an immunosuppressive manner [12, 32]. Namely, catecholamines and cortisol inhibit lymphocyte proliferation, the activity of antigen-presenting cells and macrophages, the production of some interleukins, and mediate the differentiation of T-helper (Th)1 cells into Th2 cells, to the detriment of Th1 cells. This shifts the balance toward humoral immunity and activates B cells, eosinophils, and mast cells, leading to an enhanced inflammatory and allergic response [33, 34] (Fig. 1.4).

Similar to this central HPA axis, there is also a peripheral cutaneous HPA axis in which CRH, ACTH, and their receptors are produced in skin cells [35–37]. Acute stress therefore also leads to the activation of this peripheral HPA axis, resulting in an increase in endogenous hormones. CRH is produced by several local cells, including keratinocytes, melanocytes, and mast cells. In mast cells, CRH triggers degranulation and increases vascular permeability, which promotes inflammation. In melanocytes and local fibroblasts, CRH leads to the production of ACTH, which promotes the formation of Th2 cytokines. However, in chronic stress, a persistent Th2 cytokine profile acts as a negative feedback loop to regulate HPA axis activity [24].

1.5.2 SAM Axis

In addition to activation of the central and peripheral HPA axis, stress also leads to activation of the SAM axis. SAM is a neuroendocrine system that provides a direct connection between the brain and the adrenal medulla via fibers of the sympathetic

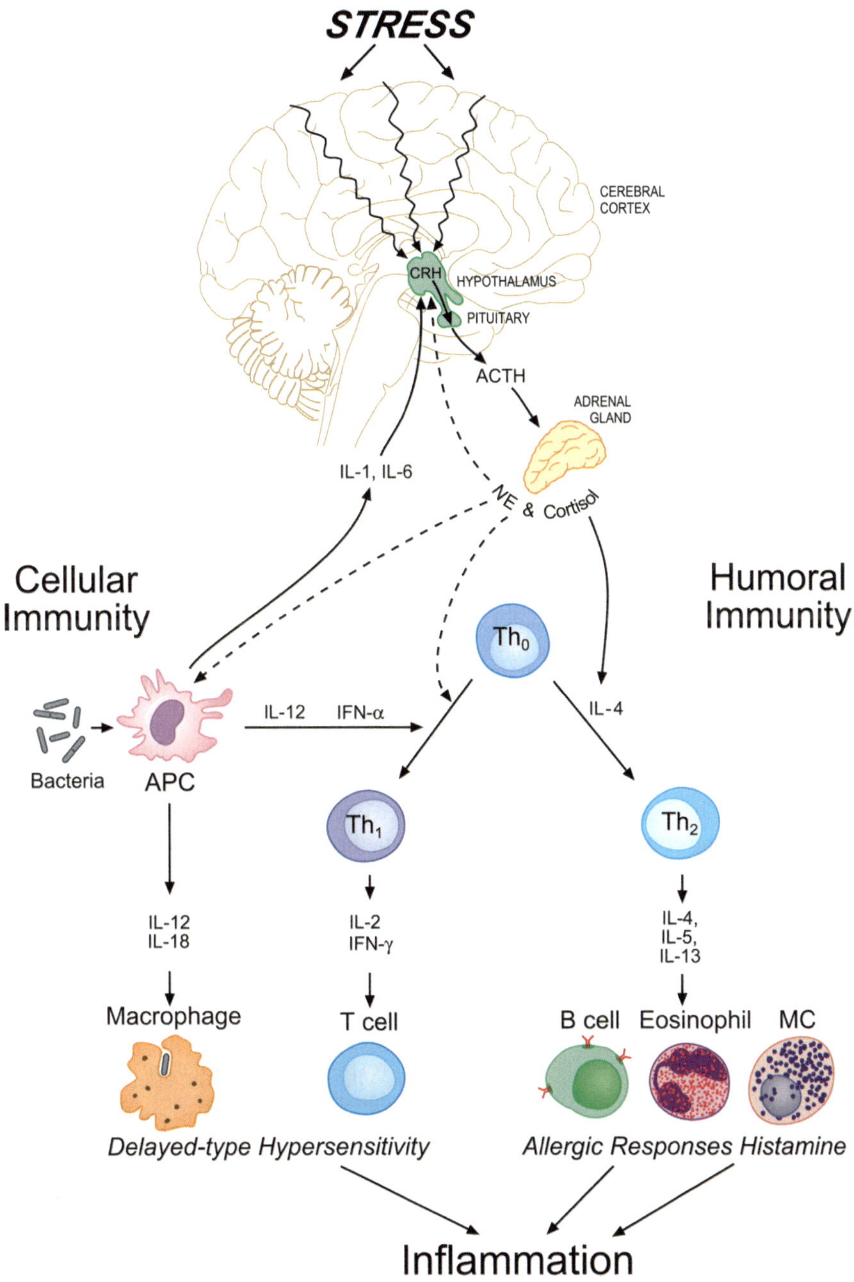

Fig. 1.4 Central HPA axis. (Reproduced from Psychoneuroimmunology by Tausk F et al. with permission from John Wiley and Sons and Copyright Clearance Center). CRH corticotropin-releasing hormone, ACTH adrenocorticotropin hormone, IL interleukin, NE norepinephrine, Th T-helper cells, APC antigen-presenting cell, INF interferon, MC mast cells

nervous system and triggers the production and release of catecholamines (such as epinephrine and norepinephrine). These hormones not only have systemic effects, as they are the primary mediators of the body's "fight or flight" response, but also affect the skin, where they compromise immune and inflammatory functions, influence cytokine production, Th1 cell response, and Th2 cell differentiation [38, 39].

In addition, sensory nerve endings innervating the skin release some neuropeptides under stress conditions, such as calcitonin and substance P gene-related peptides. These neuropeptides not only influence the local inflammatory response, but also seem to be involved in the development of psychodermatological diseases such as atopic dermatitis [40] and psoriasis [41].

1.5.3 Microbiota-Gut-Brain-Skin Axis

Stress also affects the gut level and alters the so-called microbiota-gut-brain-skin axis [42–44]. By activating the HPA axis and increasing circulating glucocorticoids, exposure to stressors significantly alters naturally occurring microbial populations in the gastrointestinal tract (especially bifidobacteria and lactobacilli) and leads to local overproduction of inflammatory mediators. The resulting increase in epithelial barrier permeability is responsible for the subsequent translocation of cytokines, endotoxins, neuroendocrine hormones, and neuropeptides from the intestinal lumen into the systemic circulation. Once these substances enter the bloodstream, they can reach various targets, such as the central nervous system (CNS) and skin, where they may play a role in the development of skin diseases. The connection between the gut and the brain should not be considered a one-way street, as the brain, in turn, can influence the composition of the microbiota through the targeted release of neurochemicals into the gut lumen [43, 45–48].

1.5.4 Immune and Inflammatory Dysregulation

Scientific evidence suggests that immune response dysregulation and a pro-inflammatory state play a role in the pathogenesis of skin diseases as well as in psychiatric disorders. In fact, literature reports that many dermatological diseases (such as dermatitis, psoriasis) originate from a dysfunction of the immune system as well as both dysimmune mechanisms and neuroinflammation are thus involved in the onset, duration, severity, and response to treatment of psychiatric disorders such as psychosis, depression, self-injuries, and attempted suicide. In particular, at the level of the CNS, microglial activation results in the release of cytokines as well as reactive forms of nitrogen and oxygen, inducing the activation of the astroglia, which in turn amplifies local inflammation. These mechanisms negatively affect the production of neurotrophic factors and neurogenesis, contributing to the onset and persistence of psychiatric disorders [49].

1.6 Assessment

Accurate and timely recognition and evaluation of psychodermatological disorders is still difficult today. This is partly because there are few specialized clinics and physicians who specialize in this area, and partly because it is difficult to identify psychiatric problems that go beyond problems that seem to affect only the skin. In clinics that do not specialize in psychodermatology, dermatologic evaluation does not routinely include an in-depth mental examination, and recognition of the disorders and subsequent referral of patients to specialized clinics sometimes fail [50, 51]. Even where psychodermatology clinics have been set up, accesses for primary psychiatric disorders with dermatological manifestations remain more frequent than those for patients with primary dermatological disorders with associated psychiatric symptoms [52]. Early recognition of the psychodermatologic disorder would result in time and cost savings by reducing the number of often unnecessary examinations performed for diagnostic classification [2, 53]. Another difficulty is that patients with psychodermatologic disorders often come to the physician believing that they have only a dermatologic problem. The physician's role is to take a detailed and comprehensive history and to have an accurate interview with the patient in order to instill confidence and increase compliance with treatment. The performance of a correct objective examination with a complete inspection of the skin and skin appendages is also fundamental in the search for signs of psychodermatological disorders, which must be described taking into account the number of lesions, the morphology of the lesion, the distribution of the lesion, the time of appearance, and the course of the lesion.

Lesions such as excoriations or excessive scratching may be observed, for example, in skin picking disorder or delusional infestations. Erosions, burns, cuts, scratches, and bites may be fictitious or self-inflicted injuries or signs of abuse. The physician must also pay special attention to the patient's excessive or, on the contrary, lack of inclination to show his own skin injuries. For example, an excessive tendency to talk about and show injuries could indicate a factitious disorder. Conversely, a remarkable reluctance is typical of patients who self-injure and try to hide their marks and scars by wearing bracelets, accessories, and covering clothing, even in the warmer months. These types of situations need to be recognized immediately by the physician to identify individuals who may be engaging in suicidal behaviors [54]. In addition to self-injury, there are other risk factors for suicide that can be identified through interview and history: previous suicide attempts, suicide planning, isolation, and recent loss of a relationship or job [50]. Indeed, assessment of the patient's mental status is mandatory [55, 56]. The mental state examination includes assessment of:

- physical appearance
- mood
- speech
- behavioral and psychomotor activity
- form and content of thought
- perception (e.g., eventual hallucinations)

- cognitive assessment (e.g., orientation, attention, and concentration)
- insight (it is worth mentioning that patients with a primary psychiatric disorder may not have insight)

A thorough examination of a patient's mental status may require several clinic visits. During these visits, it must be made clear to the patient that the entire interview is strictly confidential and that clinicians will share the information obtained with other health professionals only when necessary and useful to improve the patient's treatment.

Depending on clinical needs, the assessment may be integrated with screening questionnaires, which may be useful for assessing psychiatric symptoms commonly seen in individuals with psychodermatologic disorders. For example, the Beck's Depression Inventory [57], the Depression Anxiety Stress Scale (DASS) [58], and the hospital anxiety and depression scale [59] can be used to measure depressive and anxious symptoms. Obsessive-compulsive symptoms can be evaluated by the Dimensional Obsessive-Compulsive Scale (DOCS) [60]. In addition, there are screening instruments to measure the impact of skin disease on patients' quality of life (QoL), such as the Children's Dermatology Life Quality Index (CDLQI) [61] and the Dermatology Life Quality Index (DLQI) [62].

Based on the results of the medical history, interview, skin examination, and examination of the patient's mental state, the physician evaluates the psychodermatological disorder, the presence of psychiatric symptoms, and their severity. All these elements are carefully evaluated to establish a correct and complete treatment plan involving a multidisciplinary team (consisting of dermatologists, psychiatrists, psychologists, and social services, as well as other health professionals) [12].

1.7 Treatment

In the treatment of psychodermatologic disorders, the key element is to determine and treat the primary cause, if it can be determined, as this may lead to the disappearance or reduction of both psychiatric and dermatologic symptoms. However, if the primary cause cannot be determined and/or the severity of the symptoms warrants it, the concurrent dermatologic and psychiatric symptoms must be treated.

Finally, treatment must be directed toward the following goals [63]:

- improve the patient's functioning
- reduce stress
- manage social isolation/withdrawal
- improve self-esteem

The choice of treatment depends on three factors [50]:

- the main group into which the psychodermatologic disorder is classified (whether it is a primary dermatologic disorder with secondary psychiatric manifestations or a primary psychiatric disorder with secondary dermatologic manifestations);

- any association with anxious, depressive, obsessive-compulsive, or psychotic symptoms;
- the severity of the anxious, depressive, and obsessive-compulsive symptoms as determined by screening scales and questionnaires; and the possible identification of psychiatric risk factors (e.g., suicidal ideation).

Depending on these factors, medical evaluation, and the needs of the individual patient, both nonpharmacologic and pharmacologic therapies may be used alone or in combination. Treatment of psychodermatological disorders should always include psychoeducation, a form of intervention aimed at providing the patient with information about the disorder and strategies for coping with it. Psychotherapy, such as cognitive behavioral therapy (CBT), is one of the most widely used and well-studied nonpharmacological strategies. It is a problem-focused psychotherapy that works on the thoughts, feelings, physical symptoms, and behaviors to address the situations that precede the psychocutaneous manifestation and the consequences that maintain and reinforce the disorder. Other nonpharmacological approaches include relaxation techniques, stress management techniques, and biofeedback [64, 65].

Medications are used according to clinical practice. These include medications for psychiatric symptoms (e.g., antidepressants, anxiolytics, antipsychotics, mood stabilizers) and medications for dermatological symptoms (immunosuppressants, antihistamines, oral or systemic corticosteroids, and other topical medications) [1, 12, 65].

1.8 Conclusion and Future Direction

All the above scientific findings prove the deep and bidirectional relationship between psyche and skin. The skin can be considered as a mirror of the psyche and vice versa. Often it is not possible to determine whether the dermatological or the psychological problem occurred first, and in some cases a single stressor may condition the occurrence of both psychiatric and dermatological disorders without one necessarily causing the other. Therefore, the patient must be guaranteed a comprehensive and holistic approach. The future direction of psychodermatology aims to increase knowledge of the interaction between skin and psyche, raise awareness among health professionals through education and training, support the formation of multidisciplinary teams, and provide guidelines for appropriate diagnosis and treatment. Further development in this field could improve care and outcomes for patients and enhance their quality of life [6].

References

1. Jafferany M, Franca K. Psychodermatology: Basics concepts. Acta Derm Venereol. 2016;96:35–7.

2. Marshall C, Taylor R, Bewley A. Psychodermatology in clinical practice: main principles. Acta Derm Venereol. 2016;96:30–4.
3. Franca K, Chacon A, Ledon J, Savas J, Nouri K. Pyschodermatology: a trip through history. An Bras Dermatol. 2013;88(5):842–3.
4. Rodríguez-Cerdeira C, Pera-Grasa JT, Isa-Isa R. Psychodermatology: past, present and future. Open Dermatol J. 2011;5:21–7.
5. Shafii M, Shafii SL. Exploratory psychotherapy in the treatment of psoriasis: twelve hundred years ago. Arch Gen Psychiatry. 1979;36(11):1242–5.
6. França K, Castillo DE, Roccia MG, Lotti T, Wollina U, Fioranelli M. Psychoneurocutaneous medicine: past, present and future. Wiener Medizinische Wochenschrift. 2017;167:31–6.
7. The Holy Bible: English Standard Version. Crossway Bibles, March 3, 2006.
8. Elangasinghe V, Lee KYC, Levell NJ. An historical account of dermatology in Buddhist Sri Lankan literature. Int J Dermatol. 2014;53(3):390–2.
9. Koo JYM, Pham CT. Psychodermatology: practical guidelines on pharmacotherapy. Arch Dermatol. 1992;128(3):381–8.
10. Ingram JT. The personality of the skin. Lancet. 1933;1:889.
11. Bewley A, Taylor RE, Reichenberg JS, Magrid M. Practical pyschodermatology. West Sussex: Wiley Blackwell; 2014.
12. Munoli RN. Psychodermatology: an overview of history, concept, classification, and current status. Indian J Priv Psychiatry. 2021;14(2):85–91.
13. Tareen RS. Pediatric psychodermatology: a clinical manual of child and adolescent psychocutaneous disorders. Berlin: DeGruyter; 2013.
14. Jafferany M, França K. Geriatric psychodermatology: psychocutaneous disorders in the elderly. New York: Nova Science; 2015.
15. França K, Panchaprateep R, Tosti A. Optimal patient management of alopecia. Oxford: Gardner Healthcare Communications; 2015.
16. França K, Nouri K. Psycodermato-oncology: skin cancers in the elderly. In: Jafferany M, França K, editors. Geriatric psychodermatology: psychocutaneous disorders in the elderly. New York: Nova Science; 2015. p. 187–93.
17. Castillo D, França K, Lotti T. Psychological approach in cosmetic dermatology: clinical approach and procedures in cosmetic dermatology. In: Daily routine in cosmetic dermatology. 2016. http://link.springer.com/referenceworkentry/10.1007/978-3-319-20250-1_3-1. Accessed 26 Feb 2023.
18. Tyring S, Lupi O, Hengge U. Tropical dermatology. Edinburgh: Churchill Livingstone; 2006.
19. Freiman A, Barankin B, Elpern DJ. Sports dermatology part 1: common dermatoses. C Can Med Assoc J. 2004;171(8):851–3.
20. França K, Jafferany M. Stress and skin disorders: basic and clinical aspects. Cham: Springer; 2017. p. 1–257.
21. Gilbert SF. Developmental biology. 6th ed. Sunderland (MA): Sinauer Associates; 2000. Available from: http://www.ncbi.nlm.nih.gov/books/NBK9983/
22. Koblenzer CS. Psychosomatic concepts in dermatology. Arch Dermatol. 1983;119(6):501.
23. Mercan S, Kivanç Altunay I. Psychodermatology: a collaborative subject of psychiatry and dermatology. Turk Psikiyatr Derg. 2006;17(4):1–9.
24. Chen Y, Lyga J. Brain-skin connection: stress, inflammation and skin aging. Inflamm Allergy Drug Targets. 2014;13(3):177–90.
25. Ferreira BR, Jafferany M, Misery L. Psychodermatology in the Era of COVID-19. J Clin Aesthet Dermatol [Internet]. 2021;14(3 Suppl 1):S24–7. Available from: http://www.ncbi.nlm.nih.gov/pubmed/34188742. http://www.pubmedcentral.nih.gov/articlerender.fcgi?artid=PMC8211322
26. Kutlu Ö, Aktaş H, İmren IG, Metin A. Short-term stress-related increasing cases of alopecia areata during the COVID-19 pandemic. J Dermatolog Treat. 2022;33(2):1177.
27. Shen M, Xiao Y, Yuan Y, et al. Perceived stress links income loss and urticaria activity during the coronavirus disease 2019 pandemic. Ann Allergy Asthma Immunol. 2021;126(1):89–90.

28. Kuang Y, Shen M, Wang Q, et al. Association of outdoor activity restriction and income loss with patient-reported outcomes of psoriasis during the COVID-19 pandemic: a web-based survey. J Am Acad Dermatol. 2020;83(2):670–2.
29. Selye H. Allergy and the general adaptation syndrome. Int Arch Allergy Immunol. 1952;3(4):267–78.
30. Cannon WB. The adrenal medulla. Bull N Y Acad Med. 1940;16(1):3–13.
31. Smith SM, Vale WW. The role of the hypothalamic-pituitary-adrenal axis in neuroendocrine responses to stress. Dialogues Clin Neurosci. 2006;8(4):383–95.
32. Sapolsky RM, Romero LM, Munck AU. How do glucocorticoids influence stress responses? Integrating permissive, suppressive, stimulatory, and preparative actions. Endocr Rev. 2000;21(1):55–89.
33. Elenkov IJ, Webster EL, Torpy DJ, Chrousos GP. Stress, corticotropin-releasing hormone, glucocorticoids, and the immune/inflammatory response: acute and chronic effects. Ann N Y Acad Sci. 1999;876:1–11; discussion 11–13.
34. Tausk F, Elenkov I, Moynihan J. Psychoneuroimmunology. Dermatol Ther. 2008;21:22–31.
35. Slominski A, Zbytek B, Nikolakis G, Manna PR, Skobowiat C, Zmijewski M, Li W, Janjetovic Z, Postlethwaite A, Zouboulis CC, Tuckey RC. Steroidogenesis in the skin: implications for local immune functions. J Steroid Biochem Mol Biol. 2013;137:107–23.
36. Arck PC, Slominski A, Theoharides TC, Peters EMJ, Paus R. Neuroimmunology of stress: skin takes center stage. J Invest Dermatol [Internet]. 2006;126(8):1697–704. Available from: https://doi.org/10.1038/sj.jid.5700104
37. Kim JE, Cho BK, Cho DH, Park HJ. Expression of hypothalamic-pituitary-adrenal axis in common skin diseases: evidence of its association with stress-related disease activity. Acta Derm Venereol. 2013;93(4):387–93.
38. McCarty R, Horwatt K, Konarska M. Chronic stress and sympathetic-adrenal medullary responsiveness. Soc Sci Med. 1988;26(3):333–41.
39. Panina-Bordignon P, Mazzeo D, Di Lucia P, D'Ambrosio D, Lang R, Fabbri L, et al. β2-agonists prevent Th1 development by selective inhibition of interleukin 12. J Clin Invest. 1997;100(6):1513–9.
40. Toyoda M, Nakamura M, Makino T, Hino T, Kagoura M, Morohashi M. Nerve growth factor and substance P are useful plasma markers of disease activity in atopic dermatitis. Br J Dermatol. 2002;147(1):71–9.
41. Reich A, Szepietowski JC. Vasoactive peptides in the pathogenesis of psoriasis. G Ital Dermatol Venereol. 2008;143(5):289–98.
42. Arck P, Handjiski B, Hagen E, Pincus M, Bruenahl C, Bienenstock J, et al. Is there a "gut-brain-skin axis"? Exp Dermatol. 2010;19(5):401–5.
43. Bowe WP, Logan AC. Acne vulgaris, probiotics and the gut-brain-skin axis—back to the future? Gut Pathog [Internet]. 2011;3(1):1. Available from: http://www.gutpathogens.com/content/3/1/1
44. Vaughn AR, Notay M, Clark AK, Sivamani RK. Skin-gut axis: the relationship between intestinal bacteria and skin health. World J Dermatology. 2017;6(4):52–8.
45. Söderholm JD, Perdue MH. Stress and the gastrointestinal tract II. Stress and intestinal barrier function. Am J PhysiolGastrointest Liver Physiol. 2001;280(1 43-1):7–13.
46. Foster JA, Rinaman L, Cryan JF. Stress & the gut-brain axis: regulation by the microbiome. Neurobiol Stress [Internet]. 2017;7:124–36. Available from: https://doi.org/10.1016/j.ynstr.2017.03.001
47. Lyte M. Microbial endocrinology and the microbiota-gut-brain axis. Adv Exp Med Biol. 2014;817:3–24.
48. Rea K, Dinan TG, Cryan JF. The microbiome: a key regulator of stress and neuroinflammation. Neurobiol Stress [Internet]. 2016;4:23–33. Available from: https://doi.org/10.1016/j.ynstr.2016.03.001
49. Soria V, Uribe J, Salvat-Pujol N, Palao D, Menchón JM, Labad J. Psychoneuroimmunology of mental disorders. Rev Psiquiatr y Salud Ment (English Ed) [Internet]. 2018;11(2):115–24. Available from: https://doi.org/10.1016/j.rpsmen.2017.07.002

50. Jafferany M, Ferreira BR, Abdelmaksoud A, Mkhoyan R. Management of psychocutaneous disorders: a practical approach for dermatologists. Dermatol Ther. 2020;33(6):1–8.
51. Elpern DJ. Medically unexplained dermatologic symptoms still a problem. J Eur Acad Dermatology Venereol. 2018;32(12):e449.
52. Ferreira BR, Pio-Abreu JL, Reis JP, Figueiredo A. First psychodermatology clinic in a Portuguese Department of Dermatology. J Eur Acad Dermatology Venereol. 2019;33(3):e119–20.
53. Aguilar-Duran S, Ahmed A, Taylor R, Bewley A. How to set up a psychodermatology clinic. Clin Exp Dermatol. 2014;39(5):577–82.
54. Humphreys F, Humphreys MS. Psychiatric morbidity and skin disease: what dermatologists think they see. Br J Dermatol. 1998;139(4):679–81.
55. Srinath S, Jacob P, Sharma E, Gautam A. Clinical practice guidelines for assessment of children and adolescents. Indian J Psychiatry. 2019;61:158–75.
56. Silverman JJ, Galanter M, Jackson-Triche M, Jacobs DG, Lomax JW 2nd, Riba MB, Tong LD, Watkins KE, Fochtmann LJ, Rhoads RS, Yager J, American Psychiatric Association. The American Psychiatric Association practice guidelines for the psychiatric evaluation of adults. Am J Psychiatry. 2015;172(8):798–802. https://doi.org/10.1176/appi.ajp.2015.1720501. PMID: 26234607.
57. Beck AT, Steer RA, Brown GK. Manual for the Beck DepressionInventory-II. San Antonio: Psychological Corporation; 1996.
58. Lovibond SH, Lovibond PF. Manual for the depression anxiety stress scales. 2nd ed. Sydney: Psychology Foundation of Australia; 1995.
59. Zigmond AS, Snalth RP. The hospital anxiety and depression scale. Acta Psychiatr Scand [revista en Internet] 2014 [acceso 28 de noviembre de 2019]; 64(5):361–70. Acta Psychiatr Scand [Internet]. 1983;67(6):361–70. Available from: https://www.ncbi.nlm.nih.gov/pubmed/6880820
60. Abramowitz JS, Deacon BJ, Olatunji BO, Wheaton MG, Berman NC, Losardo D, et al. Assessment of obsessive-compulsive symptom dimensions: development and evaluation of the dimensional obsessive-compulsive scale. Psychol Assess. 2010;22(1):180–98.
61. Lewis-Jones MS, Finlay AY. The Children's Dermatology Life Quality Index (CDLQI): initial validation and practical use. Br J Dermatol. 1995;132(6):942–9.
62. Finlay AY, Khan GK. Dermatology Life Quality Index (DLQI)—a simple practical measure for routine clinical use. Clin Exp Dermatol. 1994;19(3):210–6.
63. Bewley A, Affleck A, Bundy C, Higgins E, McBride S. Psychodermatology services guidance: the report of the British Association of Dermatologists' Psychodermatology Working Party. Br J Dermatol. 2013;168(6):1149–50.
64. Van Moffaert M. Training future dermatologists in psychodermatology. Gen Hosp Psychiatry. 1986;8(2):115–8.
65. Bondade S, Hosthota A, Bindushree R, Raj P. Psychodermatology: an evolving paradigm. Dermatologica Sin. 2022;40(2):71–7.

Chapter 2
Psychocutaneous Diseases

Gianni Angelini, Aurora De Marco, and Domenico Bonamonte

The skin and the central nervous system arise from the same embryonal tissue, the ectoderm, but this particular interlink, that lasts throughout life, actually extends beyond their common embryogenic origin. In fact, there is a continual interplay among the neuroendocrine system, the immune system, and the skin [1–10].

The existence of psychocutaneous diseases has been recognized since ancient times. Aristotle (384–322 BC) claimed that the mind and body are complementary, not separate [11]. Hippocrates (460–377 BC) discussed the effects of stress on the skin and described cases of patients who tore their hair out while in prey to emotional stress [11]. The field of psychodermatology, that has a long history, has become the focus of ample studies in the last decades [12, 13]. According to Korabel and Coll., 30%–40% of dermatological patients present with psychiatric comorbidity [14]. However, although a study conducted in the United States on a sample of dermatologists showed that 61.7% of them had seen patients with known psychological disorders more than once a week, and 79% had discussed methods for reducing their stress, only 6.38% had administered a psychiatric questionnaire at each visit [15].

Given the two-way interaction between the skin and the psyche, it is really quite difficult to establish whether the primary problem is of cutaneous or psychic origin. The neuroendocrine and immune systems interactions in skin diseases are linked to psychosocial stress: the latter, whether it is mental or physical, plays an important role in the immune regulation of psychocutaneous diseases, and contributes to the

G. Angelini
Dermatology, University of Bari "Aldo Moro", Bari, Italy
e-mail: gianniang@alice.it

A. De Marco · D. Bonamonte (✉)
Department of Precision and Regenerative Medicine and Ionian Area, University of Bari "Aldo Moro", Bari, Italy
e-mail: a.demarco24@studenti.uniba.it; domenico.bonamonte@uniba.it

G. Angelini et al. (eds.), *Psychocutaneous Diseases*,
https://doi.org/10.1007/978-3-031-70296-9_2

exacerbation of the same disorders [16–18]. The mechanisms whereby stress influences the skin are not entirely understood [18–22]. The response to stress differs according to how long it lasts: in acute stress there is an immediate response, with the release of glucocorticoids, catecholamines, and neuropeptides. This triggers the release of inflammatory cells and their relative mediators, and then a rapid interruption of the response occurs as soon as the stressful event is over. Instead, in chronic stress the prolonged release of hormones leads, over time, to a dysregulation of the innate and adaptative immune systems [23, 24]. Thus, stress can induce autoimmune or autoinflammatory dermatological diseases through the altered neuroendocrine and neuroimmune regulation processes. This, in practice, means that psychosomatic disorders are actually reactive skin diseases of two-way, mutually interdependent type [25].

2.1 Classification

There are various types of classification of psychocutaneous disorders. Adopting a highly simplified model, it could be said that diseases that involve the skin and psyche can be grouped as follows [3]:

A. "Somatopsychic" disorders, when the body is primarily involved, and mental disturbances are a consequence of the physical damage.
B. "Psychosomatic" disorders, when psychological or psychiatric disorders lie at the origin of the problem, while the somatic disturbances are the secondary effect.

Actually, research into a causal relationship in the etiopathogenesis of any disease is quite complex because of the interactions among life events, conditions of the organs and different psychological states, that occur at various levels during a lifetime. Therefore, the assumption of a purely linear causal relationship, although useful in clinical practice, is not only impossible but may not even be a proper scientific model that can reveal the true interactions [3, 26–28].

Any disease can cause the patient some psychic distress. In particular, in the case of skin diseases, that are often characterized by "visible" evidence, the psychological distress is exacerbated. Naturally, the younger the age of onset and the more serious the clinical course, the worse the psychological damage.

A common classification with a prevalently psychiatric slant subdivides psychocutaneous disorders into four groups [7, 8].

A. *Psychophysiological disorders.* These include skin diseases precipitated or exacerbated by psychological stress. In this case, there is a clear chronological association between the stressful event and the exacerbation of the skin disease. Some obvious examples are alopecia areata, acne, psoriasis, atopic dermatitis, and chronic spontaneous urticaria.

B. *Dermatologic disorders with psychiatric symptoms.* The emotional component due to the presence of a skin disease is more prominent and more severe than the physical symptoms. Some examples include alopecia areata, albinism, vitiligo, hemangiomas and vascular malformations, and psoriasis.
C. *Psychiatric disorders with dermatological symptoms.* The primary problem is the mental disorder, and skin lesions may follow, and may be self-inflicted. An underlying psychopathologic or psychological disorder is the cause of the skin disorder. Conflicts of this kind are evident, for example, in cases of obsessive-compulsive disorders, factitious disorders, and delusion of parasitosis.
D. *Miscellaneous.* Various other disorders come under this group, such as skin sensory disorders and medication-related adverse effects of both psychiatric and dermatologic medications, for example.

There are other recognized classifications of psychocutaneous diseases: the Diagnostic and Statistical Manual of Mental Disorders (DSM-V), produced and regularly modified by the American Psychiatric Association [29], and the International Classification of Diseases and nomenclature system for medical and psychiatric disorders (ICD-10) published by the World Health Organization [30]. Nevertheless, these classifications, based on diagnostic criteria and largely similar, do not seem to be much consulted by dermatologists [1].

Undoubtedly, psychocutaneous disorders are in the great majority of cases correlated to mental disorders, and so they are generally included among psychiatric disorders. This is also because the treatment primarily targets the mental rather than the dermatological disorder [31–34]. Despite these valid reasons, here we prefer to adopt a classification that highlights the dermatological aspect of the problem, starting from the various skin pictures, that can, in turn, be induced by or else induce psychological or psychiatric disturbances (Table 2.1) [1, 2, 34, 35].

2.2 Management: General Remarks

Psychodermatology, a field of medicine that is in continual evolution, is a subspecialty of dermatology and psychiatry, and close interrelations between the two specialist fields are absolutely necessary to ensure high-quality integrated patient treatment [7, 8, 18, 36, 37]. In fact, various studies have highlighted the major benefit that is derived from a combined clinical approach to the management of patients with psychocutaneous disorders [38–42]. Moreover, in terms of financial implications, it has been reported that combined clinical care reduces costs, cutting to a minimum the need for multiple specialist visits, unnecessary laboratory tests, and expensive medical procedures [43–45].

The therapeutic approach to psychocutaneous disorders is based above all on an optimal doctor–patient collaboration [46–49]. The relationship must be empathic, genuine, and respectful and will require several continuous visits to make a complete evaluation, varying the approach according to the etiology of the problem.

Table 2.1 Dermatological classification of psychocutaneous diseases. (Modified, from Ref. [1])

1. Self-inflicted cutaneous disorders whose nature is denied or hidden
A. Factitious disorders without external incentives (psychiatric disorders with cutaneous symptoms)
Dermatitis artefacta
Dermatological pathomimicry (in part)
Gardner-Diamond syndrome
Münchausen syndrome
Münchausen syndrome by proxy
Dermatitis simulata
Dermatitis passivata ("Diogenes syndrome")
B. Factitious disorders with external incentives (malingering)
Malingering in adolescents
Malingering in soldiers
Occupational dermatitis artefacta
Dermatitis artefacta with patch test artefacts
Witchcraft syndrome
Secrétan syndrome (in part)
Dermatological pathomimicry (in part)
Religious stigmata as malingering artefacts
2. Cutaneous disorders with a non-denied and non-hidden behavior (impulsive/compulsive disorders)
Psychogenic pruritus
Lichen simplex
Prurigo nodularis
Acne excoriée
Trichotillomania
Trichoteiromania
Trichotemnomania
Onychophagia
Onychotillomania
Onychotemnomania
Cheilitis factitia
Morsicatio buccarum
Pseudo-knuckle pads
Rhinotillexomania
3. Cutaneous diseases precipitated or perpetuated by emotional factors (psychosomatic or psychophysiological disorders)
Acne
Hemangiomas and vascular malformations
Vitiligo
Albinism
Chronic eczema

(continued)

Table 2.1 (continued)

Atopic dermatitis
Psoriasis
Seborrheic dermatitis
Vesicular eczema of palms and soles
Alopecia areata
Hyperhidrosis
Urticaria and angioedema
Aphthosis
Flushing reactions and rosacea
4. Psychiatric disorders without significant dermatological disease
A. Delusional syndromes
Parasitosis
Smell
Impregnations and contamination
Folie à deux
Morgellons syndrome
B. Disorders of body awareness
Body dysmorphic disorders
Psychogenic pruritus
Phobias:
Venereophobia
Parasitophobia
Steroid phobia
Compulsive behaviors:
Hand washing
Pain disorders:
Glossodynia
Vulvodynia
Scrotodynia
Anodynia
Drug-dependence syndromes:
Alcohol-related syndrome
Substance abuse
Psychosis and skin cancer
Cutaneous disorders due to psychopharmacological medicaments
5. Group and mass population reactions
Sick building syndrome
Epidemic hysteria

Ideally, these patients should be assessed in a psychodermatology clinic, by an interdisciplinary team including dermatologists, psychologists, and psychiatrists [8]. The treatment aims must be not only to reduce or resolve the cutaneous symptoms, eliminate sleep disturbances, boost self-esteem, and cure anxiety and

Table 2.2 Interrelation between psychocutaneous disorders and underlying personality disorders

Psychocutaneous disorders	Personality disorders
Factitious disorders with a non-denied and non-hidden behavior	Obsessive-compulsive behavior Borderline personality disorder Narcissistic personality disorder
Factitious disorders with a denied and hidden behavior without external incentives	Borderline personality disorder
Body awareness disorders	Narcissistic personality disorder

depression, but also to improve the patient's relational life. The various treatments, both pharmacological and non pharmacological therapy, can be used alone or in combination, depending on the assessment of the individual patient and his or her individual needs.

The management of patients with personality disorders is quite challenging. However, a joint liaison between psychiatry and dermatology has proven very helpful to patients. In a study by Raikhy and Coll., 36.32% of dermatological patients presented depression, while in 18.61% of patients an anxiety disorder was diagnosed [50]. These figures underline the importance of the liaison among different specialists. There are ten specific personality disorders; in dermatological clinical practice, however, the most common are borderline, narcissistic, and obsessive-compulsive personality disorders [36]. Self-inflicted cutaneous disorders of a non-denied and non-hidden nature, such as trichotillomania, onychotillomania, face picking (acne excoriée), and rhinotillexomania, are commonly associated with compulsive-obsessive behavior although they can also be linked to borderline personality and narcissistic personality disorders [36]. Patients with factitious disorders of a denied or hidden nature and not prompted by external incentives (dermatitis artefacta), who tend firstly to resort to a visit to the dermatologist, come into the borderline personality disorder category [51–53]. Subjects who need admiration and seek grandiosity, who are often among those who request cosmetic procedures, belong to the narcissistic personality disorder category (Table 2.2) [54–59].

Based on the above considerations, and in view of the considerable percentage of dermopatients with psychiatric disturbances, it is essential that the dermatologist be familiar with the most common personality disorders, as well as working in close collaboration with psychiatrists and psychologists in order to ensure the optimal management of these patients [36, 60].

References

1. Millard LG, Millard J. Psychocutaneous disorders. In: Burns T, Brethnach S, Cox N, et al., editors. Rook's textbook of dermatology. 8th ed. Oxford: Wiley-Backwell; 2010:chap.64.1-55.

2. Rieder E, Tausk FA. Psychocutaneous skin diseases. In: Goldsmith LS, Katz SJ, Gilchrest BA, et al., editors. Fitzpratick's dermatology in general medicine. 8th ed. New York: McGraw-Hill; 2012. p. 1158–66.
3. Linder D, Bassi R. Psyche and skin. In: Giannetti A, Del Forno C, editors. Textbook of dermatology and sexually transmitted diseases. Padova: Piccin Nuova Libreria, S.P.A.; 2013. p. 431–41.
4. Bewley A, Lepping P, Taylor RE. Psychodermatology in clinical practice. Switzerland A6: Springer Nature; 2021.
5. Jafferany M. Handbook of psychodermatology. Introduction to psychocutaneous disorders. Switzerland A6: Springer Nature; 2022.
6. O'Sullivan RL, Lipper G, Lerner EA. The neuro-immuno-cutaneous-endocrine network: relationship of mind and skin. Arch Dermatol. 1998;134:1431–5.
7. Jafferany M, França K. Psychodermatology: basics concepts. Acta Derm Venereol. 2016;96:35–7.
8. Jafferany M, Ferreira BR, Abdelmaksoud A, et al. Management of psychocutaneous disorders: a practical approach for dermatologists. Dermatol Ther. 2020;33:e13969.
9. Jafferany M, Ferreira BR, Patel A. The essentials of psychodermatology. Cham: Springer International Publishing; 2020. p. 29–34.
10. Kuhn H, Mennella C, Magid M, et al. Psychocutaneous disease: clinical perspectives. J Am Acad Dermatol. 2017;76:779–91.
11. França K, Chacon A, Ledon J, Savas J, Nouri K. Psychodermatology: a trip through history. An Bras Dermatol. 2013;88:842–3.
12. Jafferany M. Psychodermatology: a guide to understanding common psychocutaneous disorders. Prim Care Companion J Clin Psychiatry. 2007;9:203–13.
13. Jafferany M, França K. The interface between geriatrics, psychiatry and dermatology. In: Jafferany M, França K, editors. Geriatric psychodermatology: psychocutaneous disorders in the elderly. New York: Nova Science Publishers; 2015. p. 3–7.
14. Korabel H, Dudek D, Jaworek A, et al. Psychodermatology: psychological and psychiatrical aspects of dermatology. Przegl Lek. 2008;65:244–8.
15. Tran A, Desir AK, Okafor LC, et al. Psychodermatology in clinical practice: an examination of physician attitudes, beliefs, and interventions toward psychocutaneous disease. Dermatol Ther. 2020;33:e13612.
16. Picari A, Albeni D. Stressful life events and skin diseases: disentangling evidence from myth. Psychother Psychosom. 2011;70:118–36.
17. Dhabhar FS. Psychological stress and immunoprotection versus immunopathology in the skin. Clin Dermatol. 2013;31:18–30.
18. Tohid H, Shenefelt PD, Burney WA, et al. Psychodermatology: an association of primary psychiatric disorders with skin. Rev Colomb Psiquiatr. 2019;48:50–7.
19. Lonne-Rahm SB, Rickberg H, El-Nour H, et al. Neuroimmune mechanisms in patients with atopic dermatitis during chronic stress. J Eur Acad Dermatol Venereol. 2008;22:11–8.
20. American Academy of Dermatology. Managing stress can help people improve their skin conditions. Available from http://www.aad.org/storics-and-news/news-releases/managing-stress-can-help-people-improve-their-skin-conditions. Accessed 2 Oct 2012.
21. Slominski A, Mihm MC. Potential mechanism of skin response to stress. Int J Dermatol. 1996;35:849–51.
22. Dave ND, Xiang L, Rehm KE, et al. Stress and allergic diseases. Immunol Allergy Clin North Am. 2011;31:55–68.
23. Jafferany M, Salimi S, Mkhoyan R, et al. Psychological aspects of aesthetic and cosmetic surgery: clinical and therapeutic implications. Dermatol Ther. 2020;33:e13727.
24. Hafi B, Uvais NA, Jafferany M, et al. Palliative psychodermatology care during COVID-19 pandemic. Dermatol Ther. 2020;3:e13732.
25. Jafferany M, Patel A. Understanding psychocutaneous disease: psychosocial and psychoneuroimmunologic perspectives. Int J Dermatol. 2019;59:8–15.

26. Engel GL. From biomedical to biopsychosocial. 1. Being scientific in the human domain. Psychother Psychosom. 1997;66:57–62.
27. White P. Biopsychosocial medicine. Oxford: Oxford University Press; 2005.
28. Koo JYM, Lee CS. General approach to evaluating psychodermatological disorders. In: Koo JYM, Lee CS, editors. Psychocutaneous medicine. New York: Marcel Dekker, Inc.; 2003. p. 1–29.
29. American Psychiatric Association. Diagnostic and statistical manual of mental disorders. DSM-V. 5th ed. Arlington: American Psychiatric Association; 2013.
30. International classification of diseases. Tenth revision (ICD-10); 2010. Available from: http://www.whp.int/classification/icd.Geneva. Cited 2022, Ang 28.
31. Koblenzer CS. Psychosomatic concepts in dermatology. A dermatologist-psychoanalyst's viewpoint. Arch Dermatol. 1983;119:501–12.
32. Gupta MA, Gupta AK. Self-induced dermatoses: a great imitator. Clin Dermatol. 2019;37:268–77.
33. Medansky RS, Handler RM. Dermatopsychosomatics: classification, physiology, and therapeutic approaches. J Am Acad Dermatol. 1981;5:125–38.
34. Musalek M, Hable B, Mossabacher U. Diagnostics in psychodermatology. Dermatol Psychosom. 2011;2:110–5.
35. Gieler U, Consoli SG, Tomás-Aragones L, et al. Self-inflicted lesions in dermatology: terminology and classification—a position paper from the European Society for Dermatology and Psychiatry (ESDaP). Acta Derm Venereol. 2013;93:4–12.
36. Jafferany M, Afrin A, Mkhoyan R, et al. Therapeutic implications of personality disorders in dermatology. Dermatol Ther. 2020;33:e13910.
37. Patel A, Jafferany M. Multidisciplinary and holistic models of care for patients with dermatologic disease and psychosocial comorbidity: a systematic review. JAMA Dermatol. 2020;156:686–94.
38. Gould WM, Gragg TM. A dermatology-psychiatry liaison clinic. J Am Acad Dermatol. 1983;9:73–7.
39. Woodruff PW, Higgins EM, du Vivier AW, et al. Psychiatric illness in patients referred to a dermatology-psychiatry clinic. Gen Hosp Psychiatry. 1997;19:29–35.
40. Fritzsche K, Ott J, Zschocke I, et al. Psychosomatic liaison service in dermatology. Need for psychotherapeutic interventions and their realization. Dermatology. 2001;203:27–31.
41. Misery L, Chastaing M. Joint consultation by psychiatrist and a dermatologist. Dermatol Psychosom. 2003;4:160–4.
42. Deshponde SS, More Y, Gokhale NR. Identification and management of psychiatric comorbidities in dermatological disorders. Malay J Psychiatry. 2015;24:1–6.
43. Altaf K, Mohandas P, Marshall C, et al. Managing patients with delusional infestations in an integrated psychodermatology clinic is much more cost-effective than a general dermatology or primary care setting. Br J Dermatol. 2017;177:544–5.
44. Goulding JMR, Harper N, Kennedy L, et al. Cost-effectiveness in psychodermatology: a case series. Acta Derm Venereol. 2017;97:663–4.
45. Seale L, Gaulding JV, Porto D, et al. Implementation of a psychodermatology clinic at a major health system in Detroit. Int J Womens Dermatol. 2018;4:227–9.
46. Franger K, Mahmud M. Doctor-patient relationship in geriatric psychodermatology. In: Jafferany M, França K, editors. Geriatric psychodermatology: psychocutaneous disorders in the elderly. New York: Nova Science Publishers; 2015. p. 9–13.
47. Kuhn H, Mennella C, Magid M, et al. Psychocutaneous disease: Pharmacotherapy and psychotherapy. J Am Acad Dermatol. 2017;76:795–808.
48. Reichenberg JS, Kroumpouzos G, Magid M. Approach to a psychodermatology patient. G Ital Dermatol Venereol. 2018;153:494–6.
49. Shah RB. Psychological assessment and interventions for people with skin disease. In: Bewley A, Taylor RE, Reichenberg JS, et al., editors. Practical psychodermatology. Oxford, UK: Wiley-Blackwell; 2014. p. 40–9.

50. Raikhy S, Gautam S, Kanodia S. Pattern and prevalence of psychiatric disorders among patients attending dermatology OPD. Asian J Psychiatr. 2017;29:85–8.
51. Briere J, Gil E. Self-mutilation in clinical and general population samples: prevalence, correlates, and functions. Am J Orthopsychiatry. 1998;68:609–20.
52. Chatterjee SS, Mitra S. Dermatitis artefacta mimicking borderline personality disorder: sometimes, skin could be misleading. Clin Psychopharmacol Neurosci. 2016;14:311–3.
53. Harth W, Mayer K, Linse R. The borderline syndrome in psychosomatic dermatology. Overview and case report. J Eur Acad Dermatol Venereol. 2004;18:503–7.
54. Loron AM, Ghaffari A, Poursafargholi N. Personality disorders among individuals seeking cosmetic botulinum toxin type A (BoNTA) injection, a cross-sectional study. Eurasian J Med. 2018;50:164–7.
55. Koblenzer CS. Body dysmorphic disorder in the dermatology patient. Clin Dermatol. 2017;35:298–301.
56. Phillips KA, Dufresne RG Jr, Wilkel CS, et al. Rate of body dysmorphic disorder in dermatology patients. J Am Acad Dermatol. 2000;42:436–41.
57. Bowe WP, Leyden JJ, Crerand CE, et al. Body dysmorphic disorder symptoms among patients with acne vulgaris. J Am Acad Dermatol. 2007;57:222–30.
58. Bjornsson AS, Didie ER, Grant JE, et al. Age at onset and clinical correlates in body dysmorphic disorder. Compr Psychiatry. 2013;54:893–903.
59. Affleck A, Stewart M. Body dysmorphic disorder in dermatology: beware of diagnostic overlabelling. Clin Exp Dermatol. 2016;41:214–5.
60. Azambuja RD. The need of dermatologists, psychiatrists and psychologists joint care in psychodermatology. An Bras Dermatol. 2017;92:63–71.

Chapter 3
Self-Inflicted Skin Disorders: Diagnosis and Management

Gianni Angelini, Aurora De Marco, and Domenico Bonamonte

Self-inflicted skin disorders (SISD) belong to the vast group of self-inflicted disorders (SID) that can be observed in all branches of specialist medicine.

SID, or factitious (from the Latin *factitious*: artificial, not natural, artful, self-induced) [1] diseases, are defined as a "falsification of physical or psychological signs or symptoms, or induction of injury or disease, associated with identified deception" [2]. Factitious disorders are, therefore, psychiatric disorders in which patients intentionally fabricate psychological or physical symptoms in order to acquire the role of patient affected by a disease [3–5].

3.1 General Clinical Remarks

In accordance with the DSM-5 and the eleventh revision of the International Classification of Diseases, most patients with SID are not, in fact, actuated by motives of external gain [2, 6]. On the contrary, in cases of malingering the self-inflicted disorder is motivated by clear external rewards or incentives, in order to avoid various duties (e.g. military service) or a prison sentence, or else to gain some advantage, usually of an occupational nature [6–13].

The motivations of patients with SID are often complex and not always entirely intelligible. In general, such subjects are driven by a more or less conscious need for

G. Angelini
Dermatology, University of Bari "Aldo Moro", Bari, Italy
e-mail: gianniang@alice.it

A. De Marco · D. Bonamonte (✉)
Department of Precision and Regenerative Medicine and Ionian Area, University of Bari "Aldo Moro", Bari, Italy
e-mail: a.demarco24@studenti.uniba.it; domenico.bonamonte@uniba.it

G. Angelini et al. (eds.), *Psychocutaneous Diseases*,
https://doi.org/10.1007/978-3-031-70296-9_3

affection and care, and so for this purpose they often have recourse to medical treatments and surgical procedures [14]. In this sense, an emblematic case is that of a patient who underwent 42 surgical procedures in the course of 850 admissions to 650 different hospitals [15]. Inevitably, such behaviour exposes them to a considerable risk of iatrogenic harm [16] and even, in rare cases, of a possible fatality [17–19]. And of course, the impact of such behaviour on health care costs is quite heavy [3, 20, 21]. Another problem is that patients with SID can have a heavy psychological impact on the hospital staff, that may feel they are being deceived in some way [22], or else that the patient is manipulating their emotions and making them feel guilty [23]. Sometimes, the patient with SID can also feel some satisfaction when observing the doctor's evident difficulties in making a diagnosis and prescribing treatment [24].

Although they have been known for centuries, the first extensive study of SID was made by Asher in the context of the Münchausen syndrome, named after the eighteenth century European aristocrat Hieronymus Karl Friedrich, Baron von Münchausen (1720–1797) [25]. Since then, the term Münchausen syndrome, that refers to a particular picture of severe, chronic SID, is often used interchangeably with factitious. Other names for SID in the literature, often mocking or derisive, are "hospital hopper syndrome", "hospital hobo syndrome", "thick chart syndrome", and "black hole syndrome" [3].

The precise prevalence of SID is not known but ranges from 0.02% to 3% in the general clinical population [26–31]. A recent study of factitious disorders, conducted in Germany and Norway in somatic hospitals from 2008 to 2016, reported a comparable incidence, of 3.71% and 3.18% per 100,000 patients, respectively [32].

Subjects with SID have been reported all over the world, but in particular in the United States and Europe [3]. Various studies show a prevalence in the female gender, with percentages ranging from 65.4%, 66.2% [3], to 73.5% [5]. Subjects with SID tend to come to medical attention already as young adults. The mean age ranges from 32 [3], 33.5 [33], to 38.4 [5] years, excluding young subjects and minors under the age of 18 years. The mean age is generally lower in females.

A number of studies show a preponderance of patients employed in the health care sector; this suggests that health care work may be a risk factor when associated with stressful life events [33–35]. Such health care work includes nursing, but also medical assistants, pharmacists, administrators, and nutritionists [4].

From the literature, a preponderance of comorbidities with personality disorders, in particular borderline personality disorders and depression, also emerges [3–5, 33, 36, 37]. Overall, these epidemiological data describe the SID phenotype: young women with health care experience and psychopathology [4, 38, 39].

In an analysis of a wide sample of patients, Yates and Feldman found that 58.7% of subjects with factitious disorders prefer to induce the illness or injury rather than simulating it (19.1%) or falsely referring (22.2%) a medical problem [3]. Therefore, these patients are at high risk of self-injury, and this risk must be taken into account in the patient management plan: family members, partners, and friends must be informed and involved in the management, so as to control the patient's access to various harmful tools and substances (drugs, poisons) that can be employed for self-injury. However, these patients sometimes use methods of self-injury that are difficult to control, such as abuse of insulin to induce hypoglycaemia, or self-venesection to provoke anaemia [3]. Once again, therefore, early detection of SID is very important to limit self-harm and promote improved outcomes. In this regard, special guidelines are needed to show how a self-inflicted injury can be diagnosed by the clinician and how such injuries can be detected early on, in the relative medical specialty field [3].

Patients with SID can induce diseases in various ways, depending on their level of imagination, medical knowledge, and on the nature of the problem they wish to produce [40]. The same patient can actually use various different methods at once to create different diseases, for example, an ulcerative dermatological lesion using metal tools or caustic substances as well as haematuria by adding blood to urine samples. In all cases, however, a certain diagnosis of a simulated disease is difficult to make and must always follow a complete series of clinical examinations and laboratory tests.

All medical specialists may find themselves in the position of needing to manage patients with an SID. In literature, the data on the predominance of cases in one specialty rather than another are conflicting. This variability may be due to a different interest in diagnosing SID in the various medical branches. Alternatively, it may be explained by the difficulties related to making a diagnosis of SID in the various specialist sectors. A simulated disease can be diagnosed more easily in dermatology, owing to the particular morphological features of self-inflicted lesions, or in endocrinology because a factitious hypoglycaemia can be revealed by laboratory tests of insulin abuse [7, 10–12, 41–47]. Clearly, the greater frequency of one type of simulation than another also depends on the fact that it is easier for the patient to induce skin damage or an endocrinological problem than to act on other organs or systems.

Whatever the true distribution of SID cases in the various specialist fields, bearing in mind the ample volume of literature on this subject it is important that all specialists be aware of this problem, and especially dermatologists, neuropsychiatrists, and endocrinologists.

In any case, it is clear from the literature that dermatology is the specialty with the highest number of cases of SID [5, 48], or at least one of the specialties with the highest incidence [3]. The lower dermatological incidence reported in some studies could depend on the patients sample enrolled: it should be remembered that patients presenting with SID in dermatology are more often under ambulatorial management. Thus, such patients would not be included in studies of only hospital patients [5]. The medical branches with the lowest incidence of SID seem to be obstetrics and gynaecology [3], as well as oncology [3, 49–51]: it is difficult to achieve simulation in the former fields, and not easy to convince the physician of the existence of a cancer unless specific imaging tests show some signs.

It is also likely that the incidence of SID is underestimated in the general population. Clinicians are led to believe the clinical history referred by the patient and, in any case, have little familiarity with SID. And even in cases of suspected SID, it remains difficult to make a definitive diagnosis of simulation, also in view of the medico-legal problems that such a diagnosis can provoke, when needing to differentiate between true simulating (malingering) and psychosomatic disease [52]. It can also be difficult to differentiate SID from a simple exaggeration or amplification of the symptoms [5]. A certain reluctance to make a diagnosis of an SID has also been reported, even in cases with strong evidence of simulation [39]. It must be remembered, however, that failure to diagnose an SID can lead to the prescription of unnecessary tests that may also be potentially harmful [5].

Other important characteristics among patients with SID are the denial of self-harm, refusal to accept a diagnosis of self-inflicted pathology, and refusal in most cases to undergo psychiatric consultation or treatment. This anomalous behaviour is inevitably accompanied by failure of all treatments and a high disease recurrence.

In conclusion, SID are one of the most challenging problems in clinical medicine and warrant further in-depth study. It is important that general practitioners and the various specialists be fully aware of this major medical problem.

3.2 Self-Inflicted Disorders in Dermatology

SISD are due to excessive manipulation of the skin and appendages, hair, and nails. This anomalous behaviour is typically repetitive, and it is this reiteration that generally leads to chronic damage. Manipulation of the skin can cause a de novo disease, or else complicate the course of a primary dermatological condition, as in the cases of pre-existing acne, psoriasis, and other itchy skin conditions [53–55].

In cases of trichotillomania and skin picking, as well as being repetitive, the nature of the behaviour is "automatic", in the sense that the patient is often unaware of doing it. These disorders are described as "stereotypic": the motor behaviour interferes with the patient's normal activity and finally results in self-inflicted injury, that is often severe enough to require medical treatment [53].

Another important aspect of the problem is the observation of several SISD together: in more than 38% of adults, skin picking is associated with trichotillomania, and in more than 20% of cases, hair pulling, or skin picking are associated with compulsive nail biting [56–58].

Self-induced dermatoses are inflicted using multiple different means, for different purposes [59–71]. They are among the most frequent self-inflicted disorders in medicine, in particular because the use of an exogenous mechanism to induce an artefact is not only easier than an endogenous mechanism, but also allows the disease to become "manifest" to all; this is the true reason motivating the whole artefactual procedure. The adoption of an exogenous mechanism, moreover, allows the patient to choose the cutaneous site very carefully, to avoid affecting the whole organism (as may occur in the case of a self-inflicted systemic disease), and to stop the harmful action when he/she wishes [7, 10, 43–45, 72–75].

In the great majority of cases, the simulation of a cutaneous disorder is dictated by psychiatric problems: in such an event, the subject desires to attract the attention of those around him, in particular the general practitioner, or else is reacting to a difficult or unfavourable environmental situation through somatization at the skin level [76]. However, as stated above, some subjects are motivated by an illicit intent: in these cases, the simulator is perfectly well aware of her/his action and hidden motivations [7, 9–13, 43–45, 70]. Therefore, these subjects do not generally suffer from any underlying psychiatric disorder.

Skin artefacts deliberately provoked by subjects with a psychiatric disorder, without any venal intent, are described as "pathomimic" (an attribute that, *stricto sensu*, identifies the faithful imitation of existing diseases but that in dermatological practice has actually acquired a wider meaning, referring specifically to irresponsible simulations of psychogenic origin). Instead, artefact skin disorders caused with illicit intent, aiming to gain various advantages, are true simulations ("malingering"). In both cases, affected subjects deny or deliberately hide their pathological behaviour.

Apart from these cases, there is also a group of body-focused repetitive behavioural disorders ("impulsive/compulsive disorders") that are inflicted by aware subjects who, in the majority of cases, are very ready to confess their urge to induce self-inflicted lesions [70, 71, 77].

Skin artefacts can also be observed in infants and in school age children: the underlying intent is in these cases, too, either of a psychological nature or else aims to achieve a very precise, non-venal purpose [7, 45, 78–80].

3.3 Classification and Incidence

As emerges from the above comments, SISD involve different medical specialties: first of all, dermatologists, but also psychiatrists, psychologists, general practitioners, and in some cases paediatricians and medico-legal specialists [3, 53, 54, 63, 70, 81–87]. This is why various classifications and terminologies referring to SISD are adopted in the literature.

Various terms, in fact, are used for overlapping clinical pictures, such as self-harm [88], auto-destructive syndrome [68], self-injury [89], self-mutilation [90], dermatitis artefacta [62, 76], neurotic excoriations [91, 92], and psychogenic excoriations [93]. According to the authors of the position paper drawn up by the European Society for Dermatology and Psychiatry (ESDaP) [70], it is necessary as far as possible to adopt uniform terminology and classification of SISD.

Self-induced dermatoses are here subdivided into two groups: disorders with a denied or hidden behaviour and disorders with a non-denied and non-hidden behaviour (Table 3.1). No account will here be taken of body-modifying behaviour (tattoos, piercing, ritualistic scars, aesthetic procedures), even if these surgical or cosmetic interventions can cause permanent skin damage. These latter, in fact, cannot be considered "self-inflicted", despite the fact that it is the subject's choice that has led to the cutaneous harm. Nor will we consider here self-mutilations that occur in primary psychiatric disorders (autistic disorders, schizophrenia, intellectual disability), nor skin damage induced by phlebotomy in suicide attempts or cutaneous

A. Cutaneous disorders with a denied or hidden pathological behaviour
1. Factitious disorders without external incentives
2. Factitious disorders with external incentives (malingering)
B. Cutaneous disorders with a non-denied and non-hidden pathological behaviour
1. Compulsive-impulsive disorders

Table 3.1 Classification of self-inflicted skin disorders. (Modified, by Ref. [70])

self-injuries observed in subjects with delusional parasitosis (scratching and picking to eliminate imagined parasites), or with a disturbed awareness of the body [70].

Owing to the paucity of empirical studies, the incidence of SISD is difficult to estimate, but it is likely more common than is widely believed [62, 68, 70, 94]. A review of 18 studies on a combined cohort of 52,000 patients reported rates of SISD ranging from 0.032% to 9.36% (weighted mean 0.9%) [68]. This wide range of prevalence is likely linked to various factors, such as the specific medical field of interest, the level of diagnostic attention paid by physicians, and the diagnostic criteria applied. Some authors believe that the incidence of SISD may rise because of the growing sociocultural acceptance of self-manipulative habits observed in certain fields, such as piercing and tattooing [94].

Except for the Münchausen syndrome, that is more frequent in men, SISD are more common in women, the M/F ratio being 1:3/1:20 [66, 76]. The age of patients ranges from 11 to 65 years, mean age being 31.5 years [68]. In a review of 455 cases with a factitious disorder made by Yates and Feldman, the patients with dermatological problems tended to be older (40.6 years) [3].

3.4 Diagnostic Criteria

The diagnosis of SISD does not generally present particular difficulties although clearly the dermatologist can neither rely on a precise medical history in many cases nor on the patient's collaboration.

3.4.1 Site

The lesions are usually localized on easily accessible areas. The most commonly affected areas are exposed sites like the face, especially the cheeks, and the back of the hands, followed by the forearms, more often of the non-dominant side. The face is affected in more than half the cases also in children [95–97].

Among the covered sites, those most frequently selected are the anterior region of the chest, the abdomen and in some cases the genitals. The back is generally exempt, unless the simulator is able to recruit a collaborator to procure lesions on this site (clearly, of the same nature as those elsewhere), in order to demonstrate the spontaneous occurrence of the clinical manifestations.

3.4.2 *Morphology*

Unlike spontaneous lesions, artefact lesions do not usually have a rounded or oval shape conforming to the skin blood supply cones. Moreover, except in situations where the patient wishes to perpetuate or mimic a known dermatosis [11–13, 42, 98–100], the lesions do not show the characteristics of known dermatological afflictions.

Artefact lesions are generally crude, irregular, sometimes with a bizarre, fantastic configuration, clear margins, intermittent lines, and acute angles. In other cases, the lesions are markedly linear and monomorphic, usually without involving the surrounding skin. In cases in which corrosive liquids have been used, signs of dripping are evident due to failure to control the application. Often, in case of ulcerations or ulcerous-escharotic manifestations, the lesions appear as prints, replicating the shape and size of the object used to inflict them. Ulcerative lesions have well-defined margins, may or may not be infiltrated at the base, and are often surrounded by erythematous or oedematous skin, a sign of inflammation due to chemical or physical aggression. In cases of simple erythema, the area is generally very inflamed and well-defined. If there is stasis oedema of a limb or finger (involvement of a single finger, generally the thumb, is characteristic) caused by constricting bands, the abrupt end at the point of ligature will be evident, and the consistency hard and identical all over the involved region. Oedema of the limbs due to constricting bands and hysterical dependent posture has also been described [101].

3.4.3 *Lesions*

Virtually, all elementary lesions can be observed, perhaps excepting gumma, primitive atrophy, and sclerosis. The number of lesions is highly variable, as also the sites involved as well as the type of presentation, as localized manifestations or else diffuse all over the body.

Erythema is frequently present, generally very red, or cyanotic with clearcut margins, whereas variously figured excoriated-vesicular lesions, instead, are uncommon apart from eczematous dermatitis, simulated using irritant or sensitizing substances to exploit occupational advantages (malingering). Bullous lesions are also infrequent but can be caused using vegetable extracts or other chemical agents (although weak irritants usually produce erythema and strong ones mostly ulcerations). These have an irregular morphology but sometimes a rounded shape because they may be induced with a suction mechanism [102]. Pustules are more often secondary to infection superimposed on the self-induced lesions, or have developed due to contact with contaminated objects, or as a result of methodical scratching with infected nails [103, 104]. Purpuric lesions with clearcut margins are often observed, obtained using various means involving suction or repeated trauma by pinching, or with different objects, such as ecchymoses produced using a wooden bat, or small sandbags.

The subcutaneous introduction of various substances (paraffin, milk, drugs, bacteria, enzymes, talc, body secretions, or other foreign bodies) [105] gives rise to infiltrating dermo-hypodermic lesions that can, over time, take on a hard, wooden consistency (paraffinoma), and possibly evolve into ulcers [44]. Pigmented lesions with linear margins are observed as the outcome of previous erythematous-desquamating lesions. Ulcerative or ulcerative-escharotic lesions are commonly observed (Figs. 3.1, 3.2, 3.3, 3.4, 3.5, 3.6, 3.7 and 3.8); these heal quite slowly and have an unpredictable clinical course, often associated with superimposed infections. Instead, gangrenous lesions are less frequent; these generally have irregular margins and tend to be localized on the legs. In such cases, the normal perilesional skin and integrity of appendages make it possible to exclude a spontaneous vascular origin of the complaint. Hard oedema of the back of the hand is also common, obtained by applying a haemostatic ligature or else by repeated contusion (Secrétan syndrome) [105]. Considerable atrophy and scarring can ensue after the resolution of such artefacts.

On the scalp, irregular areas of alopecia can be observed, with the hair clipped to various lengths (trichotillomania) (Figs. 3.9, 3.10, 3.11, 3.12, 3.13, 3.14, 3.15, 3.16, 3.17, 3.18 and 3.19); albeit rarely, this same alopecia can also involve the eyebrows, eyelashes, and suprapubic region (especially in women) (Figs. 3.20 and 3.21).

It is also possible to observe cases of subcutaneous emphysema after the injection of air, as well as psoriasiform [106] and vasculitic [107] lesions. Vitamin K

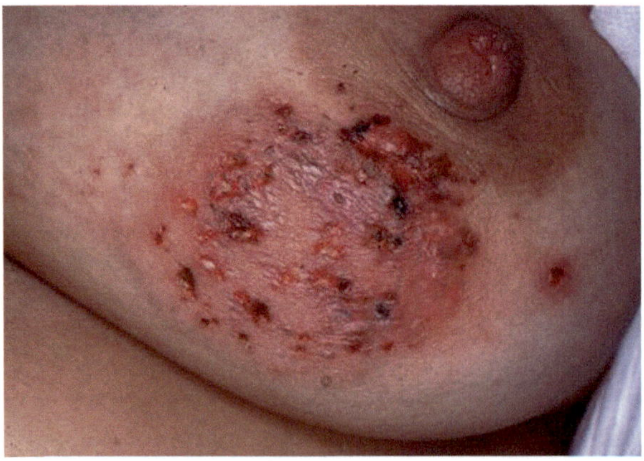

Fig. 3.1 Rounded plaque with ulcerative lesions

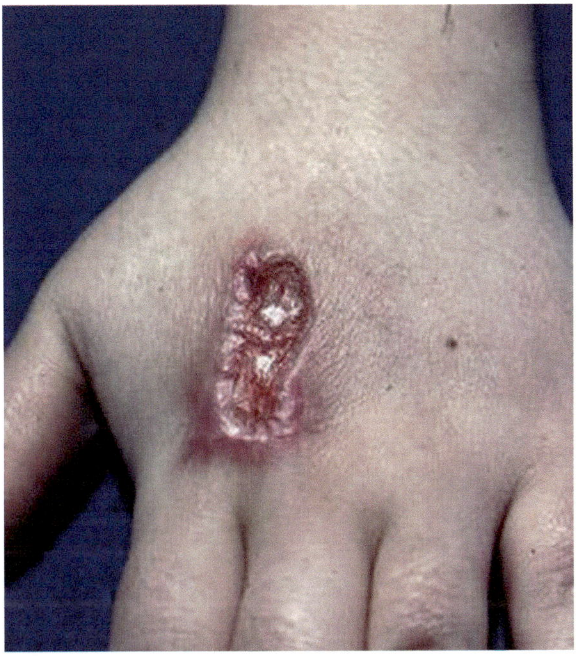

Fig. 3.2 Figured mechanically induced ulcerative lesion

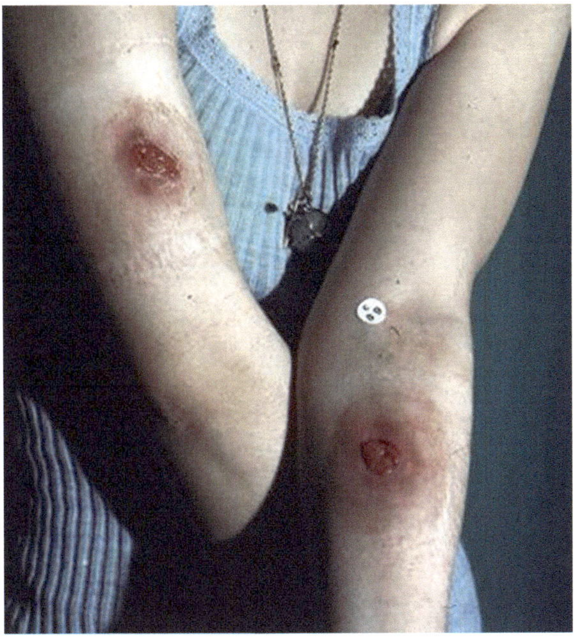

Fig. 3.3 A 35-year-old woman with ulcerative lesions. (Reproduced from Meneghini and Angelini [9]. All rights reserved)

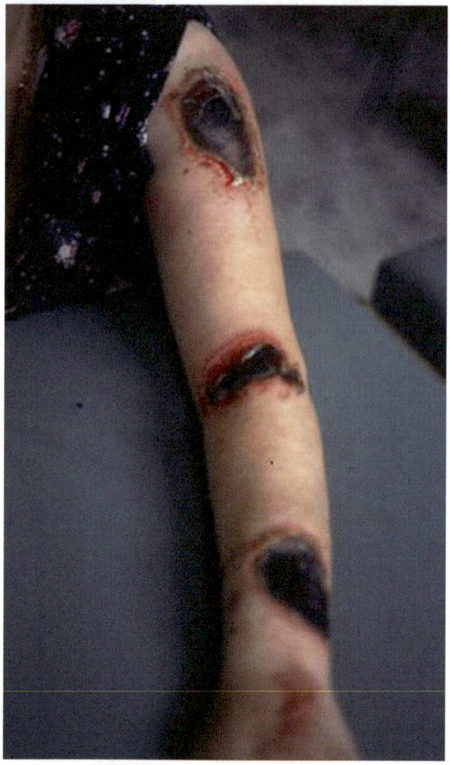

Fig. 3.4 A 50-year-old woman with multiple escharotic chemically induced lesions. (Reproduced with permission by Angelini and Bonamonte [44])

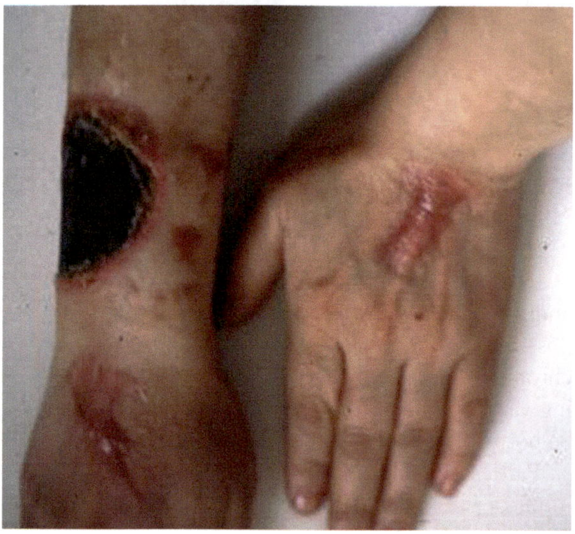

Fig. 3.5 The same patient as in Fig. 3.4. Keloid-like scars on the back of hands due to previous ulcerative lesions

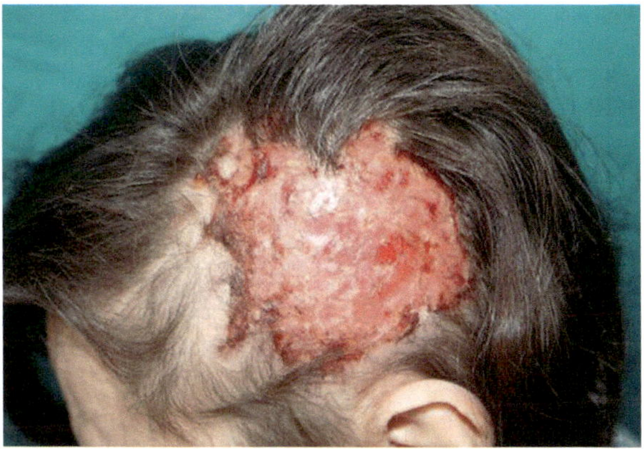

Fig. 3.6 A 70-year-old woman with an ulcerative lesion of the scalp

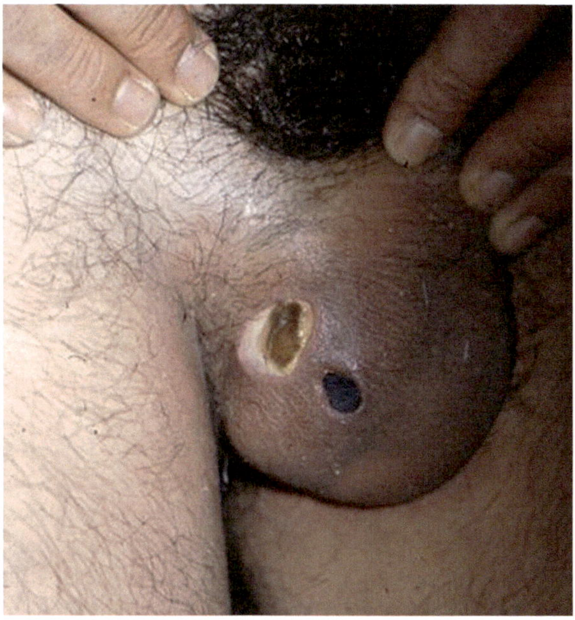

Fig. 3.7 A 30-year-old man with ulcerative lesions of the scrotum induced by incandescent metal object. (Reproduced with permission by Bonamonte et al. [45])

antagonist can aggravate the contusions and cause haemorrhage [66]. Finally, the possible association of skin lesions with other artefactual somatic signs, such as chronic fever, for example, induced by manipulating the thermometer or by injecting various substances (bacterial cultures, foreign proteins, faeces, etc.), must also be borne in mind.

Particularly imaginative subjects can sometimes produce lesions that perfectly mimic a previous spontaneous dermatosis. However, unlike a spontaneous eruption, where the course of evolution of the lesions is evident (some new lesions while others are already fully developed and mature), in simulated artefacts the lesions all appear fully formed and at the same stage of development [72]. Inability to elicit the

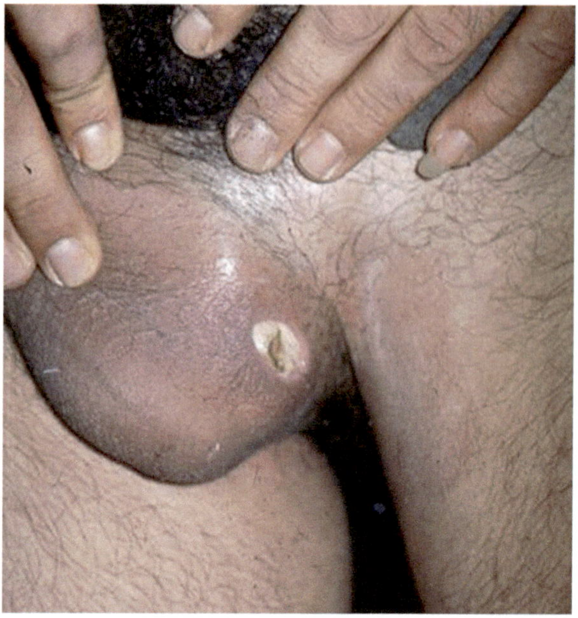

Fig. 3.8 The same patient as in Fig. 3.7. (Reproduced with permission by Bonamonte et al. [45])

clinical evolution of such skin diseases comes under the heading of a "hollow history", that is typical of subjects with SISD.

3.4.4 *Complementary Tests*

In all cases of primary rather than secondary SISD, as an aggravation of pre-existing spontaneous skin diseases, the various laboratory tests are within normal limits, except for brief peaks due to inflammation in acute cases (ESR, leukocytosis), and even the latter values normalize rapidly. Instrumental diagnostic investigations will also yield negative results in cases of artefact lesions appearing as ulcerations on the legs in the form of a pretended arterial or venous disorder.

Oedema of the limbs induced by constricting bands will regress quite rapidly although in lymphoedema due to chronic stricture, lymphography may show a specific "broken glass" aspect of the collateral lymphatic vessels [108, 109]. In cases of recurrent episodes or in ischaemic thumb, vascular scan can exclude embolic disease. Skin artefacts of pathomimic type will be supported by psychiatric clinical data.

Apart from the clinical characteristics suggestive of a simulated dermatitis, some tests on the lesions themselves can be performed to gain confirmation. The aetiological means commonly used by women include bleaches, soaps, and household cleaners, while industrial acids and automobile fluids are employed by men; in both cases, such chemicals can produce a persistent, detectable smell on the skin [84].

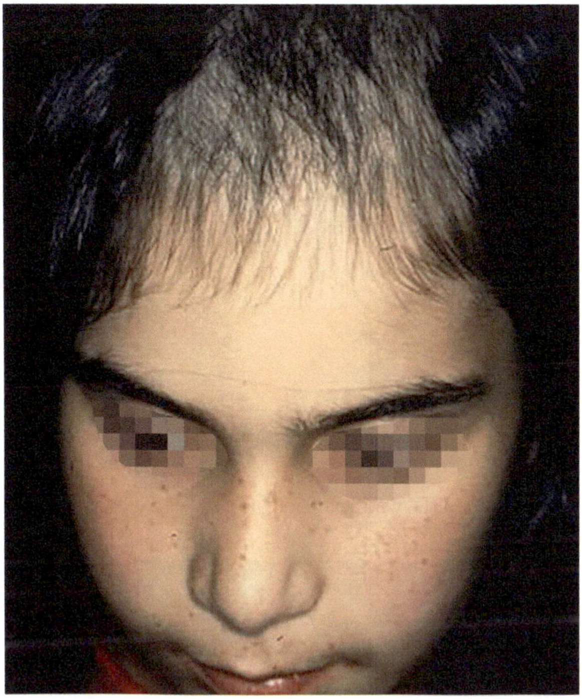

Fig. 3.9 Frontal trichotillomania in an 8-year-old girl. (Reproduced with permission by Bonamonte et al. [7])

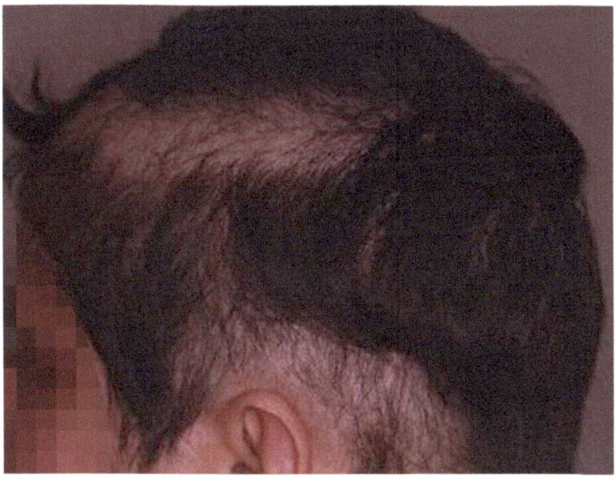

Fig. 3.10 Parietal trichotillomania in a 9-year-old boy

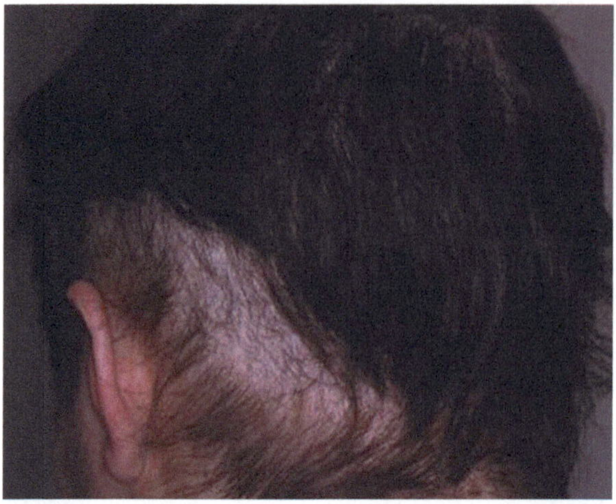

Fig. 3.11 Parietal trichotillomania in a 17-year-old boy

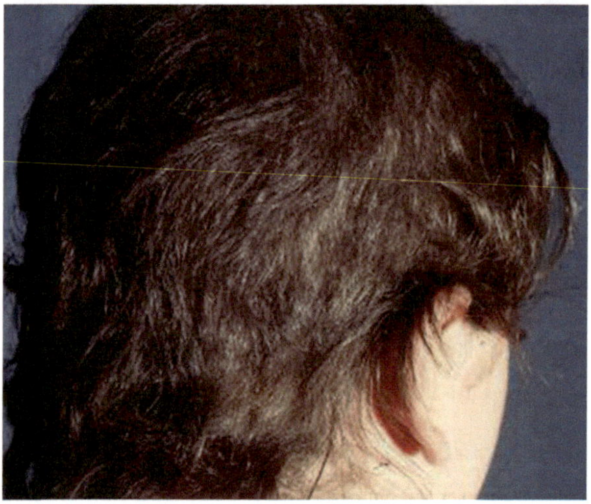

Fig. 3.12 Bilateral parietal trichotillomania in a 9-year-old boy. (Reproduced with permission by Bonamonte et al. [7])

Extraneous matter on the surface of suspect lesions can be revealed by surface biopsy in the form of stripping with a polyethylene polyester plaster made to adhere with a drop of cyanoacrylate glue; 30–60 seconds after application, the plaster is removed and the stratum corneum cells thus obtained are used for cytological tests or cultures. In cases of ulcerative lesions, light brushing of the base of the lesion may allow a fairly approximative identification of the extraneous matter used. Determining the pH can help to demonstrate the use of acid or alkaline substances applied shortly before and not washed off [11–13, 77, 98, 110].

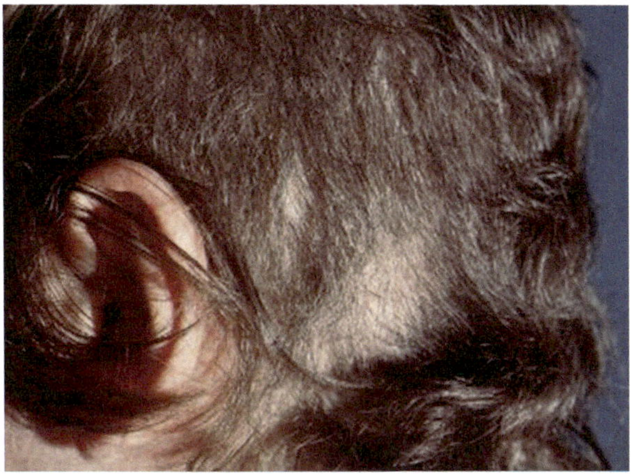

Fig. 3.13 The same patient as Fig. 3.12. (Reproduced with permission by Bonamonte et al. [7])

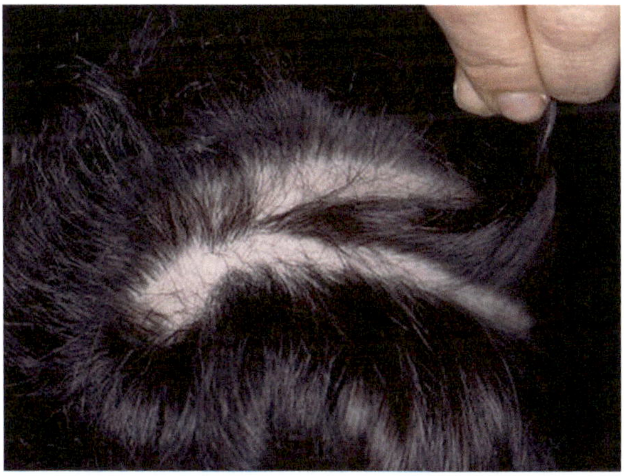

Fig. 3.14 Trichotillomania in a 15-year-old boy

Of course, in all cases histopathology testing is necessary to make a more certain differential diagnosis from spontaneous clinical forms with the same morphology. Depending on the type and duration of the artefact, various histological patterns can emerge, some of which may mimic spontaneous disorders. It is therefore very important that the clinician inform the histopathologist of the suspected artefactual nature (based on clinical or medical history data) of the lesions. In general, the histological damage is to the epidermis: in fact, the most common pattern is epidermal necrosis, with a modest inflammatory process at the derma, that is the result of exposure to thermal, chemical, or electrical aggression [110, 111].

Blisters are also common, induced by various attacks; clinically, they can mimic immunobullous disorders, but the histopathological difference is the presence of full-thickness epidermal necrosis, clearcut margins and a scarce inflammatory

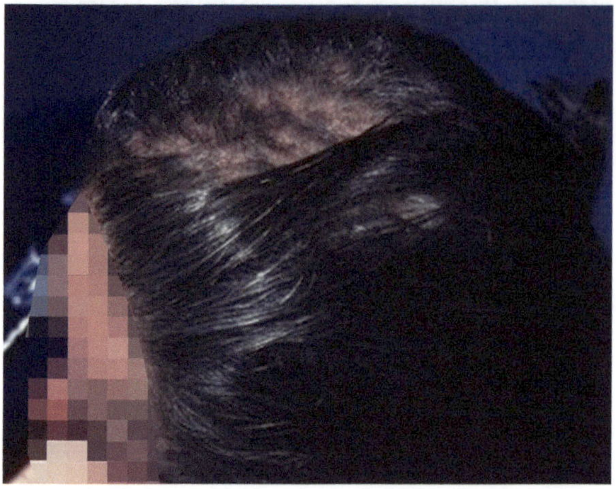

Fig. 3.15 Trichotillomania in a 52-year-old woman. (Reproduced with permission by Bonamonte et al. [7])

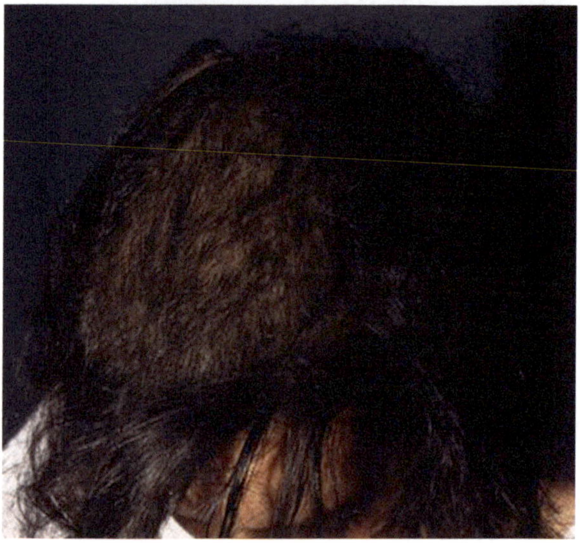

Fig. 3.16 Trichotillomania in an adult woman

infiltrate lacking eosinophils [112]. Immunofluorescence will, of course, be negative. Intraepidermal or subepidermal blisters induced by electrical burns present vertically elongated keratinocyte nuclei and homogenization of superficial dermal collagen [113, 114].

The introduction of foreign material can cause the formation of a dermic or subcutaneous foreign-body granuloma, occasionally revealing polarizable material

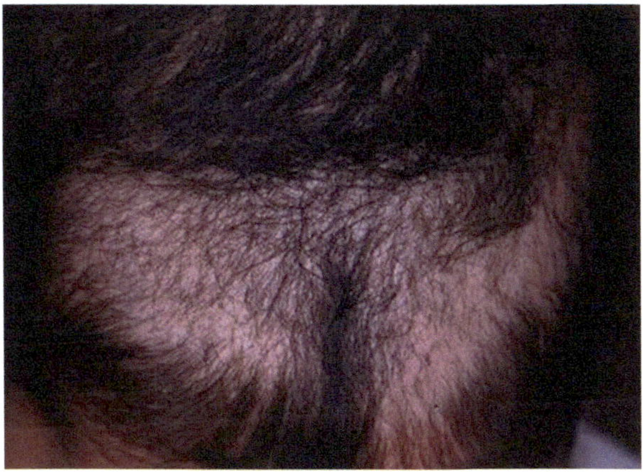

Fig. 3.17 Tonsure-like trichotillomania in an adult man

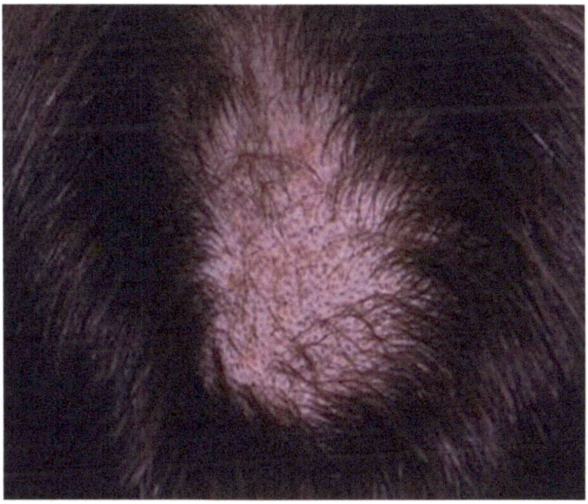

Fig. 3.18 Tonsure-like trichotillomania in an adult patient

[115]. Other possible histopathological findings include erosions, epidermal acanthosis, and neutrophilic infiltrates [116, 117].

An infrequent reported histopathological finding, but suggestive of dermatitis artefacta, is the presence of epidermal multinucleated keratinocytes, often comprising more than five nuclei [110, 111, 118, 119]. The mechanism underlying the formation of these cells remains unknown: they could be due to chronic epidermal irritation subsequent to exposure to corrosive substances or mechanical trauma, which causes cell-to-cell fusion and the disruption of cytokinesis rather than mitotic failure [111, 118]. Naturally, it is important to remember that epidermal multinucleated cells can be found in many other conditions, such as tumours, inflammatory

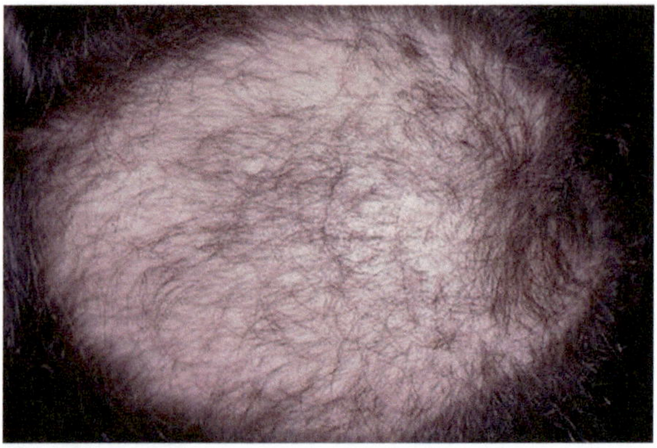

Fig. 3.19 Tonsure-like trichotillomania in a woman

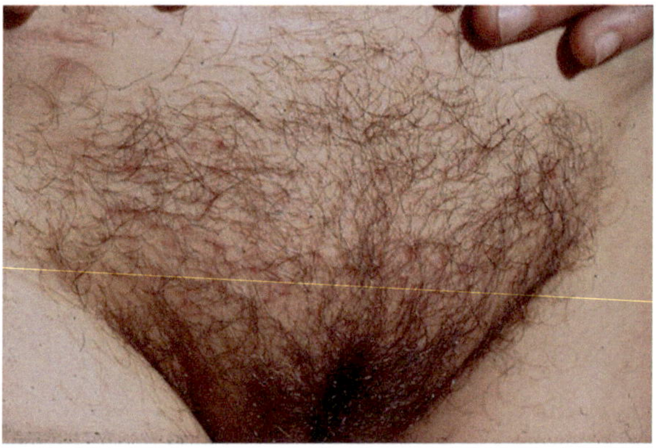

Fig. 3.20 Trichotillomania of the pubic area

disorders, acantholytic dermatoses, and herpetic infections, to name just a few. Except in cases of HSV infections, multinucleated keratinocytes of dermatitis artefacta lack the typical bright grey-blue nuclei with marginalized chromatin [110, 111, 120].

3.4.5 Clinical Course

Skin artefacts usually resolve quite fast, except in clinical pictures characterized by severe trophic disorders of the dermic-hypodermic tissues, such as ulcers, gangrene, paraffinoma. An unexpectedly slow improvement or healing and unpredictable course of a lesion is in any case elements that can guide the diagnosis. However, it

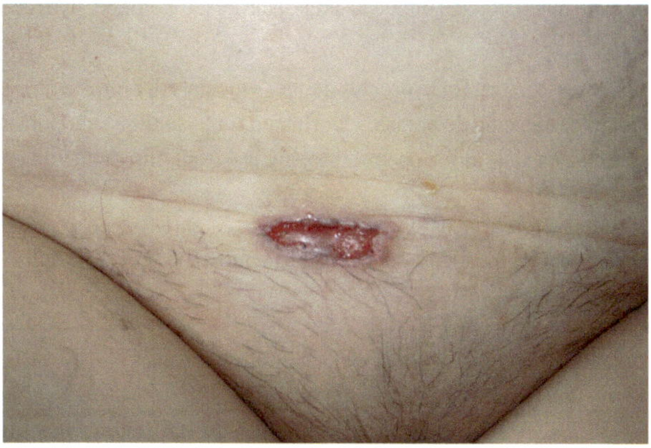

Fig. 3.21 Trichotillomania and figured ulcerative lesion of the pubic area

is essential to stress that rapid resolution can only be obtained with occlusive dressing under strict medical and paramedical control.

True complications can sometimes arise, and even iatrogenic, that are possible because a self-induced artefact can become chronic if not promptly diagnosed. The infective nature of some artefacts poses a risk of septic complications, and even fatal septicaemia [121]. Oedema and lymphoedema due to constricting bands can cause lesions of the cortical bone (thickening) and subcutaneous fibrosis. Hideous scars, cheloids, and retractions can also remain. The intentional aggravation of a post-surgical wound, if it goes undiagnosed, can lead to repetitive operative revisions, that in turn legitimize the continuity of the artefact, followed by unexpected complications (osteomyelitis, fistulae, and peritonitis) [122–124].

Only few follow-up studies of SISD have been reported in the literature. Haenel and Coll investigated a large series of 81 patients with factitious skin lesions without external incentives: the follow-up confirmed the persistence of the problem in 39 cases [125, 126]. Of these, 25 (64%) referred a difficult family situation during their childhood, 19 (48.7%) were under psychiatric treatment, and 23 (53%) suffered from a markedly depressive state. According to the authors, these patients did not have sufficient psychological resources to overcome their problems. A similar study of 43 patients followed up for many years showed that 33 of them continued to present symptoms up to 12 years after the first manifestation of self-inflicted skin lesions [127]. In 20 cases, the symptoms improved over time as a result of new family situations, while some of these patients showed marked similarities to anorexia patients.

Table 3.2 Aetiological agents of self-induced skin disorders. (Modified, by Ref. [45])

A. Chemical agents
1. Acids (acetic, chromic, formic, hydrochloric, hot vinegar, trichloroacetic)
2. Alkalis (calcium oxide, caustic potash, chlorinated lime, sodium salt, potassium salt)
3. Solvents (boiling oils and liquids, petrol, propane gas, salt, turpentine oil)
B. Physical agents
Metal objects (forks, needles, paper knives, pins, pincers, scissors, tweezers, various tools), cheese graters, fingernails, incandescent needles, haemostatic ligatures, lighted cigarettes, pumice stone, small sandbags, wire brushes
C. Biotic agents
1. Animal (caterpillars, jellyfishes, sea-anemones, salted sardines)
2. Plant (agave, cactus, ferula, fig latex, nettle, primula)
3. Miscellaneous: substances used for injections (air, bacterial cultures from laboratories, blood, faeces, foreign proteins, gasoline, industrial grease, liquid paraffin, milk, saliva, silicones, talc, urine)

3.5 Aetiological Agents

Causal agents can be of a physical, chemical, or biotic nature (Table 3.2). Those in the first two categories are more frequently adopted [13, 44, 45, 98].

Among mechanical means, those produced simply by fingernails must also be taken into account. The chemicals most commonly used are acids and alkalis. Strong acids have a corrosive action, while weak ones tend to be astringent. Hydrochloric acid provokes deep burns that may then form blisters. Sulphuric acid carbonizes the skin forming ulcers that resolve very slowly. Nitric acid has a strong oxidizing power and induces deep, intensely yellow burns. Other strong acids generally provoke ulcerative lesions with blurred margins. Strong alkaline solutions cause extensive skin destruction, exerting a solubilizing action on the tissues and causing the formation of hard escharotic lesions.

The mechanism of action of biotic agents is complex, and there are multiple types, although essentially, they can be summarized as having a pharmacological type of action that releases biochemical mediators and proteolytic enzymes.

In practice, identifying the aetiological agent can sometimes be difficult, due to the obstinate reticence of the simulator. In such cases, the dermatologist needs to rely on generic suggestive criteria: blisters are often due to vegetable agents, ecchymoses to mechanical agents, ulcers to chemical agents. However, the precise individuation of the culprit substance is sometimes impossible unless the simulator confesses. The use of salted sardines, or propane gas from a lighter, for example, as emerged in some of our cases, is difficult to image.

3.6 Concluding Diagnostic Remarks

The diagnostic criteria can be summarized as follows [7, 43, 44]:

Resumptive criteria. These serve to raise the suspicion of a self-inflicted disorder and are based above all on making as detailed as possible a diagnosis of the development of the lesions. In cases of suspected occupational artefact dermatitis, it is also wise to enquire into the employment status (loss of work, reduced working activity, and consequently reduced wages), and into possible disagreements with the employer.

Probability criteria. These are based mainly on the objective evaluation of clinical-morphological findings and on observation of the lesions over a period of time and under occlusive dressings. In many cases, the morphology of the lesions alone may provide sufficient grounds for the diagnosis of an artefact. The diagnosis is more difficult when a simulator seeks to aggravate or to prolong and perpetuate a pre-existing spontaneous dermatitis since this subject may know a lot about its aetiology. In such cases, continued observation in the hospital may be necessary to solve the diagnostic problem.

Certain criteria. These include the successful identification of residues of the agent employed (chemical or biological) at the site of the lesions, and of partial or complete admission of self-inflicted harm. The latter can be achieved by means of various reassuring, confidential discussions, combined with persuading the patient that it is useless to deny the factual evidence.

From the medico-legal standpoint, the problem is serious. It is important that the physician who suspects a self-inflicted disease should immediately share this suspicion with colleagues, fostering ample discussion and recruiting institutional management of legal services, in order to protect the physicians themselves from the possible risks of isolation and persecution.

3.7 Management

3.7.1 Assessment

Patients affected by SISD need both psychiatric and dermatological assessment.

Because SISD are clearly correlated to mental disorders, the dermatologist needs to have some familiarity with psychiatric issues, in order to ensure the best management of these patients, also as regards the basic elements involved in the treatment. This is because most patients with factitious disorders do not believe in the possible psychogenic origin of their symptoms and, in any case, are often reluctant to accept any referral to a consultation of psychiatric type.

It must be borne in mind, moreover, that the effects of these diseases on the family and social life of the patients may be very severe. Therefore, as well as psychiatric help and controlling patient compliance to medications, the dermatologist must inform the family members, who, where possible, can often be of great aid. It should also be remembered that the diagnosis of a cutaneous artefact may impair the doctor's relationship with the patient. Besides, the dermatologist may feel that he/she is being manipulated and may reflect this feeling on the patient during the visit. Finally, the dermatologist must also check for the presence of comorbidities, such as eating disorders and dependence and/or abuse of non-addictive substances, for instance, that are observed in a considerable percentage of cases [31].

Among the various dermatological diagnostic criteria, the clinical-morphological aspects are undoubtedly the most important. The type of lesions, especially their pattern and configuration, and the anatomo-functional conditions of the perilesional skin, are elements with a considerable diagnostic value. However, this criterion must not be overemphasized, given the possible occurrence of spontaneous dermatoses with equally bizarre configurations. Before diagnosing an artefact, therefore, differential diagnosis must be made with all the possible spontaneous causes of the afflictions, based on clinical data, and also taking into account the possible unfavourable influence of therapies applied before the dermatologist consultation. The diagnosis of a skin artefact must not therefore be seen as the result of a process of elimination but as a possible diagnosis among others. In cases of "irresponsible" patients, the artefact must be accepted as the expression of strong mental suffering of which the patient is unaware [67].

3.7.2 Treatment Approach

The simulation of skin artefacts not dictated by external incentives is perhaps one of the most complex problems to treat in dermatology [67].

Since most patients with psychocutaneous disorders are first, and perhaps only, seen by a dermatologist, it is extremely important that the latter should stick to an appropriate appointment schedule, limiting as much as possible the frequency of phone calls [62]. The dermatologist must plan continual contact with the patient, during frequent, not too brief (lasting at least half an hour) appointments. It will often take many weeks and many meetings to establish an optimal relationship with the patient. The physician must not become discouraged if progress is very slow and there are frequent setbacks.

It is also absolutely essential to "save the patient's face" and avoid the humiliation of direct accusations of simulation and about the aetiology of the lesions. A direct confrontation must be avoided at all costs because it is counterproductive (owing to the risk of a necessary defensive strategy), and the approach to psychiatric consultation and treatment must be introduced gently and rationally [62, 66, 128–132]. The patient may "open up" and recognize his/her behaviour only after a variable series of interviews and some simple medical treatment [68]. These patients must be visited in a quiet room, and not in the presence of many staff members or students asking questions [133].

3.7.2.1 Dermatological Treatment

Hospitalization in a dermatological ward, in particular in serious cases, can help to placate the conflict between the patient and the surrounding environment. The doctor-nurses team must act in symbiosis and establish an unvarying attitude.

Occlusive dressings are used both as a diagnostic tool and to prevent further self-mutilation. However, it is important not to insinuate that these dressings are aimed at preventing self-mutilation, nor to show triumph if the lesions heal after the use of occlusive dressings. Moreover, it must be remembered that the patient may find a way to manipulate the dressing or may transfer the site of injury to another skin area.

3.7.2.2 Psychiatric Treatment

The main therapy is psychological and based on restructuring the patient's personality and on psychotropic drugs. The former relies on analytical psychotherapy adapted to borderline personalities and must be performed by a psychoanalyst with specific experience in the field. To make a precise diagnosis of the various personality disorders, many tools are publicly available: questionnaires are clinically validated and less "subjective" than a physician's assessment [133–136]. In particular, the treatment of psychocutaneous disorders should include psychoeducation, psychotherapy, psychotropic treatment, and, if necessary, psychobiotics [135, 137]. To draw up an adequate therapeutic strategy, it is necessary to take into account the type of disorder (psychophysiological, psychiatric with dermatological symptoms, and dermatological with psychiatric symptoms), the type of comorbidity (anxiety, depression, obsessive-compulsive or psychotic symptoms), and the severity of the comorbidity, assessed with screening scales and questionnaires [135]. In practice, the management of the various types of disorders must always include psychoeducation of the patient, by means of proper information and systematic knowledge transfer of the dermatological and psychological problems involved, to allow the patient to understand and face the situation, and to collaborate with a real expectation of success of the proposed treatment [137, 138]. This is particularly important in cases of cutaneous sensory disorders (vulvodynia, burning mouth syndrome, for example), that most physicians consider "medically unexplained", thereby increasing the patient's feelings of anxiety and depression [138]. Yet again, this highlights the importance of the doctor-patient relationship; it may even be claimed that the most important treatment the physician can prescribe is her or his complete attention [135, 139].

Psychotherapy (cognitive behavioural therapy, hypnosis) and psychotropics (benzodiazepine, hydroxyzine, serotonin), must also be considered, depending on the severity of the psychopathology (anxiety, depression) linked with the cutaneous symptoms [62, 135]. In the management of psychocutaneous disorders, psychobiotics (*Lactobacillus casei*, *Lactobacillus acidophilus*, *Bifidobacterium bifidum*) are also suggested, in view of their antidepressant and anxiolytic effect [140–143]. Finally, in psychodermatology it is essential to consider psychiatric risk assessment (prior suicide attempts, suicide plans, hopelessness, isolation, and loss of a relationship or a job) that once more highlights the absolute importance of relying on a multidisciplinary team (dermatologist, psychiatrist, and psychologist). In fact, it must be borne in mind that various suicides occur during severe depression and anxiety, psychosis, and/or substances misuse, all comorbidities that can be observed also in dermatology [144–151].

From what has been stated about the management of psychocutaneous disorders, it is clear that it is essential to ensure a full awareness among dermatologists, psychiatrists, and psychologists of the problem of psychodermatology, to increase specific knowledge in the various sectors and so ensure a productive collaboration [152].

3.8 Conclusions

SISD are complex, multifactorial conditions that, on the one hand, are still in need of standardized nomenclature and classification based on diagnostic criteria, and on the other, of an individualized psychosocial approach.

Self-inflicted skin diseases contribute significantly to morbidity in the dermatologic patient and can also complicate the course of a spontaneous primary condition, such as acne and some pruritic dermatoses.

In the great majority of cases, self-inflicted dermatoses are linked to acute or chronic problems with emotional regulation and various levels of dissociation. The skin and its appendages, hair, and nails are amply innervated with a dense network of afferent sensory nerves and efferent autonomic nerves, and the skin is often the target of tension-reducing behaviour, especially in cases of overexcitement of the autonomic nervous system. For all these reasons, it is important that dermatologists, psychiatrists, and psychologists, in particular, be well aware of SISD, in order to ensure an optimal collaboration in the management of patients with psychodermatological problems.

References

1. Illustrated Stendman's Medical Dictionary. 24th ed. Baltimore/London: Williams and Wilkins; 1982:p. 508.
2. American Psychiatric Association (APA). Diagnostic and statistical manual of mental disorders. DSM-5. 5th ed. Washington, DC: APA; 2013.
3. Yates GP, Feldman MD. Factitious disorder: a systematic review of 455 cases in the professional literature. Gen Hosp Psychiatry. 2016;41:20–8.
4. Jimenez XF, Nkanginieme N, Dhand N, et al. Clinical, demographic, psychological, and behavioral features of factitious disorder: a retrospective analysis. Gen Hosp Psychiatry. 2020;62:93–5.
5. Bérar A, Bouzillé G, Jego P, et al. A descriptive, retrospective case series of patients with factitious disorder imposed on self. BMC Psychiatry. 2021;21:588.

6. ICD-11 for Mortality and Morbidity Statistics (Version: 05/2021). [Cited 2021 Sept 4]. Available from: https://icd.who.int/browse11/lm/en#/http%3a%2f%2fid.who.int%2ficd%2fentity2t790764418
7. Bonamonte D, Foti C, De Marco A, et al. Self-inflicted pathological cutaneous disorders. Part II. Ital J Dermatol Venerol. 2022;157:480–8.
8. Malingering AR. Talking sense. Bath: Pitman Press; 1973. p. 145–7.
9. Meneghini CL, Angelini G. Occupational dermatitis artefacta. Derm Beruf Umwelt. 1979;27:163–5.
10. Petruzzellis V, Angelini G, Vena GA. La dermatite artefatta. Dermatol Allergol Profes. 1988;3:23–40.
11. Lachapelle JM, Frimat P, Temstealt D, et al. Dermatoses simulées en medicine du travail. In: Dermatologie professionnelle et de l'environnement. Paris: Masson; 1922. p. 263–71.
12. Angelini G. Occupational dermatitis artefacta. In: Kanerva L, Elsner P, Wahlberg JE, et al., editors. Handbook of occupational dermatology. Berlin: Springer; 2000. p. 141–7.
13. Angelini G, Bonamonte D. Occupational dermatitis artefacta. In: Syall-Smith D, Marks R, editors. Dermatology at the millennium. The proceedings of the 19th World Congress of Dermatology. Sydney, 15-20 June, 1988. New York: The Parthenon Publishing Group Inc.; 1999. p. 508–13.
14. Lawlor A, Kirakowski J. When the lie is the truth: grounded theory analysis of an online support group for factitious disorder. Psychiatry Res. 2014;218:209–18.
15. Robertson MM, Hossain G. Münchausen's syndrome coexisting with other disorders. Br J Hosp Med. 1997;58:154–5.
16. DeWitt DE, Ward SA, Prabhu S, et al. Patient privacy versus protecting the patient and the health system from harm: a case study. Med J Aust. 2009;191:213–6.
17. Hirayama Y, Sakamaki S, Tsuji Y, et al. Fatality caused by self-bloodletting in a patient with factitious anemia. Int J Hematol. 2003;78:146–8.
18. Nichols GR, Davis GJ, Corey TS. In the shadow of the Baron: sudden death due to Münchausen syndrome. Am J Emerg Med. 1990;8:216–9.
19. Vaduganathan M, McCullough SA, Fraser TN, et al. Death due to Münchausen syndrome: a case of idiopathic recurrent right ventricular failure and a review of the literature. Psychosomatics. 2014;55:668–72.
20. Bright R, Eisendrath S, Damon L. A case of factitious aplastic anemia. Int J Psychiatry Med. 2001;31:433–41.
21. Romano A, Alqahtani S, Griffith J, et al. Factitious psychogenic nonepileptic paroxysmal episodes. Epilepsy Behav Case Rep. 2014;2:184–5.
22. Dahale AB, Hatti S, Thippeswamy H, et al. Factitious disorder-experience at a neuropsychiatric center in southern India. Indian J Psychol Med. 2014;36:62–5.
23. Chambers E, Yager J, Apfeldorf W, et al. Factitious aortic dissection leading to thoracotomy in a 20-year-old man. Psychosomatics. 2007;48:355–8.
24. Chastaing M. Pathomimie et syndrome de Münchausen. Rev Prat. 2009;59:511–7.
25. Asher R. Münchausen's syndrome. Lancet. 1951;1:339–41.
26. Sutherland AJ, Rodin GM. Factitious disorders in a general hospital setting: clinical features and a review of the literature. Psychosomatics. 1990;31:392–9.
27. Fliege H, Scholler G, Rose M, et al. Factitious disorders and pathological self-harm in a hospital population: an interdisciplinary challenge. Gen Hosp Psychiatry. 2002;24:164–71.
28. Bauer M, Boegner F. Neurological syndromes in factitious disorder. J Nerv Ment Dis. 1996;184:281–8.
29. Mailis-Gagnon A, Nicholson K, Blumberger D, et al. Characteristics and period prevalence of self-induced disorder in patients referred to a pain clinic with the diagnosis of complex regional pain syndrome. Clin J Pain. 2008;24:176–85.
30. Gieler V, Eckhardt-Henn A. Factitious disorders. Dermatol Psychosom. 2004;5:93–8.

31. Fliege H, Grimm A, Eckhardt-Henn A, et al. Frequency of ICD-10 factitious disorder: survey of senior hospital consultants and physicians in private practice. Psychosomatics. 2007;48:60–4.
32. Geile J, Aasly J, Madea B, et al. Incidence of the diagnosis of factitious disorders—Nationwide comparison study between Germany and Norway. Forensic Sci Med Pathol. 2020;16:450–6.
33. Caselli I, Poloni N, Ielmini M, et al. Epidemiology and evolution of the diagnostic classification of factitious disorders in DSM-5. Psychol Res Behav Manag. 2017;10:387–94.
34. Feldman MD, Eisendrath SJ. The spectrum of factitious disorders. 1st ed. Washington, DC: American Psychiatric Press; 1995.
35. Plassmann R. Münchausen syndromes and factitious diseases. Psychother Psychosom. 1994;62:7–26.
36. Gordon DK, Sansone RA. A relationship between factitious disorder and borderline personality disorder. Innov Clin Neurosci. 2013;10:11–3.
37. Earle JR Jr, Folks DG. Factitious disorder and coexisting depression: a report of successful psychiatric consultation and case management. Gen Hosp Psychiatry. 1986;8:448–50.
38. Bass C, Halligan P. Factitious disorders and malingering: challenges for clinical assessment and management. Lancet. 2014;383:1422–32.
39. Krahn LE, Li H, O'Connor MK. Patients who strive to be ill: factitious disorder with physical symptoms. Am J Psychiatry. 2003;160:1163–8.
40. Haddad SA, Winer KK, Gupta A, et al. A puzzling case of anemia. Transfusion. 2002;42:1610–3.
41. Chew BH, Pace KT, Honey RJ. Münchhausen syndrome presenting as gross hematuria in two women. Urology. 2002;59:601.
42. Parent DJ, Krafft T, Noel JC, et al. Cutaneous Münchausen syndrome with presentation simulating pyoderma gangrenosum. J Am Acad Dermatol. 1994;31:1072–4.
43. Angelini G, Vena GA. Dermatosi artefatte. In: Angelini G, Vena GA, editors. Dermatologia professionale e ambientale. Brescia: ISED; 1997. p. 257–68.
44. Angelini G, Bonamonte D. La dermatite artefatta. G Ital Dermatol Venereol. 1999;134:99–113.
45. Bonamonte D, Foti C, De Marco A, et al. Self-inflicted pathological cutaneous disorders. Part I. Ital J Dermatol Venerol. 2022;157:389–401.
46. Kenedi CA, Shirey KG, Hoffa M, et al. Laboratory diagnosis of factitious disorder: a systematic review of tools useful in the diagnosis of Münchausen's syndrome. N Z Med J. 2011;124:66–81.
47. Kinns H, Housley D, Freedman DB. Münchausen syndrome and factitious disorder: the role of the laboratory in its detection and diagnosis. Ann Clin Biochem. 2013;50:194–203.
48. Niforatos JD, Chaitoff A. Factitious disorder commonly presents as dermatitis factitia: a U.S. population-based study. Gen Hosp Psychiatry. 2020;64:129–30.
49. Feldman MD. Prophylactic bilateral radical mastectomy resulting from factitious disorder. Psychosomatics. 2001;42:519–21.
50. Levenson JL, Chafe W, Flanagan P. Factitious ovarian cancer: feigning via resources on the internet. Psychosomatics. 2007;48:71–3.
51. Feldman MD, Hamilton JC. Mastectomy resulting from factitious disorder. Psychosomatics. 2007;48:361.
52. Galli S, Tatu L, Bogousslavsky J, et al. Conversion, factitious disorder and malingering: a distinct pattern or a continuum? Front Neurol Neurosci. 2018;42:72–80.
53. Gupta MA. Emotional regulation, dissociation, and the self-induced dermatoses: clinical features and implications for treatment with mood stabilizers. Clin Dermatol. 2013;31:110–7.
54. Gupta MA, Gupta AK, Haberman HF. The self-inflicted dermatoses: a critical review. Gen Hosp Psychiatry. 1987;9:45–52.
55. Gupta MA, Levenson JL. Dermatology. In: Levenson JL, editor. The American psychiatric publishing textbook of psychosomatic medicine: psychiatric care of the medically ill. 2nd ed. Washington, DC: American Psychiatric Publishing Inc.; 2011. p. 667–90.

56. Odlaug BL, Grant JE. Clinical characteristics and medical complications of pathologic skin picking. Gen Hosp Psychiatry. 2008;30:61–6.
57. Flessner CA. Diagnosis and comorbidity. In: Grant JE, Stein DJ, Woods DE, et al., editors. Trichotillomania, skin picking and other body-focused repetitive behaviors. Arlington: American Psychiatry Publishing Inc.; 2012. p. 83–96.
58. Kenthen NJ, Siev JS, Reese H. Assessment of trichotillomania, pathological skin picking and stereotypic movement disorder. In: Grant JE, Stern DJ, Woods DE, et al., editors. Trichotillomania, skin picking and other body focused repetitive behaviors. Arlington: American Psychiatry Publishing Inc.; 2012. p. 129–50.
59. Koblenzer CS. Psychodermatology of women. Clin Dermatol. 1997;15:127–41.
60. Farber SK. Self-medication, traumatic re-enactment and somatic expressions in bulimic and self-mutilating behavior. Clin Soc Work J. 1997;25:87.
61. Hirsch M. The body as a transitional object. Psychother Psychosom. 1994;62:78–81.
62. Koblenzer CS, Dermatitis artefacta. Clinical features and approaches to treatment. Am J Clin Dermatol. 2000;1:47–55.
63. Koblenzer CS. Psychosomatic concepts in dermatology. A dermatologist-psychoanalyst's viewpoint. Arch Dermatol. 1983;119:501–12.
64. Panconesi E. Psychosomatic dermatology. Clin Dermatol. 1984;2:94–179.
65. Van Moffaert M, Vermander F, Kint A. Dermatitis artefacta. Int J Dermatol. 1985;24:236–8.
66. Gieler U. Factitious disease in the field of dermatology. Psychother Psychosom. 1994;62:48–55.
67. Consoli SG. Dermatitis artefacta: a general review. Eur J Dermatol. 1995;5:5–11.
68. Kocalevent RD, Fliege H, Rose M, et al. Autodestructive syndromes. Psychother Psychosom. 2005;74:202–11.
69. Harth W, Taube KM, Gieler U. Factitious disorders in dermatology. J Dtsch Dermatol Ges. 2010;8:361–72.
70. Gieler U, Consoli SG, Tomás-Aragones L, et al. Self-inflicted lesions in dermatology: terminology and classification—a position paper from the European Society for Dermatology and Psychiatry (ESDaP). Acta Derm Venereol. 2013;93:4–12.
71. Gupta MA, Gupta AK. Self-induced dermatoses: a great imitator. Clin Dermatol. 2019;37:268–77.
72. Lyell A. Cutaneous artifactual disease. A review, amplified by personal experience. J Am Acad Dermatol. 1979;1:391–407.
73. Fabisch W. What is dermatitis artefacta? Int J Dermatol. 1981;20:427–8.
74. Shelley WB. Dermatitis artefacta induced in a patient by one of her multiple personalities. Br J Dermatol. 1981;105:587–9.
75. Hänel T, Rauchfleisoh V, Schuppli R. Die Bedeutung von Haut-artefakten. Schweiz Med Wo chenschr. 1982;112:326–33.
76. Nielsen K, Jeppesen M, Simmelsgaard L, et al. Self-inflicted skin diseases. A retrospective analysis of 57 patients with dermatitis artefacta seen in a dermatology department. Acta Derm Venereol. 2005;85:512–5.
77. Krooks JA, Weatherall AG, Holland PJ. Review of epidemiology, clinical presentation, diagnosis, and treatment of common primary psychiatric causes of cutaneous disease. J Dermatol Treat. 2018;29:418–27.
78. Gelmetti G, Bonifazi E. Le patomimie cutanee nel bambino. Pediatric Dermatol News. 1985;4:146–69.
79. Ring HC, Miller IM, Benfeldt E, et al. Artefactual skin lesions in children and adolescents: review of the literature and two cases of factitious purpura. Int J Dermatol. 2015;54:27–32.
80. Alcántara Luna S, García Bravo B, Rodríguez Pichardo A, et al. Dermatitis artefacta in childhood: a retrospective analysis of 44 patients, 1976–2006. Pediatr Dermatol. 2015;32:604–8.
81. Fabisch W. Psychiatric aspects of dermatitis artefacta. Br J Dermatol. 1980;102:29–34.
82. Medansky RS, Handler RM. Dermatopsychosomatics: classification, physiology, and therapeutic approaches. J Am Acad Dermatol. 1981;5:125–36.

83. Musalek M, Hable B, Massabacher V. Diagnostics in psychodermatology. Dermatol Psychosom. 2001;2:110–5.
84. Millard LG, Millard J. Psychocutaneous disorders. In: Burns T, Brethnack S, Cox N, et al., editors. Rook's textbook of dermatology. 8th ed. Oxford: Wiley-Blacwell; 2010:chap.64.1-55.
85. Riedler E, Tanks FA. Psychocutaneous skin disorders. In: Goldsmith LS, Katz SJ, Gilchrest BA, et al., editors. Fitzpatrick's dermatology in general medicine. 8th ed. New York: McGraw-Hill; 2012. p. 1158–66.
86. Linder D, Bassi R. Psyche and skin. In: Giannetti A, Del Forno C, editors. Textbook of dermatology and sexually transmitted diseases. Padova: Piccin Nuova Libraria S.P.A; 2013. p. 431–41.
87. Kuhn H, Mennella C, Magid M, et al. Psychocutaneous disease: Clinical perspectives. J Am Acad Dermatol. 2017;76:779–91.
88. Cumming S, Covic T, Murrell E. Deliberate self-harm: have we scratched the surface? Behaviour Chance. 2006;23:186–99.
89. Klonsky ED, Moyer A. Childhood sexual abuse and non-suicidal self-injury: meta-analysis. Br J Psychiatry. 2008;192:166–70.
90. Van Moffaert M. The spectrum of dermatological self-mutilation and self-destruction including dermatitis artefacta and neurotic excoriations. In: Koo J, Lee CS, editors. Psychocutaneous medicine. New York: Marcel Dekker Inc.; 2003. p. 169–89.
91. Gupta MA, Gupta AK, Haberman HF. Neurotic excoriations: a review and some new perspectives. Compr Psychiatry. 1986;27:381–6.
92. Fruensgaard K. Psychotherapeutic strategy and neurotic excoriations. Int J Dermatol. 1991;30:198–203.
93. Arnold LM, Auchenbach MB, McElroy SL, Psychogenic excoriation. Clinical features, proposed diagnostic criteria, epidemiology and approaches to treatment. CNS Drugs. 2001;15:351–9.
94. Gieler U, Effendy I, Stangier U. Cutaneous artefacts—possibilities for treatment and their limits. Z Hautkr. 1987;62:882–90.
95. Millard L. Dermatitis artefacta in the 1990s. Br J Dermatol. 1995;135(Suppl. 47):27.
96. Rogers M, Fairley M, Santhanam R. Artefactual skin disease in children and adolescents. Australas J Dermatol. 2001;42:264–70.
97. Saez-de-Ocariz M, Orozco-Covarrubias L, Mora-Magaña I, et al. Dermatitis artefacta in pediatric patients: experience at the national institute of pediatrics. Pediatr Dermatol. 2004;21:205–11.
98. Bonamonte D, Foti C, Verni P, et al. Occupational dermatitis artefacta. In: Angelini G, Bonamonte D, Foti C, editors. Clinical contact dermatitis. A practical approach. Berlin: Springer Nature Switzerland AG; 2021. p. 583–95.
99. Levitz SM, Tan OT. Factitious dermatosis masquerading as recurrent herpes zoster. Am J Med. 1988;84:781–3.
100. Millard LG. Dermatological pathomimicry: a form of patient maladjustment. Lancet. 1984;2:969–71.
101. Smith RJ. Factitious lymphedema of the hand. J Bone Joint Surg Am. 1975;57:89–94.
102. Dufton P, Griffiths A. Suction blisters mimicking pemphigoid: an unusual case of dermatitis artefacta. Clin Exp Dermatol. 1981;6:163–6.
103. Wilhem R, Hertel G. Über Artefakte der Haut. Med Welt. 1961;2:81–6.
104. Corraze MJ. Un cas de pathomimie inhabituel: périonixys pustuleux. Bull Soc Fr Derm Syph. 1965;42:191–2.
105. Angelini G, Meneghini CL, Vena GA. Secrétan's syndrome: an artefact oedema of the hand. Contact Dermatitis. 1982;8:345–6.
106. Sneddon I, Sneddon J. Self-inflicted injury: a follow-up study of 43 patients. Br Med J. 1975;3:527–30.
107. Harper JI, Copeman PW. Dermatitis artefacta presenting as a 'vasculitis'. J R Soc Med. 1983;76:970–1.

108. Krener P. Factitious disorders and the psychosomatic continuum in children. Curr Opin Pediatr. 1994;6:418–22.
109. Flechet ML, Priollet P, Consoli S, et al. L'oedème bleu de Charcot. Une observation. Ann Med Interne. 1983;134:35–7.
110. Gutierrez D, Schowalter MK, Piliang MP, et al. Epidermal multinucleated keratinocytes: a histopathologic clue to dermatitis artefacta. J Cutan Pathol. 2016;43:880–3.
111. Tittelbach J, Peckruhn M, Elsner P. Histopathological patterns in dermatitis artefacta. J Dtsch Dermatol Ges. 2018;16:559–64.
112. Ikenaga S, Nakano H, Umegaki N, et al. A case of bullous dermatitis artefacta possibly induced by a deodorant spray. J Dermatol. 2006;33:40–2.
113. Sokumbi O, Comfere NI, McEvoy MT, et al. Bullous dermatitis artefacta. Am J Dermatopathol. 2013;35:110–2.
114. Boyd AS, Dewan A. Dermatitis artefacta in an adolescent female. J Cutan Pathol. 2015;42:660–1.
115. Kwon EJ, Dans M, Koblenzer CS, et al. Dermatitis artefacta. J Cutan Med Surg. 2006;10:108–13.
116. Ilter N, Adişen E, Gürer MA, et al. Dermatitis artefacta masquerading as pyoderma gangrenosum. Int J Dermatol. 2008;47:975–7.
117. Gattu S, Rashid RM, Khachemoune A. Self-induced skin lesions: a review of dermatitis artefacta. Cutis. 2009;84:247–51.
118. Winters C, Machan M, Liu D, et al. Multinucleated giant cells in factitial dermatitis. J Cutan Pathol. 2013;40:205–8.
119. Sweeney SA, Sulit DJ, Adams EG, et al. Grape cells (multinucleated keratinocytes) in noninfectious dermatoses: case series and review of the literature. Am J Dermatopathol. 2015;37:143–6.
120. Amin SM, Yélamos O, Martinez-Escala ME, et al. Epidermal necrosis with multinucleated keratinocytes: a possible diagnostic clue for dermatitis artefacta in children. J Eur Acad Dermatol Venereol. 2016;30:101–2.
121. Reich P, Gottfried LA. Factitious disorders in a teaching hospital. Ann Intern Med. 1983;99:240–7.
122. Angus J, Affleck A, Leich IH, et al. Factitious disease presenting as non-healing wounds. J Eur Acad Dermatol Venereol. 2005;19:70.
123. Reed DH, Martin I. Dermatitis artefacta complicated by a cerebral abscess. Postgrad Med J. 1988;64:976–7.
124. Murray SJ, Ross JB, Murray AH. Life-threatening dermatitis artefacta. Cutis. 1987;39:387–8.
125. Haenel T, Rauchfleisch U, Schuppli R, et al. The psychiatric significance of dermatitis artefacta. Eur Arch Psychiatry Neurol Sci. 1984;234:38–41.
126. Rauchfleisch U, Schuppli R, Haenel T. Zur Persönlichkeit von Patienten mit dermatologischen Artefakten. Z Psychosom Med Psychoanal. 1983;29:76–84.
127. Sneddon IB. The presentation of psychiatric illness to the dermatologist. Acta Derm Venereol. (Suppl). 1979;59:177–9.
128. Koblenzer CS. Psychocutaneous disease. Orlando (FL): Grune Stratton; 1987.
129. Sneddon IB. Simulated disease: problems in diagnosis and management. Br J Hosp Med. 1983;17:199–205.
130. Cotterill JA. Self-stigmatization: artefact dermatitis. Br J Hosp Med. 1992;47:115–9.
131. Plassmann R. Inpatient and outpatient long-term psychotherapy of patients suffering from factitious disorders. Psychother Psychosom. 1994;62:96–107.
132. Friedman B, Yaffe B, Blankstein A, et al. Self-inflicted hand injuries: diagnostic challenge and treatment. Ann Plast Surg. 1988;20:345–50.
133. Reichenberg JS, Kroumpouzos G, Magid M. Approach to a psychodermatology patient. G Ital Dermatol Venereol. 2018;153:494–6.
134. Jafferany M, França K. Psychodermatology: basics concepts. Acta Derm Venereol. 2016;96:35–7.

135. Jafferany M, Ferreira BR, Abdelmaksoud A, et al. Management of psychocutaneous disorders: a practical approach for dermatologists. Dermatol Ther. 2020;33:e13969–76.
136. Torales J, Melgarejo O, González I, et al. Psychopharmacology in dermatology: treatment of primary psychiatric conditions in dermatology. Dermatol Ther. 2020;33:e13577–82.
137. Jafferany M, Ferreira BR, Patel A. The essentials of psychodermatology. Cham: Springer International Publishing; 2020. p. 29–34.
138. Ferreira BR, Pio-Abreu JL, Reis JP, et al. Medically unexplained dermatologic symptoms and psychodermatology. J Eur Acad Dermatol Venereol. 2018;32:447–8.
139. Elpern DJ. Medically unexplained dermatologic symptoms still a problem. J Eur Acad Dermatol Venereol. 2018;32:e449.
140. Ansari F, Pourjafar H, Tabrizi A, et al. The effects of probiotics and prebiotics on mental disorders: a review on depression, anxiety, Alzheimer, and autism spectrum disorders. Curr Pharm Biotechnol. 2020;21:555–65.
141. Tohid H, Shenefelt PD, Burney WA, et al. Psychodermatology: an association of primary psychiatric disorders with skin. Rev Colomb Psiquiatr. 2019;48:50–7.
142. Jafferany M, Afrin A, Mkhoyan R, et al. Therapeutic implications of personality disorders in dermatology. Dermatol Ther. 2020;33:e13910–3.
143. Patel A, Jafferany M. Multidisciplinary and holistic models of care for patients with dermatologic disease and psychosocial comorbidity: a systematic review. JAMA Dermatol. 2020;156:686–94.
144. Gupta MA, Pur DR, Vujcic B, et al. Suicidal behaviors in the dermatology patient. Clin Dermatol. 2017;35:302–11.
145. Gupta MA. Suicide risk and skin diseases. In: Berman AL, Pompili M, editors. Medical conditions associated with suicide risk. Washington: American Association of Suicidology; 2011. p. 251–73.
146. Cotterill JA, Cunliffe WJ. Suicide in dermatological patients. Br J Dermatol. 1997;137:246–50.
147. Picardi A, Lega I, Tarolla E. Suicide risk in skin disorders. Clin Dermatol. 2013;31:47–56.
148. Gupta MA, Gupta AK. Depression and suicidal ideation in dermatology patients with acne, alopecia areata, atopic dermatitis and psoriasis. Br J Dermatol. 1998;139:846–50.
149. Phillips KA, Coles ME, Menard W, et al. Suicidal ideation and suicide attempts in body dysmorphic disorder. J Clin Psychiatry. 2005;66:717–25.
150. Reid WH, Kirwin S. Risk and risk management in psychodermatology. In: Bewley A, Taylor RE, Reichenberg JS, et al., editors. Practical psychodermatology. UK: Wiley Blackwell; 2014. p. 50–9.
151. Osman OT, Souid AK, Al-Mugaddam F, et al. Attentiveness of dermatologists in the middle east to psychocutaneous medicine. Prim Care Companion CNS Disord. 2017;19(2):22854.
152. Levine AZ, Aljabari R, Dalrymple K, et al. Non suicidal self-injury and suicide: differences between those with and without borderline personality disorder. J Pers Disord. 2020;34:131–44.

Chapter 4
Factitious Skin Disorders Without External Incentives

Domenico Bonamonte, Aurora De Marco, and Gianni Angelini

Factitious cutaneous disorders without external incentives come under the classification of self-inflicted skin diseases (SISD) with a denied or hidden behaviour (Table 4.1) [1–19].

SISD are conditions in which patients consciously induce, feign, or exaggerate physical or psychiatric symptoms. They are rare, but well known to dermatologists; however, they often remain undiagnosed for some time before the unusual or bizarre clinical morphology of the lesions, combined with normal blood tests and non-specific histology, lead to the correct diagnosis [20].

From the psychological standpoint, the anomalous behaviour of subjects with self-inflicted disorders can be linked to various factors of both an "internal" and an "interpersonal" nature [11]. Internal factors include various dysmorphic symptoms, like tension, loneliness, anxiety, and aggression: in these cases, the self-injury is followed by a sense of relief and calm [21]. Other possible factors are to protect against the external world through pain [22], to interrupt feelings of derealization and dissociation, self-punishment, and reduce feelings of guilt [23], as well as to enhance self-esteem [11, 24]. In the latter case, the patient feels proud of the sense of power over his/her own body and of presenting to the doctor as an enigmatic, difficult case. Among "interpersonal" factors, the predominant one is the need for attention, in particular by the medical system, and the need to escape from problematic relationships and attacks [11].

D. Bonamonte (✉) · A. De Marco
Department of Precision and Regenerative Medicine and Ionian Area, University of Bari "Aldo Moro", Bari, Italy
e-mail: domenico.bonamonte@uniba.it; a.demarco24@studenti.uniba.it

G. Angelini
Dermatology, University of Bari "Aldo Moro", Bari, Italy
e-mail: gianniang@alice.it

G. Angelini et al. (eds.), *Psychocutaneous Diseases*,
https://doi.org/10.1007/978-3-031-70296-9_4

Table 4.1 Self-inflicted skin disorders with a denied or hidden behaviour

1. Factitious skin disorders without external incentives
Dermatitis artefacta
Dermatological pathomimicry (in part)
Gardner-Diamond syndrome
Münchausen syndrome
Münchausen syndrome by proxy
Dermatitis simulata
Dermatitis passivata ("Diogenes syndrome")
Morgellons syndrome
Secrétan syndrome (in part)
2. Factitious skin disorder with external incentives (malingering)

Table 4.2 Some clues that may raise a suspicion of deception

1. Reticent and inconsistent information by the patient
2. Symptoms dramatically reported and inconsistent with the suspected diagnosis
3. Symptoms inconsistent with the examination findings
4. Symptoms inconsistent with anatomy and physiology
5. Atypical evolution of the disease according to the usual course of the suspected somatic illness
6. Extensive medical history with invasive procedures and surgeries
7. Interference with treatment
8. Refusal of psychiatric consultation and treatment

It must be borne in mind that in addition to some personality disorders (obsessive-compulsive behaviour, borderline personality disorders and narcissistic personality disorders being the most common), many patients also have comorbidities, such as eating disorders (bulimia, anorexia nervosa), and dependence on and/or misuse of non-addictive substances [11, 24].

Patients with SISD can produce the symptoms artificially using various means (see Table 4.1, Chap. 3), ranging from mechanical injuries to self-induced infections and the application of toxic substances to the skin [12].

4.1 Diagnostic Clues

As well as clinical and laboratory criteria (see "Diagnostic Criteria", Chap. 3), the diagnosis of SISD may rely on some clues that can help a lot (Table 4.2) [1, 25–27]. Above all, an extremely detailed medical history is essential, as well as an accurate physical examination. The patient will generally provide inconsistent information and refer highly dramatic symptoms that are disproportionate to the suspected diagnosis. These are often inconsistent with anatomy and physiology, as well as with the results of the tests, unless the patient has a good medical knowledge, as in Münchausen syndrome, for example.

The patient may resist the release of the medical records, but more often will present with an extensive medical history, detailing numerous disorders and surgical procedures. The inconsistency of the various laboratory tests with the reported symptoms may raise the suspicion of deception and falsification of a medical or psychiatric condition.

Other possible elements that can aid the diagnosis of deception are a close search of the patient's hospital room to find possible means of inducing the symptoms, such as syringes, medications for blood pressure, laxatives, and sedatives. The patient appears excessively anxious to start treatment, even if he/she may actually interfere with this, by not taking the prescribed drugs, for instance.

Despite the above clues, however, in many cases definitive evidence is lacking. It should also be borne in mind that most of these patients tend to exaggerate their symptoms to gain more attention: this can complicate the diagnosis because there is not always a clear limit between what is considered normal or pathological [25].

4.2 Management and Prognosis

General rules for the management of subjects with SISD are reported in Chap. 3. It is important to be aware that only in few cases and with restricted symptoms will medical treatment significantly improve the symptoms of factitious disorders. Such patients often present psychiatric comorbidities and so the only treatment that could be efficacious is appropriate psychotherapy [28, 29].

The problem for clinicians is the approach to the start of treatment since the greatest barrier to this is, in fact, the patient's unwillingness to cooperate. It is therefore necessary to develop a strategy before facing the patient, also in order to minimize embarrassment and accusations. In most cases, patients with SISD refuse treatment, especially psychiatric: it is necessary therefore to create a trusting relationship with the patient before introducing the conclusions.

Patients with SISD generally have a poor prognosis. Even when they become convinced to start the treatment, various dropouts will occur although patients who agree to long-term treatment can have a favourable outcome [28]. Patients with a psychiatric comorbidity, like depression and a borderline personality disorder, have a poor prognosis, while those affected by anxiety, mood, and substance abuse disorders generally have a better prognosis.

In short, a factitious disorder is not a benign disease, is associated with important comorbidities, and can also lead to risky surgical procedures, and potentially lethal self-injury.

4.3 Dermatitis Artefacta

Dermatitis artefacta (factitial dermatitis, dermatitis factitia) is a disorder linked to fully aware actions of the patient, consisting of continual self-manipulation of the skin, appendices (hair, nails), and mucosae. The patient denies any responsibility for the problem but presents a clinical history that is inconsistent with the laboratory findings and physical examination [3–5, 12, 15–17, 30–49].

The term dermatitis artefacta was coined in 1908 by the writer Paul Bourget following the request by the dermatologist Dieulafoy to define the particular behaviour of one of his patients. This patient, aged in his 30s, had self-inflicted gangrenous skin lesions on his arms and one foot, obtained using potassium hydroxide, and had kept these actions hidden from various doctors for more than 2 1/2 years [38, 50].

The term dermatitis artefacta can also be used to refer to SISD. The European Society for Dermatology and Psychiatry suggests that this affliction should be included among factitious skin disorders, i.e. self-inflicted lesions produced without external incentives [13].

4.3.1 Aetiopathogenesis

There is no rational reason for this behaviour, so it is accounted as a psychological disturbance with secondary skin involvement [10, 36, 42, 49, 50].

Dermatitis artefacta is classified in DSM-V as a factitious disorder imposed on the self: the subject poses as ill, an invalid, or injured, and there can be evidence of deceptive behaviour in the absence of obvious external incentives [1]. Apart from the physical signs, characteristically there is a "hollow history" since the clinical history is actually a compendium of lies [16, 51].

The patient does not refer to the genesis of the skin lesions but describes them as manifestations with an abrupt onset and no prodromic stage. The lesions, generally symmetrical, in crops or groups, and all at the same clinical stage, are "discovered" by chance by the patient during working or leisure activities in the day. In rare cases, the patient adopts different methods and substances to produce the affliction; in addition, he/she affects nonchalance, in the sense of a "belle indifference" to the lesions, wearing an enigmatic "Monna Lisa smile" [16].

The prevalence of dermatitis artefacta ranges from 0.04% to 1.5% in dermatology clinics [16]. It is certainly the most common manifestation among factitious disorders: in a very large case series of 13,330 patients with an umbrella diagnosis of factitious disorders, dermatitis artefacta accounted for 61% of the cases [40]. There is a remarkable female preponderance, the F/M ratio being 20:1 [20, 52]. Although it can be observed at any age, dermatitis artefacta is more frequent in patients of around 20–30 years of age [38, 53], and exceptional after the age of 50–60 years.

From the pathophysiological standpoint, dermatitis artefacta is an enigma. A variety of dysphoric states lies at the basis of the self-harmful behaviour [11, 14, 18, 35, 39, 54–56]. Self-injury can serve to relieve tension or may be a self-punitive function exerted to mitigate guilt feelings. It has also been suggested that the self-harm serves to enhance self-esteem: the patient is proud to present as an enigmatic case and at the same time is complacent about his/her power over the body and the ability to support pain [56, 57]. From the interpersonal perspective, self-injury can be a way to escape from problematic relations or else a cry for help [11]. According to Wilkinson, it can be a phenomenon of flying a "flag of desperation, although the captain of the ship does not know that the flag has been hoisted" [58].

Many events can precipitate a self-harm disorder. Age is an important factor: school, sex, and work are the most frequent in young people from adolescence up to the age of 25, while in later years, although work problems persist, the most frequent other issues are familial and especially matrimonial problems, severe disease, and bereavement.

The psychological aspects in cases of self-injury without external incentives need to be clarified by the psychologist or psychiatrist. The type of personality, neurotic, psychotic or borderline is an important prognostic factor. Another is the age at onset of the factitious disorder: there are greater chances of recovery among adolescents and young adults although even in these patients a skin artefact can turn into a true “lifestyle” accessory.

In cases of male subjects, although these are less common, the personality is often of paranoid type. Such men are intolerant, rigid in their attitudes, diffident and afraid of being tricked. Behind a mask of false modesty or pride, they suffer from a great vulnerability that can become delusional [49]. In women, the problem is more often of hysterical type; the lesions are readily shown and indeed, often exhibited [59]. In any case, the most frequent type is a borderline personality in which the conflict of their inner world with the outside world causes the patient to feel insecure and vacillating [60].

Patients with self-inflicted harm share the following characteristics: a marked masochism (a tendency to actively re-enact situations of physical or mental suffering), poor social and affective relations (“an affective desert”), and at the same time an intense affective dependence and consequent narcissistic fragility (insecurity and poor self-esteem). These subjects often suffered from little affection in childhood, due to parental abandonment, long separation or long hospital stay. Sometimes they develop an ambivalent attitude, a love-hate relationship with the people around them and also with their general practitioner. In the first case, the skin artefact is a call for love, but at the same time a means of keeping others at a distance, a way of distancing themselves from those felt to be unworthy of trust or even dangerous. In the case of the general practitioner, an initial close relationship and insistent demands for attention and treatment will degenerate, and the patient will accuse the doctor of causing this “rejection” [49]. Depression is also a common characteristic in these subjects, being the primary cause of the behavioural disorder [61–63].

Adebanjo and Coll. described the case of a woman affected by mood and anxiety disorders for many years, who presented, during the recent COVID-19 pandemic, self-inflicted cutaneous lesions on several parts of the body. The authors believed that fear of a possible contagion, combined with the insistent media information and the lockdown condition, induced an increased anxiety state in the patient, that led to her self-harm behaviour [64].

4.3.2 Clinical Features

The situation that develops as soon as a subject with a self-inflicted injury enters the ambulatory is unmistakable: the atmosphere is tense, the patient ostentates the lesions and calmly waits to greet the physician [44, 63]. By contrast, the family members who accompany the patient are anxious and suspicious, impatient to show the thick dossier about the various visits and repeated laboratory controls and show anger and disappointment in the physicians consulted before [44, 65].

From the clinical standpoint, the lesions are morphologically varied (see "Diagnostic Criteria", Chap. 3), depending on the simulator's creativity and the methods employed [6]. Sometimes the simulator will perpetuate or mimic a known dermatosis [66–70] but in most cases, the lesions have no recognizable characteristics of any known skin disease.

The lesions are often in easily accessible areas (face, hands, arms, upper trunk, and legs), have a bizarre appearance with irregular, geometric, and angular borders that do not conform to any spontaneous pathological process. They are usually surrounded by completely healthy skin. In cases where corrosive liquids have been used there are characteristic linear tracks. Particularly creative pathomimics can reproduce, as stated above, the lesions of a previous dermatosis, now resolved, or those seen in another person. Unlike what is observed in cases of spontaneous disorders, in which the lesions are at different stages of evolution, in dermatitis artefacta the lesions all appear fully formed and at the same stage of development [6]. This is characteristic of self-injury behaviour due to the obvious inability to elicit the evidence of evolutionary changes (a "hollow history") [44]. More than one person can be involved, as in cases of "folie à deux" in two patients with factitious ulcers [71].

The most common lesions are deep excoriations produced with the fingernails or sharp instruments, scarifications with a knife or a fragment of glass, erosions, scabs, and ulcers due to the use of caustic chemicals, and burning, in general with cigarettes [72, 73] (Figs. 4.1, 4.2, 4.3, 4.4, 4.5, 4.6, 4.7, 4.8, 4.9, 4.10, 4.11, 4.12, 4.13, 4.14, 4.15 and 4.16). In cases where the target organ is the subcutaneous tissue, the diagnosis can be very difficult, as occurs in cases of chronic paraffinomas and panniculitis due to the insertion of various chemicals deep into the skin.

Sometimes the types of lesions can be due to different aetiological agents. For example, blisters can be induced by applying various vegetable substances to the skin, or by a suction mechanism using rubber teats with a stiffened rim [74]. Burns, while rare, are linked to various aetiological agents: flame, fire, scalding, contact with a hot object, chemicals, electrical equipment, excessive cold [75].

It is not always easy to discover the aetiological agent, and the motivations leading to self-harm are often quite unthinkable. A woman aged 40 years with no previous history of disease attended many dermatological and otorhinolaryngological specialists about an erythemato-vesicular dermatitis on the face that was particularly intense at the level of the meati and ear pavilions. The affliction improved gradually until the Friday and had worsened dramatically by the Monday. A complex psychopathological situation was behind the self-injury. The patient knew she was allergic to nickel and each weekend she rubbed her facial skin with a metal watch and ear canals with a metal paper clip to achieve her purpose. The patient's attitude was unusual: passivity, indifference, and lack of interest in any form of examination or treatment. She was perpetuating the dermatitis to avoid, or at least postpone, a marriage already agreed to, but unwanted. It was important for her that her fiancé should find her in disastrous skin conditions every time he came to visit on Sundays [76].

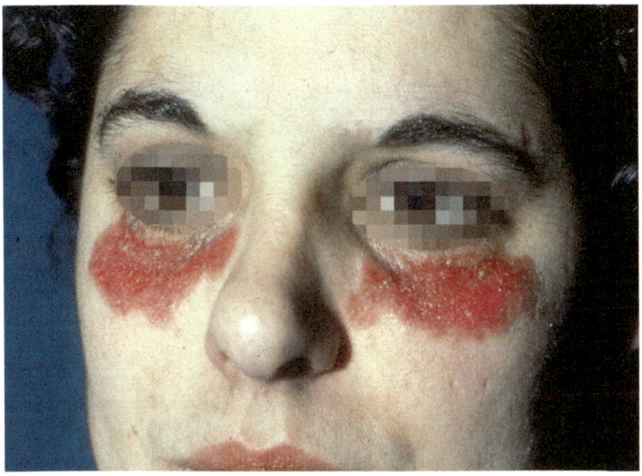

Fig. 4.1 Self-artefact by acids. (Reproduced with permission by Foti et al. [72])

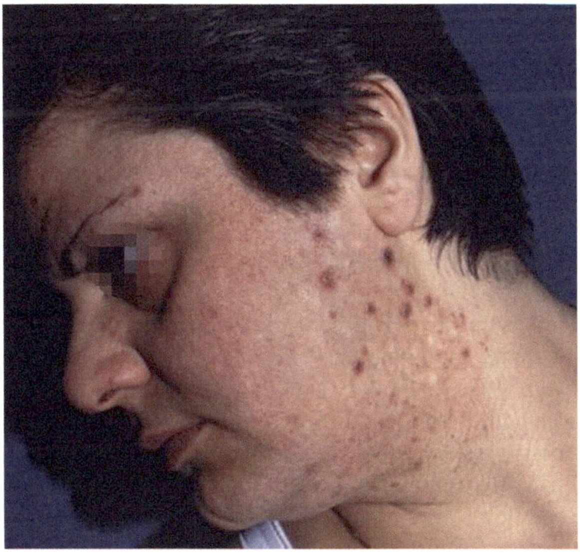

Fig. 4.2 Excoriations in a 45-year-old patient

A 60-year-old married woman presented for 6 months with shallow ulcers on the left leg and calf, with no signs of inflammation. The patient said that the lesions developed suddenly, without any pre-existing symptoms. On the X-ray, radio-opaque images of many intact and broken sewing needles were seen at various depths of the lower limb soft tissues. The patient claimed that nobody had inserted the needles in her body and said she was certain it was the result of witchcraft. But finally, she reluctantly admitted that she had acted in order to receive more attention from her husband, who was extremely short-tempered and had frequent bursts of anger that frightened and intimidated her. In fact, the patient urged the psychiatrist

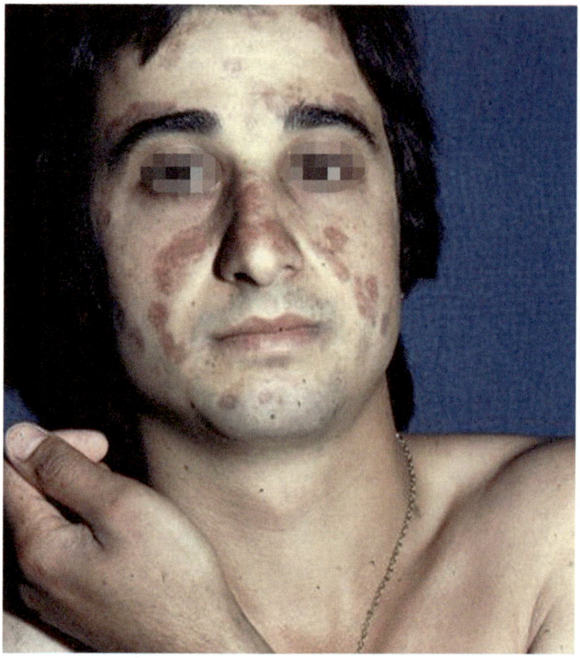

Fig. 4.3 Excoriations in a 27-year-old patient. (Reproduced with permission by Bonamonte et al. [73])

to consider the revelation confidential because she was afraid her husband would leave her [77].

Makeup products can also be used for self-inflicted injuries, as in the case of a 26-year-old woman, single mother and nursing professional. The patient presented numerous diffuse red, violet, and blue skin discolorations on the face and neck and complained of pain and difficulty in moving. For this reason, she had presented at a police station and denounced unknown individuals, in the form of two men who had attacked and beaten her. The skin discolorations appeared as fresh bruises, and there were no petechial bleedings in the skin, conjunctiva, or mucous membranes. Confirming the forensic expert's suspicion, surprisingly, all the skin discolorations were eliminated with white cotton pads, which remained stained with red, blue, green, and yellow paint. The psychiatrist noted emotionally unstable personality traits and dissociative symptoms. Further police investigations disclosed frequent reports against unknown individuals, filed in the past by the woman. This case, featuring injuries claimed to be due to third-party-interference, is interesting because it touches on the field of forensic medicine [78].

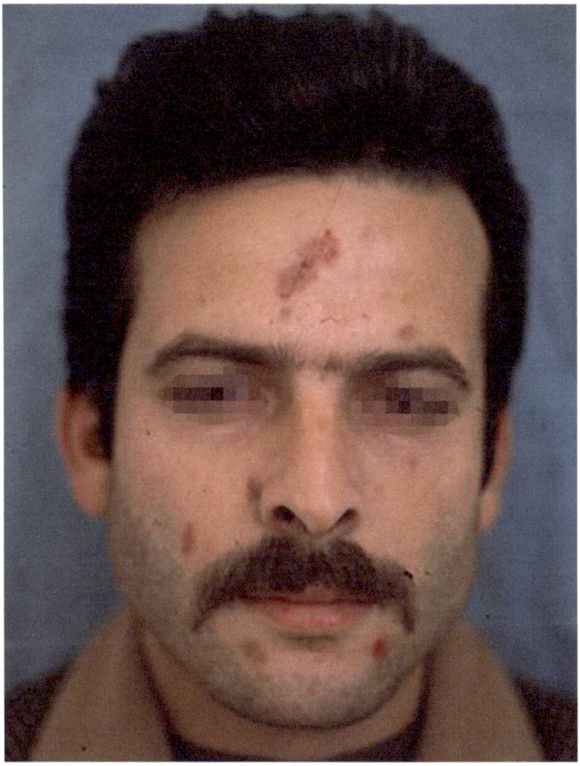

Fig. 4.4 Excoriations in a 32-year-old patient

4.3.3 Differential Diagnosis

A differential dermatological diagnosis of dermatitis artefacta depends on the age and gender of the patient, and on some peculiar characteristics like a "hollow history", the patient's insouciance when confronted with the lesions (that are generally subjectively asymptomatic), a possible thick file of prior consultations all resulting normal, of medications, tests, and examinations, and finally the bizarre morphology of the lesions.

The most common afflictions with which differential diagnosis must be made are vasculitis, pyoderma gangrenosum (histological findings are important for the diagnosis), chronic lupus erythematosus (histological examination and immunofluorescence will confirm or rule out the diagnosis), panniculitis (to be differentiated from Weber-Christian disease; the presence of haemosiderin within the nodules points to dermatitis artefacta [79]), granulomas, vascular ulcers of the legs, and arthropod bites (Table 4.3).

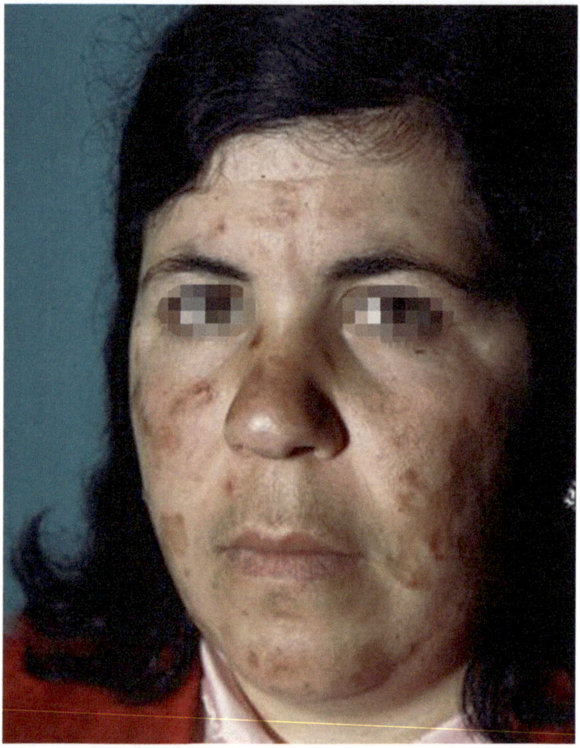

Fig. 4.5 Hyperchromic sequelae of previous excoriations in a 35-year-old woman. (Reproduced with permission by Angelini and Bonamonte [5])

Blisters and crusty lesions may simulate ecthyma, herpes simplex, and bullous disorders (immunofluorescence will be negative). Facial blisters may simulate porphyria cutanea tarda. Drug addiction causes the development of extensive ulcerations and scarring at the injection site. Purpura and tissue purpuric reactions, that can be difficult to differentiate, must be excluded. Forms with a linear and reticulate pattern must be differentiated from Nékam's disease [79–81]. Penile cellulitis can be secondary to self-injury: in this case, it is necessary to exclude various diseases of the genitals and a possible factitious dermatitis malignancy in the case of soldiers [82].

4.3.4 Dermatitis Artefacta in Children

In children, factitious skin disorders are rare, observed in approximately 1 in 23,000 paediatric consultations [83]. In a series of 201 patients with dermatitis artefacta, observed from 1976 to 2006, 44 (21.9%) were children, with a mean age of 12.9 years [84].

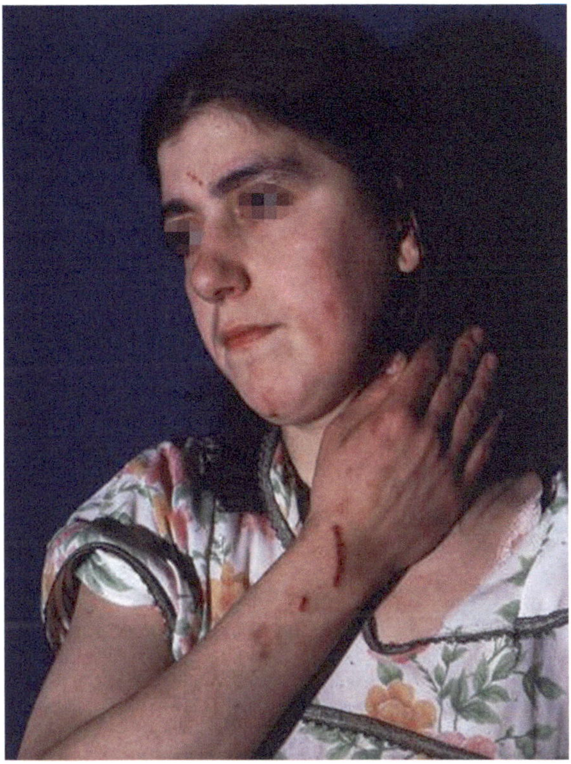

Fig. 4.6 Excoriations in a 23-year-old patient

Also in childhood, skin artefacts are more common in girls than boys. Considering all paediatric cases of factitious skin disorders gathered from the three largest case series, excoriations are the most frequent lesions (27%) (Figs. 4.17, 4.18 and 4.19), followed by purpura (7%), miscellaneous lesions (erythema, desquamation, oedema, bullae, eschars) (16%), and contact dermatitis (11%) [84–86]. The lesions are generally localized on the head and neck, followed by the arms, legs, and trunk. The observation in the same subject of various clinical forms of compulsive disorders is quite common, for example, excoriations due to dermatillomania and pseudo-knuckle pads due to repetitive sucking or continuous picking of the tissue overlying the finger joints (Figs. 4.20 and 4.21). Another common complaint is the cheilitis factitial, also known as self-inflicted cheilitis: the constant lip-licking leads to eczematous lesions ("lick eczema") and painful skin fissures (Figs. 4.22, 4.23, 4.24, 4.25, 4.26 and 4.27) [87].

Based on the pattern of the lesions, the causative instrument or material used can be deduced; sometimes a firm identification can be made by the child's parents. As in adults, the injury can be of a physical (sandpaper, screwdriver, nail brush, the sharp point of a compass, pumice stone), chemical (irritant or caustic substances, paint or pigment), or thermal nature (car cigarette lighter, lighted matches) [88, 89].

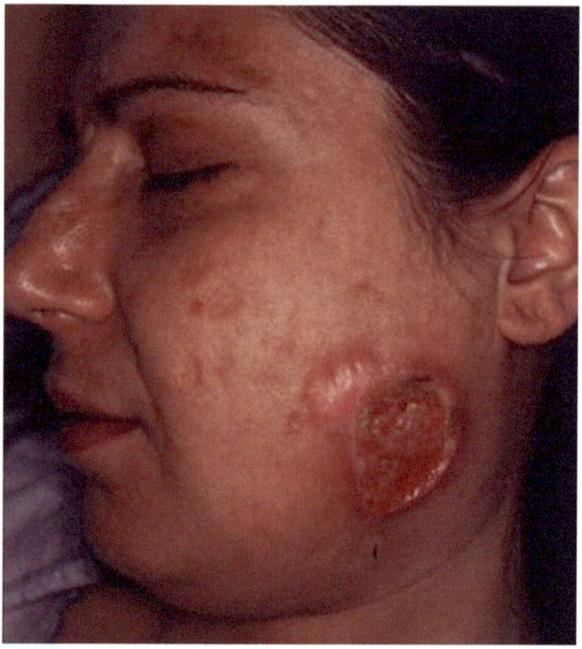

Fig. 4.7 Excoriations and rounded ulcerative lesion in a 40-year-old woman. (Reproduced with permission by Angelini and Bonamonte [5])

A particularly dangerous form of factitious disorders, observed mostly in adolescence, is the so-called choking dermatitis: a neologism describing self-asphyxial behaviour to achieve a brief euphoric state caused by cerebral hypoxia [90, 91]. This disorder, described in North America, France, and Columbia, presents as skin lesions usually localized on the front of the neck: pigmented and lichenified patches with possible ulcerated nodules on the laryngeal prominence. Histological examination reveals spongiosis and necrosis with nuclear dust in the epidermis, and mild fibrosis, infiltration of histiocytes and lymphocytes with no apparent vasculitis in the dermis. Different means are adopted to achieve strangulation, including bare hands, pens, and telephone wires. The behaviour is often attributable to peer pressure, curiosity, and the addictive nature of euphoria, thus suggesting a psychiatric disorder [92].

The risk of developing self-injuries in children can derive from a combination of psychological stress and exposure to a chronic disease. In the presence of these triggering factors, the self-inflicted behaviour could be interpreted as an emotional escape valve [93, 94]. Indeed, unlike adults, children rarely show features of significant psychiatric disturbance and do not use the artefact to gain the benefits of "patient status", but rather they adopt it to resolve a current predicament in their life [95].

Children and adolescents do not complain of discomfort or pain from lesions and, even more than adults, exhibit a "belle indifference", a Monna Lisa-like

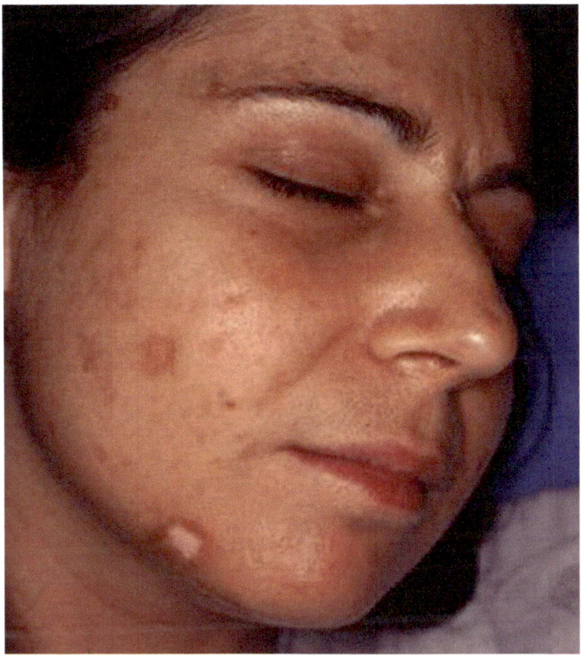

Fig. 4.8 The same patient as in Fig. 4.7 with excoriations in various evolutive phase. (Reproduced with permission by Bonamonte et al. [33])

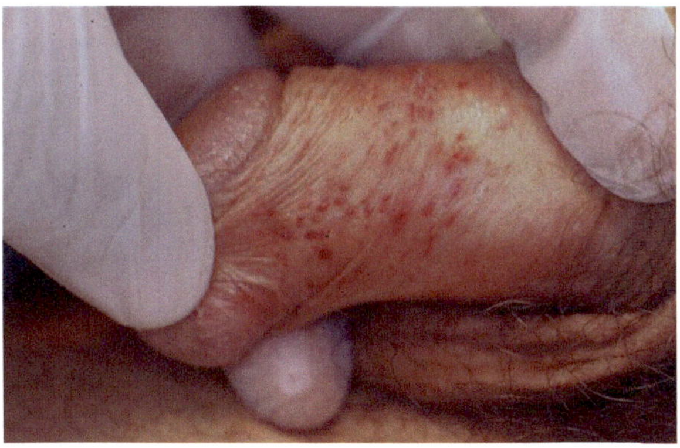

Fig. 4.9 A 35-year-old patient with self-produced excoriations by sandpaper

expression of artful innocence, a dissimulating attitude, as well as a tendency to show off the lesions at all costs [83, 93].

Once the diagnosis has been made, the dermatologist must explain the reason for the lesions to the child's parents, who often vacillate between acceptance and denial of the diagnosis but must also carefully avoid confrontation with the child. Occlusive medication must not be applied to "prove" that the lesions are self-inflicted, nor

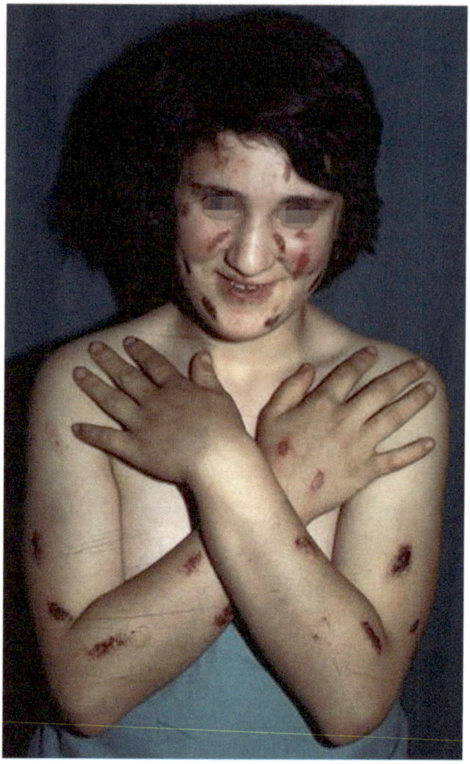

Fig. 4.10 Excoriations in a 15-year-old patient. (Reproduced with permission by Bonamonte et al. [73])

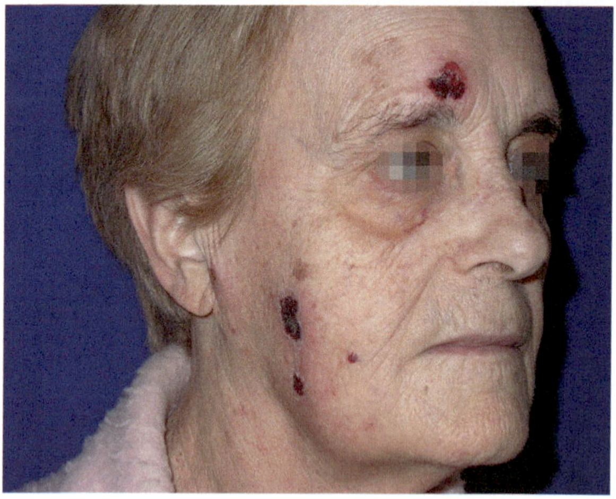

Fig. 4.11 Excoriations in a 75-year-old patient

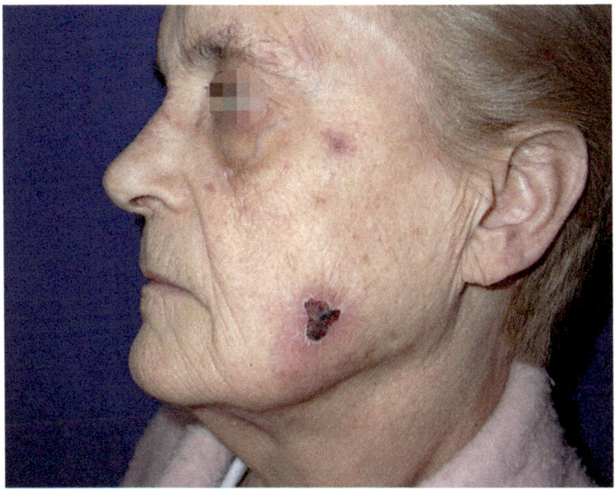

Fig. 4.12 The same patient as in Fig. 4.11

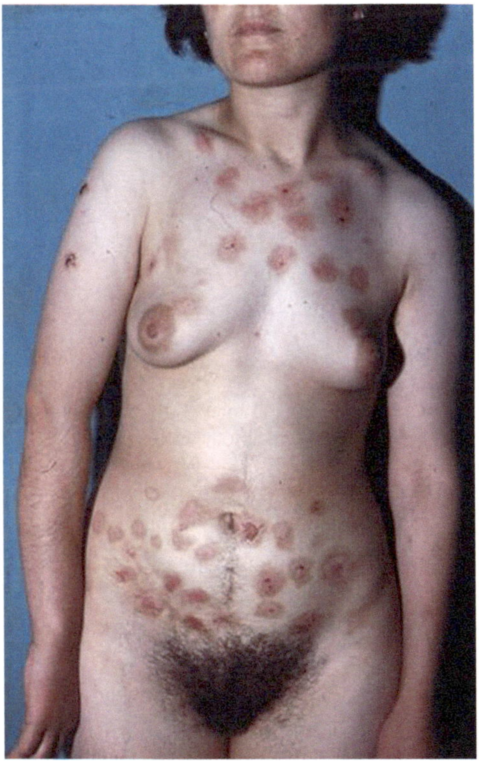

Fig. 4.13 A 35-year-old woman with rounded erosive, ulcerative, and hyperchromic lesions induced by incandescent metal object. (Reproduced with permission by Angelini and Bonamonte [5])

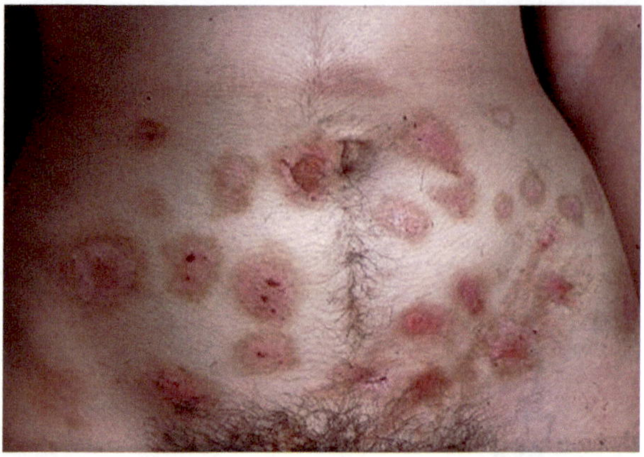

Fig. 4.14 The same patient as in Fig. 4.13. (Reproduced with permission by Bonamonte et al. [33])

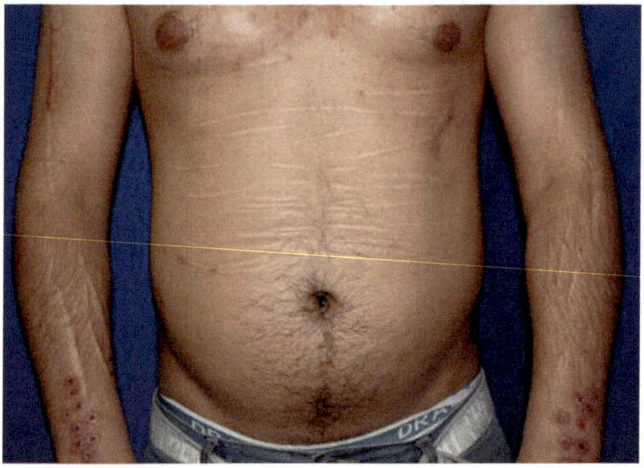

Fig. 4.15 A 28-year-old man with linear cutting scars on abdomen and forearms. (Reproduced with permission by Bonamonte et al. [33])

must the child be insistently questioned about "how" and "why", nor accused of deliberately producing the lesions. Such reactions are unproductive and can cause the child to feel alienated, thus delaying the possibility of forming a trusting alliance [85, 90, 96–101].

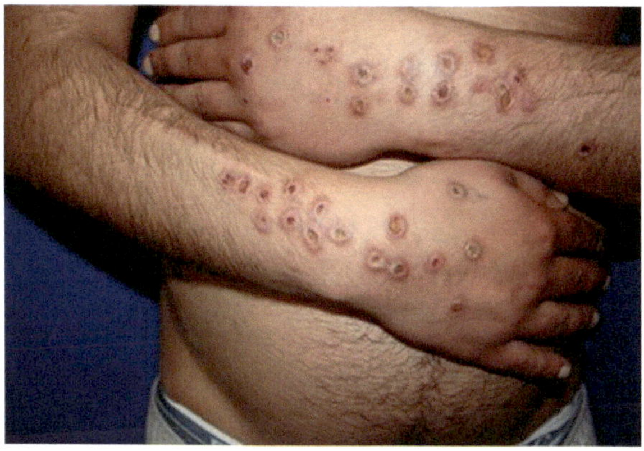

Fig. 4.16 The same patient as in Fig. 4.15 with rounded lesions on the back of hands and forearms induced by lighted cigarette. (Reproduced with permission by Bonamonte et al. [33])

Table 4.3 Common differential diagnosis of dermatitis artefacta

Irritant/allergic contact dermatitis
Vasculitis
Pyoderma gangrenosum
Chronic lupus erythematosus
Panniculitis
Granulomas
Arthropod bites
Bullous disorders
Drug eruptions
Purpura
Sexual/physical abuse (especially in children)
Bacterial infections
Viral infections
Nékam's disease

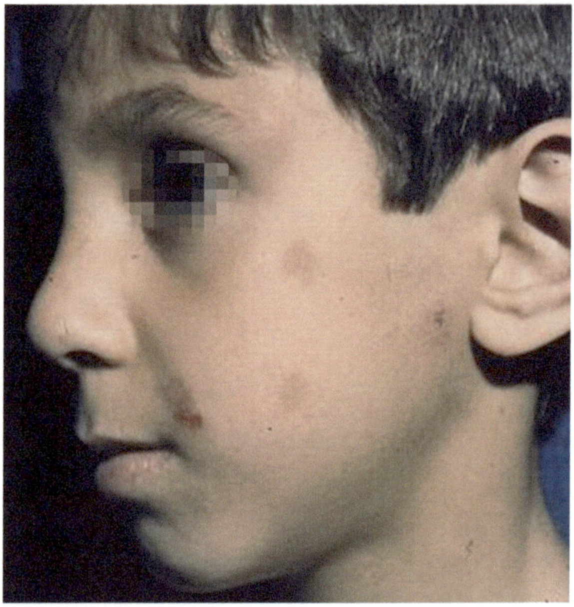

Fig. 4.17 Excoriations in a 7-year-old boy

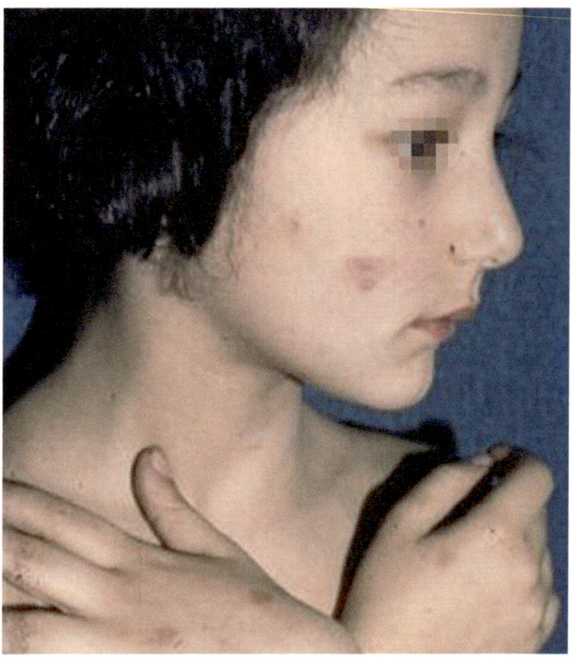

Fig. 4.18 Excoriations in an 8-year-old boy

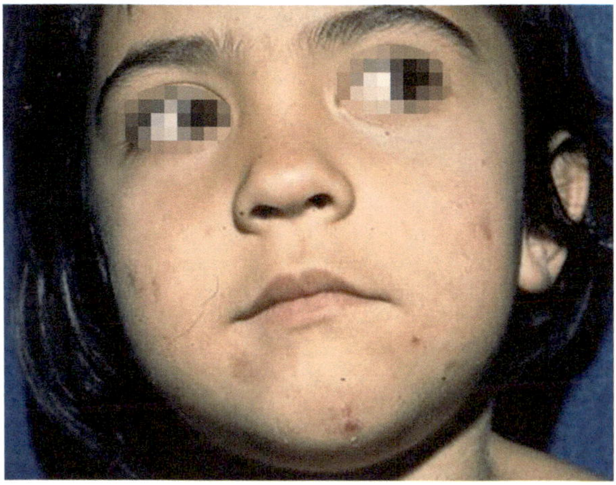

Fig. 4.19 Excoriations in a 4-year-old girl

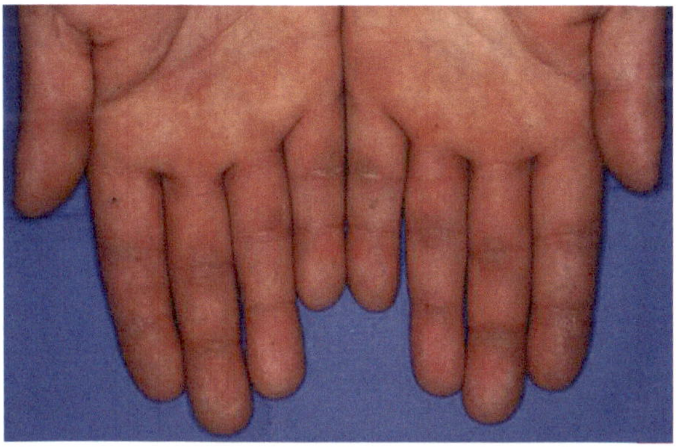

Fig. 4.20 Pseudo-knuckle pads on the palmar region of the fingers. (Reproduced with permission by Bonamonte et al. [73])

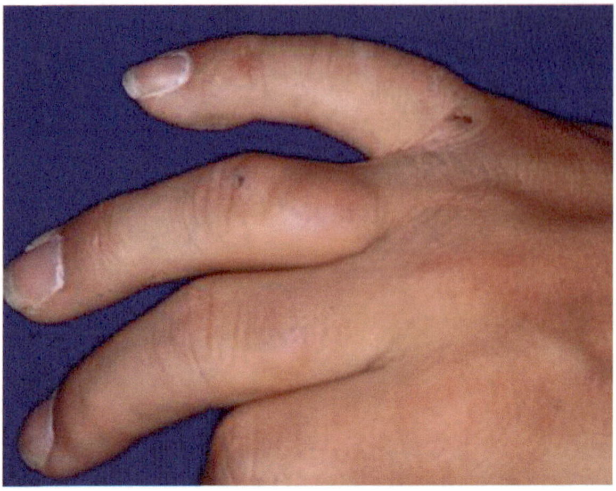

Fig. 4.21 Pseudo-knuckle pads on the dorsal finger joints. (Reproduced with permission by Bonamonte et al. [73])

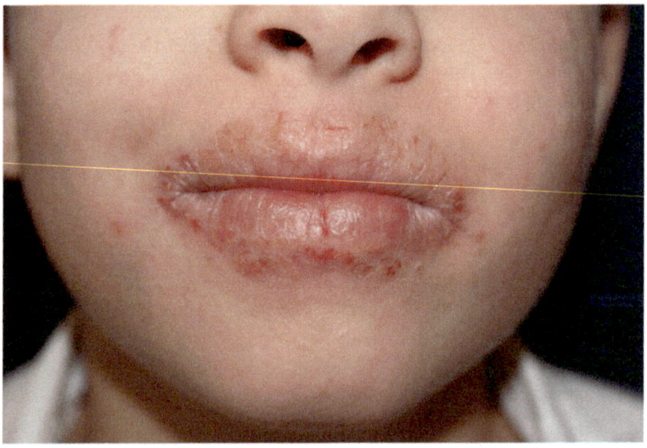

Fig. 4.22 Cheilitis and perioral dermatitis induced by saliva. (Reproduced with permission by Bonamonte et al. [87])

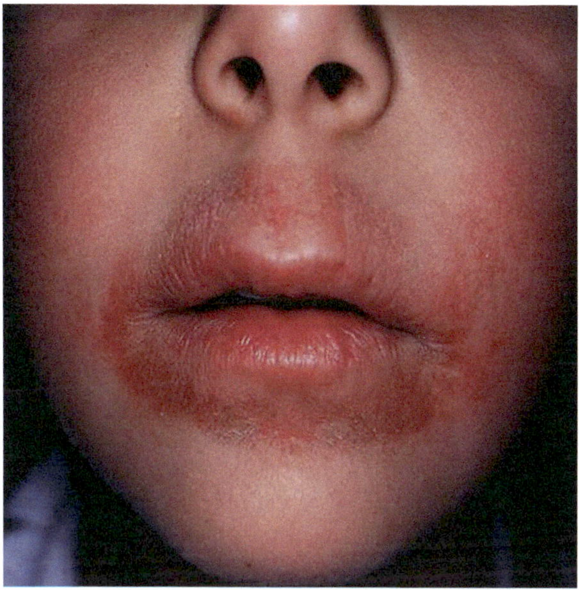

Fig. 4.23 Cheilitis and perioral dermatitis induced by saliva. (Reproduced with permission by Bonamonte et al. [87])

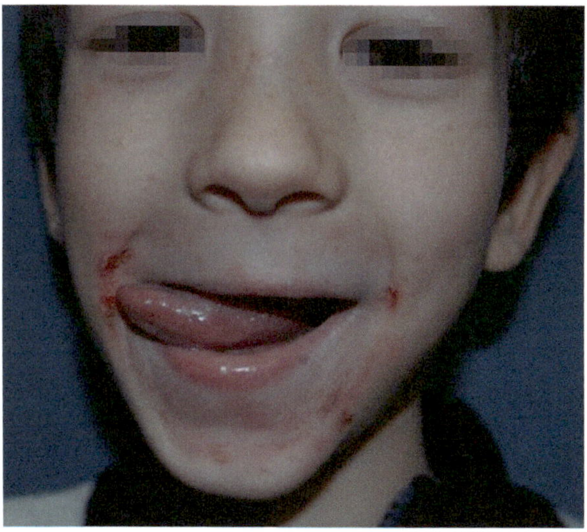

Fig. 4.24 "Lick eczema". (Reproduced with permission by Bonamonte et al. [87])

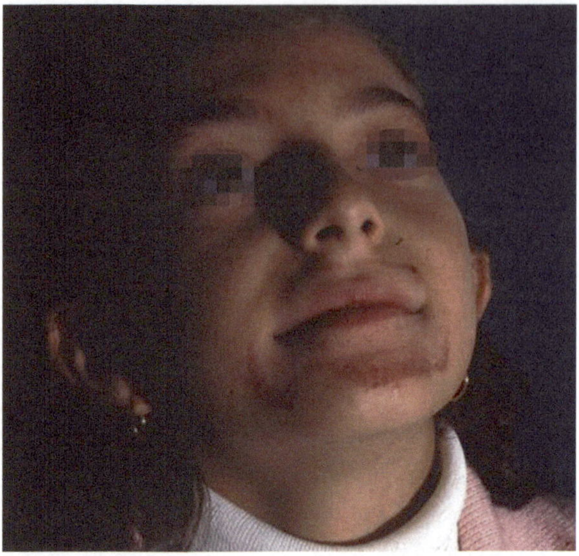

Fig. 4.25 "Lick eczema". (Reproduced with permission by Bonamonte et al. [87])

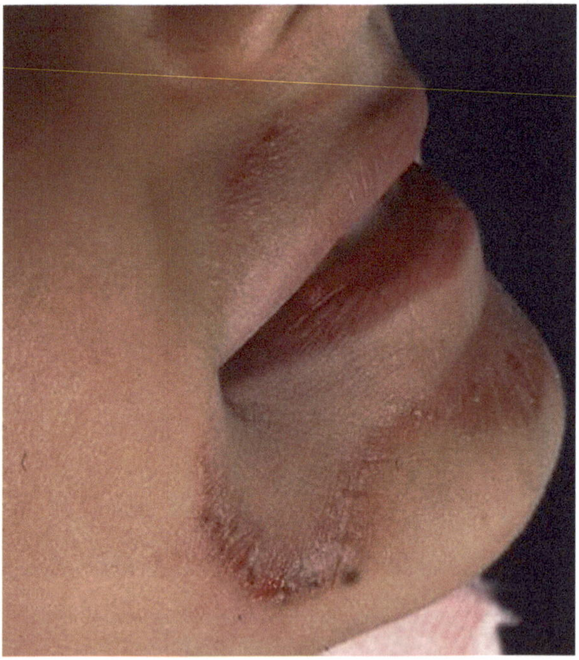

Fig. 4.26 The same patient as in Fig. 4.25. (Reproduced with permission by Bonamonte et al. [73])

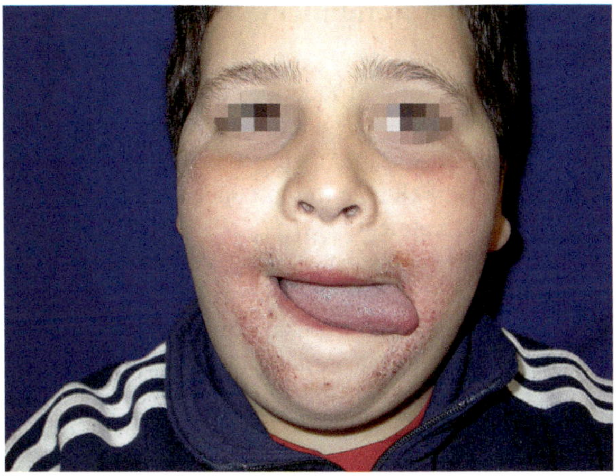

Fig. 4.27 "Lick eczema"

4.4 Dermatitis Simulata

In particularly ingenuous individuals, the use of makeup or topical printing dyes to produce a rash or a birthmark can be observed. This so-called dermatitis simulata is most common in children [102]. In this case, the skin is not badly damaged: in fact, the signs can often be removed simply by an aqueous or alcoholic swab and analysed if necessary [103].

For this purpose, glue and crystallized sugar can be used to produce a desquamating rash, and various dyes to simulate discolorations [104, 105]. Differential diagnosis is made in particular with apocrine and eccrine chromhidrosis or pseudochromhidrosis after accidental cutaneous absorption of dyes [16].

4.5 Dermatitis Passivata

This dermatitis, also called dermatitis neglecta, can be observed in adolescents and adults, as a result of a deliberate failure to wash specific areas of the body, such as the face, scalp, or arms [16, 98, 106, 107]. In the extreme form, it is also known as "Diogenes syndrome" [108, 109]. In these cases, a build-up of sebum, dirt, and keratin accumulates on the skin. The appearance is similar to that seen in vagrants, or in geriatric or demented patients, in whom the lesions are usually found on the upper central back chest and/or in the groin.

The material can easily be removed with an alcohol-soaked swab. Such subjects are affected by various personality disorders.

4.6 Dermatological Pathomimicry

Pathomimicry is a particular form of factitious disorder, featuring the provocation of outbreaks of a known disease, triggered by voluntary exposure to the specific agent responsible. The patients mimic their original spontaneous disease that they know a lot about and so are well able to reproduce the physiopathological mechanisms or interfere with the treatment.

The term "pathomimicry" was first used by Millard in 1984 in a study of 13 patients who had self-inflicted exacerbations or recurrences of their own spontaneous skin diseases, achieved through exposure by contact or ingestion to the same agent that had provoked the disease. Among them, six patients had provoked the recurrence of contact dermatitis by using substances they knew they were allergic to; four had provoked toxidermia by taking the incriminated drugs again, and three had aggravated their leg ulcers by not using the local treatments [68]. Most of these patients were young women with familial problems. Direct confrontation proved helpful, unlike in the situation of dermatitis artefacta.

The distinction between dermatitis artefacta and pathomimicry is that in the first case the lesions are atypical, and do not evoke any known dermatitis, while in the second they are those of a known complaint. Moreover, pathomimicry is achieved in a conscious state, then completely dissimulated, but with no hidden motivation or expected benefit [49, 110]. This form of self-harm must also be differentiated from self-inflicted delayed healing of surgical or traumatic wounds, which is achieved by external damage [16].

The clinical suspicion of pathomimicry must arise in the presence of unexplained exacerbations of a known disease or when patients are unexpectedly unresponsive to the adequate supervised treatment. According to the literature, the easiest diseases to reproduce are atopic dermatitis (by introducing animal danders, for example, or the topical use of notoriously irritant substances), irritant and allergical contact dermatitis (by using known irritants and allergens on the skin), and systemic drug sensitivities (due to ingestion of the implicated drug). In the latter case, it should be remembered that the presence of the drug can be revealed in the blood or urine. In cases of leg ulcers, known irritants or contaminated materials can be used [76, 111–113]. It must also be borne in mind, however, that dermatological pathomimicry can be induced for illicit purposes, too [13].

4.7 Gardner-Diamond Syndrome

Gardner-Diamond syndrome (GDS) (also known as psychogenic purpura, autoerythrocyte sensitization syndrome, or painful bruising syndrome), is a rare clinical condition characterized by recurrent atraumatic spontaneous, tender skin lesions that develop into ecchymosis, closely correlated with episodes of severe, psychiatric disorders [13, 16, 33, 114–124].

Described in 1955 by Frank Gardner and Louis Diamond [114], the complaint is more common in adult women, but can also affect men and young adolescents [125, 126]. Usually, an episode starts with prodromic burning, pain, or a tingling sensation of the skin, followed a few hours later by oedema and erythema. A day or so later, the ecchymotic lesions appear, and will take days or weeks to regress. The complaint may present in various locations, especially the extremities and face. Additional symptoms are nausea, arthralgia, fatigue, headaches, and abdominal pain [127, 128]. Occasionally, additional bleeding symptoms occur in unusual sites (eyes, ears, etc.). Since GDS predominantly develops in women, it has been suggested that oestrogen may play a role in the different frequency. Some subjects affected by GDS have a medical history of hysterectomy, amenorrhea, irregular menses, or menorrhagia [129].

The pathophysiology of this affliction is unknown. In all cases, however, there is a closely correlated psychological condition: typically, patients have a comorbid psychiatric disorder, or the first episode may be triggered by severe stressors (home conflicts, such as marital or parental conflicts, death of family members, health issues of a family member; abuse, abortion, alcoholism) [116]. A careful case history is therefore important and also psychiatric assessment. The most common associated psychiatric disorder is depression, and such patients can suffer from anxiety, personality disorders, conversion or bipolar disorders, or obsessive-compulsive disorders [130, 131].

In all cases, the various laboratory tests must be made to exclude other common haematological diseases responsible for purpura and ecchymosis. These tests must include erythrocyte sedimentation rate, bleeding time, coagulation factors, prothrombin time, partial thromboplastin time, and platelet count, but they are usually all negative. A complete investigation will include direct and indirect Coombs test, antinuclear antibodies, antidouble-stranded DNA, complement levels, and rheumatoid factor [126]. There may also be a history of bleeding disorders or platelet dysfunction [132].

The gold standard for the diagnosis of GDS is intradermal injection of autologous washed erythrocytes: within 24 h after the injection, ecchymotic lesions are observed. An intradermal injection of saline will be done as a control, in which no lesions will develop. Studies have suggested an autosensitization to the phosphoglyceride component of the blood cell membrane, and there may also be an atypical organization of erythrocyte phosphatidylserine or the cell membrane of red blood cells; this elicits a response to the autologous washed erythrocyte injection [133]. However, in some cases of GDS the response to the injection is negative [116, 134]. Ultimately, GDS is a diagnosis of exclusion after all other coagulopathies and causes of purpura have been ruled out [115, 116]. Finally, a possible relationship to religious stigmatization has been proposed [135–137].

As well as the laboratory tests, biopsy of the ecchymotic lesions may prove useful for the diagnosis: typical histological findings include extravasation of erythrocytes into the dermis, a perivascular infiltrate of lymphocytes or neutrophils, and dermal and subcutaneous haemorrhages [115, 116, 132, 138, 139].

The prognosis of GDS is good following combined symptomatic treatment although there is still no consensus about an optimal therapy. The best results are obtained by associating psychotherapy, reassurance therapy, selective serotonin reuptake inhibitors, corticosteroids, and tricyclic antidepressants [115, 116, 132, 134, 140]. Other treatments include immunosuppressive drugs and benzodiazepines that achieve better results in association with the former drugs. Moreover, a positive correlation has been observed between a psychological improvement and resolution of the physical symptoms. Other symptomatic treatments that can be associated are antihistamines and hormonal contraceptives [140, 141].

4.8 Purpura Factitia

GDS must be differentiated from purpura factitia although some overlap is possible. Bleeding, bruising, and purpuric lesions can also be observed in the course of dermatitis artefacta, with or without external incentives. In the former case, malingerers can use dicoumarol and warfarin to produce bruising and bleeding [138, 139]. High doses of aspirin can be taken to produce similar but milder effects. Adults can reproduce purpura also using machinery [140, 141]. A case of autoerythrocyte sensitization associated with dermatitis artefacta has been reported in the literature [142].

The common denominator between GDS and purpura factitia is that the lesions can occur during or in the aftermath of stressful life events, trauma, or surgery. In both cases, the diagnosis is by exclusion, after all other possible causes have been excluded. Histology can support the diagnosis: in purpura factitia, there is evident disruption of collagen fibre bundles (due specifically to the application of an external force) and extravasated red blood cells in the dermis [94].

Purpura factitia is peculiarly observed in adolescents, usually on the chin, due to sucking on a cup or glass, or pinching [85, 93, 94, 99, 101, 143]. Some authors reported stereotypical linear symmetric purpuric streaks on the extensor sides of both arms [100]: the patients were mostly females, aged 6–14 years. They had a psychiatric history or were undergoing a stressful time period. The patients presented with multiple oval or square purpuric macules, forming a discontinuous linear band. Laboratory exams were normal and there was no vasculitis at the skin histology. One of the adolescents declared that the lesions were induced by classmates using suction. In all cases, in children it is essential to make a differential diagnosis between factitious purpura and child abuse [95, 100, 142, 143].

Finally, it should be noted that there are various ways of inducing purpura, whose manifestations, not necessarily associated to psychological disturbances, can even be caused simply by boredom. In this case, the diagnosis falls outside the scope of self-inflicted skin diseases.

4.9 Morgellons Syndrome

Sir Thomas Browne in 1674 described the Morgellons as a population in the Languedoc, characterized by the development of a hairy back. Despite that fact, this misnomer has been coined to name a syndrome, Morgellons disease [16, 96, 144].

The clinical picture is classic. The patient is particularly anxious and obsessively focused on the symptoms and may bring "specimens" of the offending agent they believe to be the cause of the skin infection or infestation: he or she finds unusual structures on or under the skin lesions, which can be fibre-like filaments, granules, and crystals. In general, the patient offers up a logical explanation for the onset of the presumed infection, and adopts external measures to combat and prevent infection, such as burning their clothes and refusing any kind of close physical contact, in particular with their children [145–149].

The clinical-morphological picture is characteristic of: multiple superficial ulcerations, linear excoriations, excoriated papulous nodules, and scars on the extremities and trunk. Associated symptoms are feelings of crawling, stinging, and biting under the skin, fibromyalgia, joint and muscle pain, debilitating chronic fatigue, cognitive dysfunction, and poor concentration and memory [150–152].

Usually, patients are females in their 40s and 50s, who learned about the disease from friends or the internet [35]. In fact, an internet search for "bugs in the skin" brings up a relevant web site: "The Morgellons Research Foundation", an organization devoted to "researching an emerging infectious disease" [153]. Some authors have pointed out that the information therein is very misleading to someone who suffers from delusions of parasitosis [150]. The Centers for Disease Control and Prevention have failed to identify an infectious or medical cause [154].

The aetiology of this complaint is still debated. Due to the absence of a primary dermatitis or evidence of infestation, the syndrome may be diagnosed as delusions of parasitosis, but it may, in fact, be associated with various psychiatric conditions, including bipolar disorder, schizophrenia, depression, drug abuse, and paranoia [146]. Alternatively, Reichenberg and Coll. in their retrospective study of 47 patients, suggested that the syndrome is more consistent with a somatic symptom disorder [155].

Further study is needed to differentiate between patients' symptoms as more consistent with a delusional or a somatic disorder, and this distinction needs to be made on an individual basis. The distinction is essential for the first-line treatment that consists of antipsychotics in cases of delusional symptoms and of antidepressants in cases of a somatic disorder [35, 145, 156].

4.10 Münchausen Syndrome

This syndrome is a chronic, severe subtype of factitious disease, observed in patients who constantly demand medical care, and have a characteristic record of passing from one hospital to a series of other, different hospitals. The diseases simulated by such patients are esoteric and rare, and often accompanied by an ample patient dossier.

The syndrome was named by the British physician Richard Asher, in 1951, after the eighteenth century European aristocrat Hieronymus Karl Friedrich Baron von Münchausen (1720–1797), who entertained audiences with stories of fantastic, impossible undertakings in which he had played the starring role [157].

The complaint is defined as the triad of: chronic factitious symptoms, hospital or doctor shopping (peregrination, hospital hopping), and pseudologia fantastica (pathological lying) [13, 16, 158–162]. Table 4.4 lists the synonyms for Münchhausen syndrome and for patients with the syndrome [162, 163].

Patients with this syndrome present to hospitals with acute, often spectacular complaints, generally late at night and at weekends, likely because at that time the staff on duty are usually less experienced [164]. The patients are frequently intelligent, very interested in their problem and have a remarkable medical culture [165]. They are particularly insistent with the medical staff, continually demanding medications, consultations, laboratory tests, and surgery [166]. The number of hospitalizations can be amazing: one patient had been admitted to 650 hospitals, hospitalized more than 850 times, and had undergone 42 laparotomies [167].

The aetiology of the disorder is unknown; however, some psychosocial factors seem to be frequent, such as a traumatic childhood, death of a loved one at a young age, sexual abuse, and abandonment. These patients may sometimes exhibit psychopathic tendencies, criminality, vagrancy, and impostership [168]. Those few patients who accept the diagnosis generally attribute it to their desire to feel a sense of importance and find a place of "belonging" [161].

It is quite difficult to determine the incidence of this disorder, also because of the obvious difficulties in confirming the diagnosis. Patients mostly reject it, can

Table 4.4 Synonyms for Münchausen syndrome and subjects with the syndrome. (Modified, from Refs. [160, 161])

Mythomania
Hospital addition syndrome
Hospital-hopper syndrome
Hospital toxicomania syndrome
Hospital black-book patients
Hospital hoboes
Frater Hospitalis
Peregrinating problem patients
Ahasuerus syndrome
Van Gogh syndrome
Peregrinating patients
Doctor shoppers

become hostile, and may change hospital. In cases of female patients, these are generally middle-aged spinsters, and often work in a health care environment although it is estimated that less than 1% of patients in the clinical sector have this syndrome [169]. In a National Hospital Discharge Survey, the incidence was 6.8 cases of factitious disorder per 100,000 patients [170].

The clinical presentation of Münchausen disorder varies remarkably. The most common symptoms include chest pain, abdominal pain, vomiting and/or diarrhoea, anaemia, infections, weakness, hypoglycaemia, vision loss, skin wounds, and arthralgias. It is also quite common for a patient with a benign known medical anomaly (e.g. a chronic abnormal ECG) to present with factitious symptoms that correlate with the findings [161]. In most cases, the referred symptoms are not confirmed by laboratory or radiographic tests. And the patient may be proud of being a "medical mystery" and confounding physicians.

As regards diagnosis, it is important to distinguish Münchausen syndrome from other conditions. The disease is incompatible with suicidal ideas: these patients do not wish to die of their condition. Hysteria or conversion signs can be reported but will disappear during the medical visit [171]. It is also possible to encounter malingering patients with some form of secondary gain, the administration of narcotics, for instance but there are no cases with external incentives such as monetary gain [164].

Skin manifestations are rare, and the disease must be considered when the lesions are spectacular, difficult to diagnose, and not supported by routine investigative techniques [164, 165, 168, 172–179]. Most patients have injected foreign materials into the skin and soft tissue, causing necrosis and ulcerations [162], and may have fever, hypertension, and sepsis, depending on what they have injected [177, 179]. The skin lesions show erythema, swelling, necrosis, and tissue breakdown. Histological examination of the cutaneous lesions due to injections of material is aspecific and shows an inflammatory infiltrate with neutrophils, lymphocytes, histiocytes, foreign body giant cells, and lipophages, but no signs of primary vasculitis [168]. The subcutaneous fat is in many cases necrotic, sometimes with haemorrhage [166]. It is subcutaneous injection of organic solvents that most often causes inflammatory reactions because these substances dissolve the subcutaneous fat [180, 181]. Foreign materials may be revealed under polarized light [164, 175]. In cases of a superimposed infection, there will be Gram stains positivity.

Because the diagnosis of Münchausen syndrome is so difficult, in addition to underdiagnosis there are many cases of misdiagnosis [182]. There are many reasons for this: above all, most patients run away when they meet a suspicious doctor, while those few patients who stay in contact refuse to collaborate and only exceptionally do they acknowledge the diagnosis and accept psychiatric treatment. The clinical presentation of the disorder is also highly varied, featuring a very wide spectrum of conditions and possibly falsified test results. Moreover, it is not rare for physicians themselves to be reluctant to identify simulations. However, it should be remembered in this context that this is the most serious among factitious disorders and that these patients may expose themselves to life-threatening surgical procedures, invasive examinations, and unnecessary treatments [182].

Münchhausen syndrome is also difficult to treat, and even in those patients who are motivated to undergo medical and psychiatric treatment the probabilities of success are very low. There is also little information in the literature about the long-term prognosis of these patients, owing to the vicious circle that the condition creates with the continual passage from one physician to another and one hospital to another [182].

4.11 Münchausen Syndrome by Proxy

Described by Professor Roy Meadow in 1977, the Münchausen syndrome by proxy refers to illness induced in children by a parent, often the mother, for the purpose of indirectly acting out the sick role [181]. This syndrome is observed almost exclusively in children whose parent or caregiver is responsible and may be a manifestation of the battered child syndrome. Data in literature show that 90% of the perpetrators are the biological mothers, 5% are other female caregivers, and 5% are the fathers [162, 184–193]. In addition, the mothers are generally white and aged between 20 and 30 years old; 80% of the perpetrators have a history of psychiatric treatment and 80% were themselves victims. Studies by Hughes and Corbo-Richert [192] demonstrate that all the mothers felt unwanted as a child. Many of these mothers hate their children and are jealous of their happy childhoods because their own childhood had been so miserable (lack of maternal attention or love during infancy) [186].

The Münchausen syndrome by proxy may be also observed in adults, who are usually elderly or mentally unstable [194].

Three subtypes of caregivers have been described: those who actually induce the injury in the child, those who invent the child's symptoms, and those who invent the symptoms and manhandle the blood and urine samples to support the credibility of the symptoms [162, 186]. Mothers are predominant in cases of Münchhausen syndrome by proxy in children, while the father is generally absent, disinterested, or distant [162]. In general, the mother uses correct medical terminology, and she often has a background in the medical field. Her attention to the child is often intense and even bizarre, and she will rarely leave the patient's room for more than a few minutes. She will fill the room with many toys and/or stuffed animals [162]. Moreover, the perpetrators seem to enjoy, or at least welcome, invasive tests and procedures practised on the child, and show little emotion when the child manifests discomfort or pain [186]. When faced by physicians and nurses with a suspected diagnosis of a factitious disorder, however, typically the parent will react angrily and leave the hospital [194]. Skin manifestations are rarely observed, but can consist of bruising, blistering, and burns, mostly on the lower legs and the arms. In babies under 1 year of age, the face and head may be affected, while the buttocks/lower back and outer thighs can be "punishment" sites. The pattern of bruising is highly various: rounded marks or striped areas; in cases of kicks to the lower body the bruises are irregular, large, and deep. Crude forms of skin lesions are procured by heat burns or caustic corrosives [162, 183, 184, 194–197].

The management of Münchausen syndrome by proxy is extremely complex. There are many steps, procedures, and guidelines described in this regard [198–207]. In order to protect children, it is imperative to create a full awareness of this syndrome among members of paediatric health care teams, employees in child protective services, law enforcement officers, members of the legal community, and of child abuse in general [186].

References

1. American Psychiatric Association (APA). Diagnostic and statistical manual of mental disorders. DSM-5. 5th ed. Washington, DC: APA; 2013.
2. International Classification of Diseases (ICD-11) (Version 05/2021). [cited 2021 Sept 4]. Available from: https://icd.who.int
3. Yates GP, Feldman MD. Factitious disorder: a systematic review of 455 cases in the professional literature. Gen Hosp Psychiatry. 2016;41:20–8.
4. Angelini G, Vena GA. Dermatosi artefatte. In: Angelini G, Vena GA, editors. Dermatologia professionale e ambientale. Brescia: ISED; 1997. p. 257–68.
5. Angelini G, Bonamonte D. La dermatite artefatta. G Ital Dermatol Venereol. 1999;134:99–113.
6. Lyell A. Cutaneous artefactual disease. A review, amplified by personal experience. J Am Acad Dermatol. 1979;1:391–407.
7. Hähel T, Rauchfleisch V, Schuppli R. Die Bedentung von Haut-artefakten. Schweiz Med Wochenschr. 1982;112:326–33.
8. Koblenzer CS. Psychosomatic concepts in dermatology. A dermatologist-psychoanalyst's viewpoint. Arch Dermatol. 1983;119:501–12.
9. Panconesi E. Psychosomatic dermatology. Philadelphia: Lippincott; 1984.
10. Gieler U. Factitious disease in the field of dermatology. Psychother Psychosom. 1994;62:48–55.
11. Kocalevent RD, Fliege H, Rose M, et al. Autodestructive syndromes. Psychother Psychosom. 2005;74:202–11.
12. Harth W, Taube KM, Gieler U. Factitious disorders in dermatology. J Dtsch Dermatol Ges. 2010;8:361–72.
13. Gieler U, Consoli SG, Tomás-Aragones L, et al. Self-inflicted lesions in dermatology: terminology and classification—a position paper from the European Society for Dermatology and Psychiatry (ESDaP). Acta Derm Venereol. 2013;93:4–12.
14. Gupta MA, Gupta AK. Self-induced dermatoses: a great imitator. Clin Dermatol. 2019;37:268–77.
15. Petruzzelli V, Angelini G, Vena GA. La dermatite artefatta. Dermat Allerg Profes. 1988;3:23–40.
16. Millard LG, Millard J. Psychocutaneous disorders. In: Burns T, Brethnach S, Cox N, et al., editors. Rook's textbook of dermatology. 8th ed. Oxford: Wiley-Blackwell; 2010:chap.64.1-55.
17. Rieder E, Tausk FA. Psychocutaneous skin diseases. In: Goldsmith LS, Katz SJ, Gilchrest BA, et al., editors. Fitzpatrick's dermatology in general medicine. 8th ed. New York: McGraw-Hill; 2012. p. 1158–66.
18. Kuhn H, Mennella C, Magid M, et al. Psychocutaneous disease: clinical perspectives. J Am Acad Dermatol. 2017;76:779–91.
19. Gieler U, Effendy I, Stangier U. Cutaneous artefacts—possibilities for treatment and their limits. Z Hautkr. 1987;62:882–90. [German].
20. Nielsen K, Jeppesen M, Simmelsgaard L, et al. Self-inflicted skin diseases. A retrospective analysis of 57 patients with dermatitis artefacta seen in a dermatology department. Acta Derm Venereol. 2005;85:512–5.

21. Favazza AR, Conterio K. The plight of chronic self-mutilators. Community Ment Health J. 1988;24:22–30.
22. Klonoff EA, Youngner SJ, Moore DJ, et al. Chronic factitious illness: a behavioral approach. Int J Psychiatry Med. 1983;13:173–83.
23. Justus PG, Kreutziger SS, Kitchens CS. Probing the dynamics of Münchausen's syndrome. Detailed analysis of a case. Ann Intern Med. 1980;93:120–7.
24. Tohid H, Shenefelt PD, Burney WA, et al. Psychodermatology: an association of primary psychiatric disorders with skin. Rev Colomb Psiquiatr. 2019;48:50–7.
25. Bass C, Halligan P. Factitious disorders and malingering: challenges for clinical assessment and management. Lancet. 2014;383:1422–32.
26. Krahn LE, Li H, O'Connor MK. Patients who strive to be ill: factitious disorder with physical symptoms. Am J Psychiatry. 2003;160:1163–8.
27. Cormahan KT, Jha A. Factitious disease. NCBY Book-Shelf. A service of the National Library of Medicine National Institutes of Health. StatPearls [Internet]. Treasure Island (Fl): StarPearls Publishing; 2022.
28. Plassmann R. Inpatient and outpatient long-term psychotherapy of patients suffering from factitious disorders. Psychother Psychosom. 1994;62:96–107.
29. Earle JR Jr, Folks DG. Factitious disorder and coexisting depression: a report of successful psychiatric consultation and case management. Gen Hosp Psychiatry. 1986;8:448–50.
30. Torales J, Melgarejo O, González I, et al. Psychopharmacology in dermatology: treatment of primary psychiatric conditions in dermatology. Dermatol Ther. 2020;33:e13557–612.
31. Mohandas P, Bewley A, Taylor R. Dermatitis artefacta and artefactual skin disease: the need for a psychodermatology multidisciplinary team to treat a difficult condition. Br J Dermatol. 2013;169:600–6.
32. Jafferany M, Stamu-O'Brien C, Mkhoyan R, et al. Psychotropic drugs in dermatology: a dermatologist's approach and choice of medications. Dermatol Ther. 2020;33:e13385.
33. Bonamonte D, Foti C, De Marco A, et al. Self-inflicted pathological cutaneous disorders. Part I. Ital J Dermatol Venerol. 2022;157:389–401.
34. Passarini B, Ismaili A, Passaretti G, et al. Factitious syndromes: a possible classification. Dermatol Experiences. 2008;10:115–20.
35. Krooks JA, Weatherall AG, Holland PJ. Review of epidemiology, clinical presentation, diagnosis, and treatment of common primary psychiatric causes of cutaneous disease. J Dermatolog Treat. 2018;29:418–27.
36. Obermayer ME. Dynamics and management of self-induced eruptions. Calif Med. 1961;94:61–5.
37. Shivakumar S, Jafferany M, Kumar SV, et al. A brief review of dermatitis artefacta and management strategies for physicians. Prim Care Companion CNS Disord. 2021;23:20nr02858.
38. Saha A, Seth J, Gorai S, et al. Dermatitis artefacta: a review of five cases: a diagnostic and therapeutic challenge. Indian J Dermatol. 2015;60:613–5.
39. Verraes-Derancourt S, Derancourt C, Poot F, et al. Pathomimie: étude rétrospective de 31 malades. Ann Dermatol Venereol. 2006;133:235–8.
40. Niforatos JD, Chaitoff A. Factitious disorder commonly presents as dermatitis factitia: a U.S. population-based study. Gen Hosp Psychiatry. 2020;64:129–30.
41. Van Moffaert M, Vermander F, Kint A. Dermatitis artefacta. Int J Dermatol. 1985;24:236–8.
42. Fabisch W. Psychiatric aspects of dermatitis artefacta. Br J Dermatol. 1980;102:29–34.
43. Walker TD, Nusbaum KB, Gilkey TW, et al. Factitial dermatitis in the hospital setting. Arch Dermatol Res. 2023;315:617–20.
44. Koblenzer CS. Dermatitis artefacta. Clinical features and approaches to treatment. Am J Clin Dermatol. 2000;1:47–55.
45. Koblenzer CS. Neurotic excoriations and dermatitis artefacta. Dermatol Clin. 1996;14:447–55.
46. Lavery MJ, Stull C, McCaw I, et al. Dermatitis artefacta. Clin Dermatol. 2018;36:719–22.
47. Chandran V, Kurien G. Dermatitis artefacta. In: StatPearls [Internet]. Treasure Island (FL): StatPearls Publishing; 2022.

48. Jafferany M, França K. Psychodermatology: basics concepts. Acta Derm Venereol. 2016;96(Suppl. 217):35–7.
49. Consoli SG. Dermatitis artefacta: a general review. Eur J Dermatol. 1995;5:5–11.
50. Dieulafoy G. Escarres multiple et récidivantes depuis deux ans et demi aux deux bras et au pied. Ambutation du bras gauche. Discussion sur la nature de ces escarres. Pathomimie. La Presse Med. 1908;47:369–72.
51. Vrij A, Mam S. Non verbal and verbal characteristics of lying. In: Halligan P, Bass C, Oakley D, editors. Malingering and illness deception. Oxford: Oxford University Press; 2003. p. 351–4.
52. Sheppard NP, O'Loughlin S, Malone JP. Psychogenic skin disease: a review of 35 cases. Br J Psychiatry. 1986;149:636–43.
53. Rodríguez Pichardo A, García BB. Dermatitis artefacta: a review. Actas Dermosifiliogr. 2013;104:854–66.
54. Fekih-Romdhane F, Homri W, Labbane R. Troubles factices en dermatologie: intérêt du concept d'état dissociatif. Ann Dermatol Venereol. 2016;143:210–4.
55. Ahmed A, Bewley A, Taylor R. Dermatitis artefacta in a vulnerable adult with a dissociative state. Clin Exp Dermatol. 2013;38:921–3.
56. Ehlers W, Plassmann R. Diagnosis of narcissistic self-esteem regulation in patients with factitious illness (Münchausen syndrome). Psychother Psychosom. 1994;62:69–77.
57. Danzer G, Klapp BF. Zur Anthropologie und Tiefelpsychologie der Aggression: Modelle und Konzepte. In: Studtt HH, editor. Aggression und Autoaggression. Leipzig/Heidelberg: Barth; 1996. p. 9–19.
58. Lachapelle JM, Frimat P, Temstealt D, et al. Dermatoses simulées en medicine due travail. In: Dermatologie professionnelle et de l'environnement. Paris: Masson; 1992. p. 263–71.
59. Cotterill JA. Self-stigmatization: artefact dermatitis. Br J Hosp Med. 1992;47:115–9.
60. Schaffer CB, Carroll J, Abramowitz SI. Self-mutilation and the borderline personality. J Nerv Ment Dis. 1982;170:468–73.
61. Fabisch W. What is dermatitis artefacta? Int J Dermatol. 1981;20:427–8.
62. Gupta MA, Gupta AK, Ellis CN. Antidepressant drugs in dermatology. An update. Arch Dermatol. 1987;123:647–52.
63. Koblenzer CS. Psychocutaneous disease. Orlando (FL): Grune and Stratton; 1987.
64. Adebanjo GAR, Parisella FR, Cittadini A, et al. A case of dermatitis artefacta during a pandemic. Dermatol Ther. 2020;33:e14235.
65. Favazza AR, Conterio K. Female habitual self-mutilators. Acta Psychiatr Scand. 1989;79:283–9.
66. Harper JI, Copeman PW. Dermatitis artefacta presenting as a 'vasculitis'. J R Soc Med. 1983;76:970–1.
67. Levitz SM, Tan OT. Factitious dermatosis masquerading as recurrent herpes zoster. Am J Med. 1988;84:781–3.
68. Millard LG. Dermatological pathomimicry: a form of patient maladjustment. Lancet. 1984;2:969–71.
69. Thomas JR 3rd, Greene SL, Dicken CH. Factitious cheilitis. J Am Acad Dermatol. 1983;8:368–72.
70. Gandy DT. The concept and clinical aspects of factitial dermatitis. South Med J. 1953;46:551–4.
71. Hubler WR Jr, Hubler WR Sr. Folie à deux. Factitious ulcers. Arch Dermatol. 1980;116:1303–4.
72. Foti C, Bonamonte D, Ambrogio F, et al. Irritant contact dermatitis. In: Angelini G, Bonamonte D, Foti C, editors. Clinical contact dermatitis. A practical approach. Berlin: Springer Nature Switzerland AG; 2021. p. 57–94.
73. Bonamonte D, Foti C, De Marco A, et al. Self-inflicted pathological cutaneous disorders. Part II. Ital J Dermatol Venerol. 2022;157:480–8.
74. Dufton P, Griffiths A. Suction blisters mimicking pemphigoid: an unusual case of dermatitis artefacta. Clin Exp Dermatol. 1981;6:163–6.

75. Mushin OP, Esquenazi MD, Ayazi S, et al. Self-inflicted burn injuries: etiologies, risk factors and impact on institutional resources. Burns. 2019;45:213–9.
76. Goitre M, Roncarolo G, Bedello PG, et al. Contact psychodermatitis. Contact Dermatitis. 1985;13:270.
77. Canuto MJ, Martins ACGP, Dwan AJ, et al. Extraordinary findings in a case of self-inflicted cutaneous lesions. Acta Derm Venereol. 2017;97:967–8.
78. Mauf S, Martinez RM, Thali MJ, et al. Made up by makeup—A case report about an exceptional kind of self-inflicted "injuries". Forensic Sci Int. 2015;257:e32–7.
79. Nékam L. Sur la question du lichen moniliformis. Press Med. 1938;46:1000.
80. Böer A. Keratosis lichenoides chronica: proposal of a concept. Am J Dermatopathol. 2006;28:260–75.
81. Patrizi A, Neri I, Passarini B, et al. Keratosis lichenoides chronica: a pediatric case. Dermatology. 1995;191:264–7.
82. Finne HA, Heal JK. Urological manifestation of cryptic severe psychiatric illness. Mil Med. 2019;184:e489–91.
83. Sneddon I, Sneddon J. Self-inflicted injury: a follow-up study of 43 patients. Br Med J. 1975;3:527–30.
84. Alcántara Luna S, García Bravo B, Rodríguez Pichardo A, et al. Dermatitis artefacta in childhood: a retrospective analysis of 44 patients, 1976-2006. Pediatr Dermatol. 2015;32:604–8.
85. Saez-de-Ocariz M, Orozco-Covarrubias L, Mora-Magaña I, et al. Dermatitis artefacta in pediatric patients: experience at the national institute of pediatrics. Pediatr Dermatol. 2004;21:205–11.
86. Libow JA. Child and adolescent illness falsification. Pediatrics. 2000;105:336–42.
87. Bonamonte D, Foti C, Gullo G, et al. Contact dermatitis in children. In: Angelini G, Bonamonte D, Foti C, editors. Clinical contact dermatitis. A practical approach. Berlin: Springer Nature Switzerland AG; 2021. p. 395–413.
88. Gelmetti G, Bonifazi E. Le patomimie cutanee nel bambino. Pediatric Dermatol News. 1985;4:146–69.
89. Rogers M, Fairly M, Santhanam R. Artefactual skin disease in children and adolescents. Australas J Dermatol. 2001;42:264–70.
90. Kwon O, Chung H, Park J. Choking dermatitis: a neologism alerting the nature of factitious dermatitis acquired from self-asphyxial behaviors. J Dermatol. 2018;45:e29–30.
91. Busse H, Harrop T, Gunnell D, et al. Prevalence and associated harm of engagement in self-asphyxial behaviours ('choking game') in young people: a systematic review. Arch Dis Child. 2015;100:1106–14.
92. Dake JA, Price JH, Kolm-Valdivia N, et al. Association of adolescent choking game activity with selected risk behaviors. Acad Pediatr. 2010;10:410–6.
93. Ring HC, Miller IM, Benfeldt E, et al. Artefactual skin lesions in children and adolescents: review of the literature and two cases of factitious purpura. Int J Dermatol. 2015;54:e27–32.
94. Yamada K, Sakurai Y, Shibata M, et al. Factitious purpura in a 10-year-old girl. Pediatr Dermatol. 2009;26:597–600.
95. Kos L, Shwayder T. Cutaneous manifestations of child abuse. Pediatr Dermatol. 2006;23:311–20.
96. Swerdlin A, Berkowitz C, Craft N, et al. Cutaneous signs of child abuse. J Am Acad Dermatol. 2007;57:371–92.
97. Van Moffaert M. Localization of self-inflicted dermatological lesions: what do they tell the dermatologist? Acta Derm Venereol Suppl (Stockh). 1991;156:23–7.
98. Garralda ME. A selective review of child psychiatric syndromes with a somatic presentation. Br J Psychiatry. 1992;161:759–73.
99. Rogers M, Fairley M, Santhanam R. Artefactual skin disease in children and adolescents. Australas J Dermatol. 2001;42:264–70.
100. Hosteing S, Uthurraiague C, Boralein F, et al. À propos de 6 cas de purpura linèaire des bras e l'enfant: une presentation clinique stéréotypée. Arch Pediatr. 2017;24:45–51.

101. Isiyel E, Ersoy Evans S, Akar HT, et al. Challenging diagnosis and rare disease in children: dermatitis artefacta. J Paediatr Child Health. 2021;57:1710–2.
102. King CM, Chalmers RJ. Another aspect of contrived disease: "dermatitis simulata". Cutis. 1984;34:463–4.
103. MacSween RM, Millard LG. A green man. Arch Dermatol. 2000;136:115–8.
104. Singal A, Thani G. Red pseudochromatosis of the neck. Clin Exp Dermatol. 2004;29:548–9.
105. Heydendael VM, Hoekzema R. Acute blue patch on the forearm. Arch Dermatol. 2007;143:937–42.
106. Poskitt L, Wayte J, Wojnarowska F, et al. 'Dermatitis neglecta': unwashed dermatosis. Br J Dermatol. 1995;132:827–9.
107. Clark AN, Mankikar GD, Gray I, Diogenes syndrome. A clinical study of gross neglect in old age. Lancet. 1975;1:366–8.
108. Hanon C, Pinquier C, Gaddour N, et al. Diogenes syndrome: a transnosographic approach. Encephale. 2004;30:315–22.
109. Reyes-Ortiz CA. Diogenes syndrome: the self-neglect elderly. Compr Ther. 2001;27:117–21.
110. Marzouki-Zerouali A, Schoeffler A, Liegeon AL, et al. Lésions auto-provoquées dans un contexte d'hidradénite suppurée : un cas de pathomimicrie. Ann Dermatol Venereol. 2019;146:135–40.
111. Millard LG. Dermatological pathomimicry—a follow up study. In: Proceedings of the first International Symposium on Dermatology and Psychiatry. Vienna: ESDaP; 1987.
112. Condé-Salazar L, Gomez J, Meza B, et al. Artefactual irritant contact dermatitis. Contact Dermatitis. 1993;28:246.
113. Cunha A, Barros M, Azevado F. Perianal contact eczema: an unusual presentation of dermatitis artefacta. Derm Psychosomatics. 2003;4:219–22.
114. Gardner F, Diamond L. Autoerythrocyte sensitization; a form of purpura producing painful bruising following autosensitization to red blood cells in certain women. Blood. 1955;10:675–90.
115. Sridharan M, Ali U, Hook CC, et al. The Mayo Clinic experience with psychogenic purpura (Gardner-Diamond syndrome). Am J Med Sci. 2019;357:411–20.
116. Block ME, Sitenga JL, Lehrer M, et al. Gardner-Diamond syndrome: a systematic review of treatment options for a rare psychodermatological disorder. Int J Dermatol. 2019;58:782–7.
117. Ferizi M, Gercari A, Ferizi M. Psychogenic purpura. Postepy Dermatol Alergol. 2019;36:643–5.
118. Priyam P, Mandal US, Sil A. Psychiatric profile and response to combined pharmacologic and psychotherapeutic treatment in psychogenic purpura. Prim Care Companion CNS Disord. 2021;23:20m02870.
119. Behrendt C, Goos M, Thiel H, et al. Painful bruising syndrome. Hautarzt. 2001;52:634–7.
120. Uthman IW, Moukarbel GV, Salman SM, et al. Autoerythrocyte sensitization (Gardner-Diamond) syndrome. Eur J Haematol. 2000;65:144–7.
121. Berman DA, Roenigk HH, Green D. Autoerythrocyte sensitization syndrome (psychogenic purpura). J Am Acad Dermatol. 1992;27:829–32.
122. Verstraete M. Psychogenic hemorrhages. Verh K Acad Geneeskd Belg. 1991;53:5–28.
123. Ingen S, Viguier M, Guitera P, et al. Painful bruising resembling cellulites of the leg. Am Dermatol Venereol. 2002;129:1029–32.
124. Boussault P, Doutre MS, Beylot-Barry M, et al. Painful bruising syndrome: a psychogenic disease. Rev Med Interne. 2005;26:744–7.
125. Ingber A, Alcalay J, Feuerman EJ. Autoerythrocyte sensitization (Gardner-Diamond syndrome) in men: a case report and review of the literature. Postgrad Med J. 1985;61:823–6.
126. Sorensen RU, Newman AJ, Gordon EM. Psychogenic purpura in adolescent patients. Clin Pediatr (Phila). 1985;24:700–4.
127. Tainwala RR, Phiske M, Raghuwanshi A, et al. Perplexing purpura in two females: rare case of autoerythrocyte sensitization syndrome. Indian Dermatol Online J. 2013;4:305–8.

128. Settle EC Jr. Autoerythrocyte sensitization successfully treated with antidepressants. JAMA. 1983;250:1749–50.
129. Durmazlar SP, Atacan D, Cemil B, et al. Is Gardner-Diamond syndrome associated with hormonal influences along with psychosocial problems? A delayed diagnosis. Eur J Dermatol. 2009;19:259–60.
130. Ratnoff OD. Psychogenic purpura (autoerythrocyte sensitization): an unsolved dilemma. Am J Med. 1989;87:16N–21N.
131. Hällström T, Hersle K, Mobacken H. Mental symptoms and personality structure in autoerythrocyte sensitization syndrome. Br J Psychiatry. 1969;115:1269–76.
132. Okur M, Turan H, Ozkan A, et al. An extremely rare cause of bruising in children: autoerythrocyte sensitization syndrome. Turk J Haematol. 2012;29:201–3.
133. Strunecká A, Krpejsová L, Palecek J, et al. Transbilayer redistribution of phosphatidylserine in erythrocytes of a patient with autoerythrocyte sensitization syndrome (psychogenic purpura). Folia Haematol Int Mag Klin Morphol Blutforsch. 1990;117:829–41.
134. Jafferany M, Bhattacharya G. Psychogenic purpura (Gardner-Diamond syndrome). Prim Care Companion CNS Disord. 2015:17. https://doi.org/10.4088/PCC.14br01697.
135. Ratnoff OD. The psychogenic purpuras: a review of autoerythrocyte sensitization, autosensitization to DNA, "hysterical" and factitial bleeding, and the religious stigmata. Semin Hematol. 1980;17:192–213.
136. Panconesi E, Hautmann G. Stress, stigmatization and psychosomatic purpuras. Int Angiol. 1995;14:130–7.
137. Whitlock FA. In: Witlock FA, editor. Self-inflicted and related dermatoses. London: WB Saunders; 1976. p. 98–107.
138. Agle DP, Ratnoff OD, Spring GK. The anticoagulant malingerer. Psychiatric studies of three patients. Ann Intern Med. 1970;73:67–72.
139. O'Reilly RA, Aggeler PM. Covert anticoagulant ingestion: study of 25 patients and review of world literature. Medicine (Baltimore). 1976;55:389–99.
140. Sneddon IB. Simulated disease: problems in diagnosis and management. J R Coll Physicians Lond. 1983;17:199–205.
141. Yates VM. Factitious purpura. Clin Exp Dermatol. 1992;17:238–9.
142. Sawhney MP, Arora G, Arora S, et al. Undiagnosed purpura: a case of autoerythrocyte sensitization syndrome associated with dermatitis artefacta and pseudo-ainhum. Indian J Dermatol Venereol Leprol. 2006;72:379–81.
143. Legano L, McHugh MT, Palusci VJ. Child abuse and neglect. Curr Probl Pediatr Adolesc Health Care. 2009;39:31.e1–e26.
144. Kellett CE. Sir Thomas Browne and the disease called the Morgellons. Ann Med Hist. 1935;7:467–79.
145. Koblenzer CS. The challenge of Morgellons disease. J Am Acad Dermatol. 2006;55:920–2.
146. Musalek M. Delusional parasitosis. In: Koo JYM, Lee CS, editors. Psychocutaneous medicine. New York: Marcel Dekker, Inc.; 2002. p. 143–52.
147. Ranka N, Godse K, Nadkarni N, et al. Morgellons disease: a myth or reality? Indian Dermatol Online J. 2016;7:430–2.
148. Laupland KB, Valiquette L. Delusional infestation. Can J Infect Dis Med Microbiol. 2016;2016:9091838.
149. Paquette M. Morgellons: disease or delusions? Perspect Psychiatr Care. 2007;43:67–8.
150. Murase JE, Wu JJ, Koo J. Morgellons disease: a rapport-enhancing term for delusions of parasitosis. J Am Acad Dermatol. 2006;55:913–4.
151. Elkan D. Morgellons disease: real or delusion. New Scientist. 2007;195:45–9.
152. Waddell AG, Burke WA. Morgellons disease? J Am Acad Dermatol. 2006;55:914–5.
153. Morgellons research Foundation Web site. Available at: http://www.morgellons.org/
154. Pearson ML, Selby JV, Katz KA, et al. Clinical, epidemiologic, histopathologic and molecular features of an unexplained dermopathy. PLoS One. 2012;7:e29908.
155. Reichenberg JS, Magid M, Jesser CA, et al. Patients labeled with delusions of parasitosis compose a heterogenous group: a retrospective study from a referral center. J Am Acad Dermatol. 2013;68(41-6):46.e1–2.

156. Savely VR, Leitao MM, Striker RB. The mystery of Morgellons disease. Infection or delusion? Am J Clin Dermatol. 2005;7:1–5.
157. Asher R. Munchausen's syndrome. Lancet. 1951;1:339–41.
158. Menninger K. Polysurgery and polysurgical addiction. Psychosomal Quart. 1934;4:173–99.
159. Newmark N, Adityanjee KJ. Pseudologia fantastica and factitious disorder: review of the literature and a case report. Compr Psychiatry. 1999;40:89–95.
160. Feldman MD. Munchausen by Internet: detecting factitious illness and crisis on the Internet. South Med J. 2000;93:669–72.
161. Weber B, Gokarakonda SB, Doyle MQ. Münchausen syndrome. In: StatPearls [Internet]. Treasure Island (FL): StatPearls Publishing; 2022.
162. Boyd AS, Ritchie C, Likhari S. Münchhausen syndrome and Munchausen syndrome by proxy in dermatology. J Am Acad Dermatol. 2014;71:376–81.
163. Samuels MP, Southall DP. Münchausen syndrome by proxy. Br J Hosp Med. 1992;47:759–62.
164. Robertson MM, Cervilla JA. Münchausen's syndrome. Br J Hosp Med. 1997;58:308–12.
165. Falagas ME, Christopoulou M, Rosmarakis ES, et al. Münchausen's syndrome presenting as severe panniculitis. Int J Clin Pract. 2004;58:720–2.
166. Huffman JC, Stern TA. The diagnosis and treatment of Münchausen's syndrome. Gen Hosp Psychiatry. 2003;25:358–63.
167. Robertson MM, Hossain G. Münchausen's syndrome coexisting with other disorders. Br J Hosp Med. 1997;58:154–5.
168. Parent DJ, Krafft T, Noel JC, et al. Cutaneous Münchausen syndrome with presentation simulating pyoderma gangrenosum. J Am Acad Dermatol. 1994;31:1072–4.
169. Ferrara P, Vitelli O, Bottaro G, et al. Factitious disorders and Münchausen syndrome: the tip of the iceberg. J Child Health Care. 2013;17:366–74.
170. Hamilton JC, Eger M, Razzak S, et al. Somatoform, factitious, and related diagnoses in the national hospital discharge survey: addressing the proposed DSM-5 revision. Psychosomatics. 2013;54:142–8.
171. Mehta P, Bussing R. Factitious coagulopathy due to Münchausen syndrome by proxy. Am J Pediatr Hematol Oncol. 1993;15:124–5.
172. Sullivan M, Trosow A. Multiple subcutaneous abscesses produced by the hypodermic injection of feces. South Med J. 1949;42:402–4.
173. Tunbridge WM. Unusual Münchausen's syndrome. Br Med J. 1969;2:312.
174. Oh C, Ginsberg-Fellner F, Dolger H. Factitial panniculitis and necrotizing fasciitis in juvenile diabetes. Diabetes. 1975;24:856–8.
175. Steinman R, Mendelson J, Portnoy J. Self-inoculation with milk as a cause of recurrent cellulitis. Can Med Assoc J. 1975;112:605–6.
176. Jackson RM, Tucker SB, Abraham JL, et al. Factitial cutaneous ulcers and nodules: the use of electron-probe microanalysis in diagnosis. J Am Acad Dermatol. 1984;11:1065–9.
177. Ackerman AB, Mosher DT, Schwamm HA. Factitial Weber-Christian syndrome. JAMA. 1966;198:731–6.
178. Okuniewska A, Walczuk BI, Czubek M, et al. Recurrent deep ulcers resembling rare cancers as a form of factitious disorder. Acta Derm Venereol. 2011;91:341–2.
179. Tochigi M, Hara H, Goshima J, et al. Cutaneous Münchausen's syndrome caused by self-injections of fermented beans. J Eur Acad Dermatol Venereol. 2008;22:886–7.
180. Mrvos R, Dean BS, Krenzelok EP. High pressure injection injuries: a serious occupational hazard. J Toxicol Clin Toxicol. 1987;25:297–304.
181. Hogan CJ, Ruland RT. High-pressure injection injuries to the upper extremity: a review of the literature. J Orthop Trauma. 2006;20:503–11.
182. Schrader H, Bøhmer T, Aasly J. The incidence of diagnosis of Münchausen syndrome, other factitious disorders, and malingering. Behav Neurol. 2019;2019:3891809.
183. Sugandhan S, Gupta S, Khandpur S, et al. 'Münchausen syndrome by proxy' presenting as battered child syndrome: a report of two cases. Int J Dermatol. 2010;49:679–83.
184. Sirka CS, Pradhan S, Mohapatra D, et al. Cutaneous Münchausen syndrome by proxy: a diagnostic challenge for dermatologist. Indian Dermatol Online J. 2018;9:435–7.

185. Paulk D. Münchausen syndrome by proxy: tall tales and real hurts. Clin Reviews. 2001;11:51–7.
186. Thomas K. Münchausen syndrome by proxy: identification and diagnosis. J Pediatr Nurs. 2003;18:174–80.
187. Sung C, Salem S, Nguyen E, et al. Pediatric factitious disorder perpetuated by others: a dermatologist's duty beyond the skin. J Clin Aesthet Dermatol. 2021;14:22–4.
188. Walters IC, MacIntosh R, Blake KD. A case report and literature review: factitious disorder imposed on another and malingering by proxy. Paediatr Child Health. 2019;25:345–8.
189. Bursch B, Emerson ND, Sanders MJ. Evaluation and management of factitious disorder imposed on another. J Clin Psychol Med Settings. 2021;28:67–77.
190. Nico MMS, Dwan AJ. Cutaneous ulcers, delusional disorders and Münchausen by proxy: from somatic to psychological diagnosis and approach. Acta Derm Venereol. 2022;102:adv00654.
191. Babu AK, Mohamed A, Das N. Münchausen syndrome by proxy. Indian Dermatol Online J. 2019;10:496–7.
192. Hughes LM, Corbo-Richert B. Münchausen syndrome by proxy: literature review and implications for critical care nurses. Crit Care Nurse. 1999;19:71–8.
193. Verity CM, Winckworth C, Burman D, et al. Polle syndrome: children of Münchausen. Br Med J. 1979;2:422–3.
194. Deimel GW 4th, Burton MC, Raza SS, et al. Münchausen syndrome by proxy: an adult dyad. Psychosomatics. 2012;53:294–9.
195. Vennemann B, Perdekamp MG, Weinmann W, et al. A case of Münchausen syndrome by proxy with subsequent suicide of the mother. Forensic Sci Int. 2006;158:195–9.
196. Weston WL, Morelli JG. "Painful and disabling granuloma annulare": a case of Münchausen by proxy. Pediatr Dermatol. 1997;14:363–4.
197. Tamay Z, Akcay A, Kilic G, et al. Corrosive poisoning mimicking cicatricial pemphigoid: Münchausen by proxy. Child Care Health Dev. 2007;33:496–9.
198. Manarch K. Reporting suspected child abuse: the first, not final steps toward prevention. Mother Baby J. 1997;2:39–42.
199. Souid AK, Keith DV, Cunningham AS. Münchausen syndrome by proxy. Clin Pediatr (Phila). 1998;37:497–503.
200. Guidelines for suspecting and identifying Münchausen syndrome by proxy. Available at: http://www.bcpl.net/agravels/Profile.htm. Accessed 5 Oct 1999.
201. Bosch JJ. Münchausen syndrome by proxy. J Pediatr Health Care. 1997;11:242.
202. Schreier HA, Libow JA. Hurting for love. New York: Guilprol; 1993.
203. Taskforce APSAC. APSAC practice guidelines: Münchausen by proxy: clinical and case management guidance. The APSAC Advisor. 2018;30:8–21.
204. Yates G, Bass C. The perpetrators of medical child abuse (Münchausen syndrome by proxy). A systematic review of 796 cases. Child Abuse and Neglect. 2017;72:45–53.
205. Rogers R. Diagnostic, explanatory, and detection models of Münchausen syndrome by proxy: extrapolations from malingering and deception. Child Abuse and Neglect. 2004;28:225–38.
206. Horwath J. Inter-agency practice in suspected cases of Münchausen syndrome by proxy (factitious illness by proxy): dilemmas for professionals. Child Family social Work. 1999;4:109–18.
207. Wilde JA, Pedroni AT. Privacy rights in Münchausen syndrome. Contemporary Pediatric. 1993;10:83–91.

Chapter 5
Factitious Skin Disorders with External Incentives

Domenico Bonamonte, Aurora De Marco, and Gianni Angelini

In most cases, self-inflicted skin artefacts are caused by psychiatric disorders. However, there are also some subjects whose simulations are motivated by illicit intent (malingering): in these cases, the simulators are well aware of their actions and hidden motivations. In short, these subjects do not suffer from underlying psychiatric disorders.

5.1 Malingering

5.1.1 General Remarks

Asher coined the term "malingering" to define the deliberate imitation, production, or encouragement of illness for a precise purpose [1]. The term is derived from the French word "malinger" ("mal": "wrongly or improperly", and "hangre": "sickly") [2]. The malingering phenomenon had already been reported in ancient Greek and Biblical literature [3].

Generally, malingering is defined as "intentionally fabricating or exaggerating the symptoms of mental or physical disorders for secondary gains including financial compensation, avoiding school, work, or military service, as well as obtaining drugs, getting lighter criminal sentences, or simply wishing to attract attention or

D. Bonamonte (✉) · A. De Marco
Department of Precision and Regenerative Medicine and Ionian Area, University of Bari "Aldo Moro", Bari, Italy
e-mail: domenico.bonamonte@uniba.it; a.demarco24@studenti.uniba.it

G. Angelini
Dermatology, University of Bari "Aldo Moro", Bari, Italy
e-mail: gianniang@alice.it

G. Angelini et al. (eds.), *Psychocutaneous Diseases*,
https://doi.org/10.1007/978-3-031-70296-9_5

sympathy" [4]. Data in the literature reveal that the most common incentives are attempts to evade various duties (in soldiers, to avoid duty shifts or a transfer, or to escape military service) or prison detention, or to gain advantages of an occupational nature, or else to obtain drugs [5–13].

It is quite difficult to estimate the prevalence of malingering. Mittemberg and Coll. report an estimated prevalence in civil (i.e. personal injury cases) and criminal legal settings in the range of 10–30% [14]. According to Udoetuk and Coll. malingering is actually a fairly rare diagnosis, with a prevalence of 0.1% in both inpatient and emergency department sites [5].

A diagnosis of malingering is more often formulated in inpatient stays than in emergency department visits. This is quite reasonable, both because hospitalized patients tend to receive more exhaustive and conclusive treatments and because inpatients are more likely to build a confidential relationship with the doctors than outpatients or emergency room patients.

Malingering can have a significant financial impact on the health service and economic finances of the country [2, 7]. In fact, it has been calculated that in the United States the cost to insurers is about $ 150 billion dollars each year [15]. A review of Social Security Disability data suggests that malingering occurs in 45–59% of adult mental disorder cases, at a cost of at least $ 20 billion per year [16]. Owing to these data, from an economic standpoint, too, since malingering is more common in emergency departments (where many decisions about the need for hospitalizations and treatments are taken), it is important that emergency clinicians be aware and prepared to recognize and manage malingering patients.

It is also important to understand that malingering is generally a diagnosis of exclusion. Malingering must be suspected only when the presenting symptoms do not point to an objective aetiology, and known external motivations for its presentation emerge. The diagnosis of malingering can be made only after all physical and psychological factors contributing to the patient's presentation have been accurately considered, explored, and eliminated [5]. Such a diagnosis has been extensively studied in forensic settings, with the aid of psychometric measures and tests. Nevertheless, even in such circumstances the diagnosis needs to be made with caution, and only after clear and ample evidence is available [5, 7, 9, 17–20].

The DSM-5 states various signs which may indicate malingering: when the medicolegal context of a presentation shows a marked discrepancy with the symptoms and objective findings, lack of cooperation, and the presence of an antisocial personality disorder [4]. In addition, the symptoms referred may contradict other elements of the medical history [21–23]. Malingerers are not in general familiar with subtle aspects of the symptomatology and so report improbable symptoms. The duration of the visit may also be an important component of the assessment: simulating symptoms often requires significant effort, and malingerers are likely to grow tired as the interview progresses. Repeated questioning by multiple team members and by serial assessments over an extended period can contribute to reveal inconsistencies in a patient's history [7, 24].

Malingering must clearly also be differentiated from factitious presentations associated with personality disorders [25–30]. One of the differential parameters is the time the simulation has lasted: usually, factitial behaviour without external incentives is chronic and persistent (for various reasons such as previous failures to diagnose the disorder, the fact that many physicians and hospitals have been consulted, refusal to accept the diagnosis and psychiatric treatment), whereas malingering is episodic, opportunistic, and short-lasting. However, this parameter may not be valid in cases of a first episode of factitious behaviour due to psychological or psychiatric disorders. Another differential parameter is the evidence of "external rewards" although even this parameter is questionable, both empirically and conceptually. Conceptually, the "absence" of external rewards cannot be equated with the "presence" of a strong internal motivation: the external rewards may sometimes be so banal that they do not seem important; moreover, the external rewards may be overshadowed by strong internal motivations [25]. On this point, other authors also believe that the presence of obvious external gain should not alone disqualify a diagnosis of a factitious disorder: a male patient, for example, could be engaging in deceptive behaviour, with exaggerated pain, for both external rewards (e.g. to obtain a narcotic to feed an addiction) and internal needs (e.g. to avoid chronic conflicts with the partner) [31]. In both cases, the diagnosis must be based on very challenging clinical and human constructs.

Malingering must also be differentiated from lesions due to abuse, torture, and tribal or cultural practices [19, 20, 32–37]. Malingering can involve any medical specialty. Fear, desire, and escape are the three most important motives to self-produce false or exaggerated physical or psychological skin lesions or to impose them on another person [12]. In dermatology, a subject can intentionally induce de novo skin lesions or else aggravate the symptoms of a spontaneous pre-existing disease (Table 5.1). Some examples of this behaviour are chronic, non-healing, post-operative scars that are manipulated with instruments, or faecal injection to maintain sepsis [38, 39]. Another possibility is an irritant or allergic hand contact dermatitis perpetuated to seek higher compensation awards [40, 41]. Even in this case, however, malingering must be differentiated from more or less involuntary actions or a deliberate lack of compliance to medical prescriptions [13].

Table 5.1 Factitious disorders with external incentives: malingering

Malingering in adolescents
Malingering in soldiers
Occupational dermatitis artefacta
Dermatitis artefacta with patch test artefacts
Witchcraft syndrome
Secrétan syndrome (in part)
Dermatological pathomimicry (in part)
Religious stigmata as malingering artefacts

5.1.2 Malingering in Adolescents

Malingering can also rarely be observed in adolescents: for example, a subject with atopic dermatitis can aggravate the lesions by using a steel brush, so as to remain at home and miss an interrogation or a class test. In an editorial about cutaneous artefacts in children, Gelmetti and Bonifazi present an episode of "curious" psychological malingering by some students in the third year of middle school in Bari. At the level of the chin and jugular area, erythematous and ecchymotic lesions were present in all of them (Fig. 5.1). The dermatitis did not worry the pupils and some of them smilingly exhibited it. This evidence of dermatitis in several subjects at the same school and the same time, and exhibited with a smile, immediately led to the diagnosis of artefacts. After a few days one of the pupils confessed their self-inflicted behaviour: during lessons, the pupils rubbed and pinched their skin, at unobserved moments, on the chin and jugular area with their thumb and index finger. The aim was to evade lessons with a teacher they disliked. The stratagem was

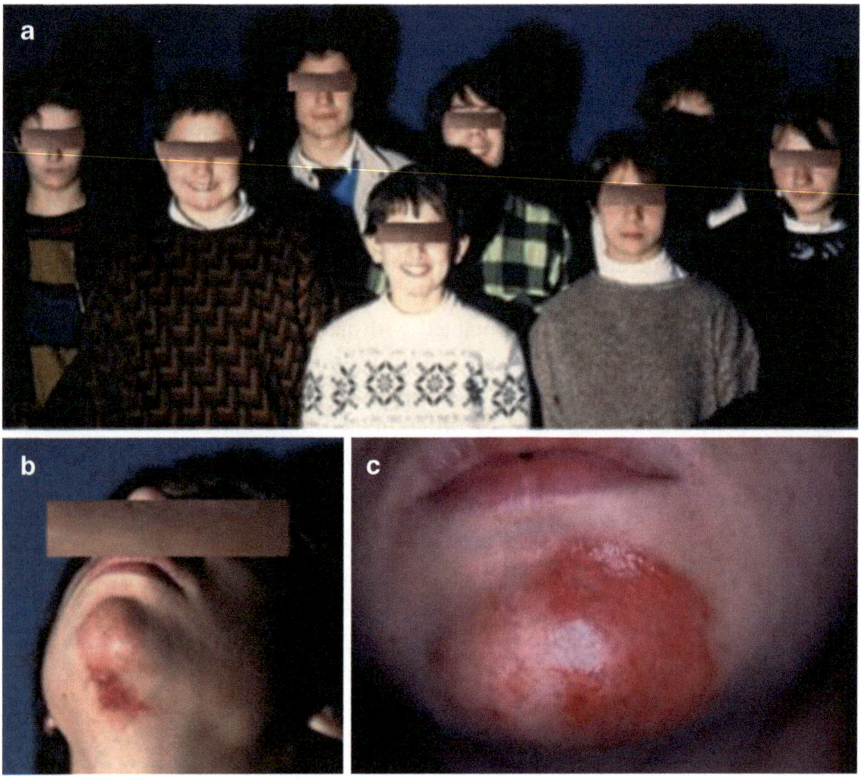

Fig. 5.1 (**a–c**) Collective dermatitis artefacta in a group of pupils: erythematous and ecchymotic lesion on the chin induced by rubbing and pinching the skin. (Courtesy of Prof. Ernesto Bonifazi. Reproduced with permission by Bonamonte et al. [10])

suggested by a pupil who had already adopted it 15 days before to avoid sitting an exam [42].

5.1.3 Malingering in Soldiers

One area which is closely linked with malingering has always been the military [2]. Odysseus is said to have affected madness to avoid fighting in the Trojan War [43]. For the same reason, Achilles dressed up in female clothing (following the decision made by his mother, Thetis), to hide among the 11 daughters of Lycomedes, King of the island of Skyros [44].

Military malingering may be triggered by fear or desire [45] and is different in times of peace and war. Soldiers feign diseases or disability to avoid duties/a mission, obtain optimal job placement, suspend a transfer or be discharged from the service [45–47]. Various self-inflicted disorders are chosen, ranging from direct self-mutilation with weapons or other means to a variety of ingenious and dangerous methods.

As regards soldiers, some of our team observed 11 men doing compulsory military service, aged between 21 and 24 years, and 1 fully signed-up career soldier, with skin artefacts of a comparatively mild degree [10, 48]. The afflictions involved the insteps (5 cases), legs and forearms (2 cases), scrotum (1 case), and trunk (4 cases). In 5 cases with bullous and ulcerative lesions the etiological agent was not discovered, whereas in 7, uncommon agents emerged, including latex from the leaves of *Agave americana* (papulous lesions), hot vinegar compresses (erosions), propane gas, salted sardines, and nettle soap (erythema and blisters) [49] (Figs. 5.2,

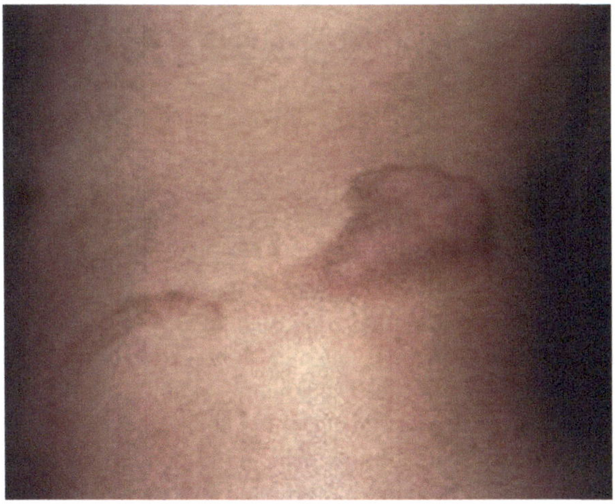

Fig. 5.2 A 21-year-old man with figured hyperchromic lesions as outcome of dermatitis induced by propane gas from a cigarette lighter. (Reproduced with permission by Bonamonte et al. [10])

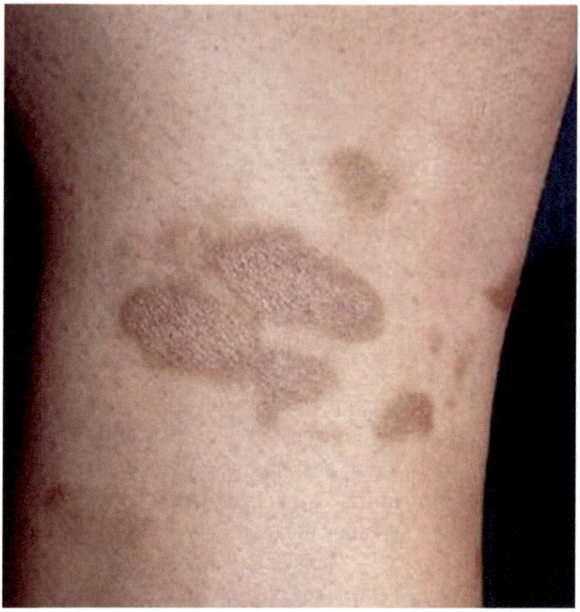

Fig. 5.3 The same patient as in Fig. 5.2. (Reproduced with permission by Bonamonte et al. [10])

5.3, 5.4, 5.5, 5.6, 5.7, 5.8, 5.9, 5.10, 5.11 and 5.12). In the cases that admitted their actions, the purpose of the artefacts was to obtain convalescence leave. Naturally, in such cases it is equally necessary to differentiate true simulation from that induced by a psychological disorder [50].

5.2 Occupational Dermatitis Artefacta

In the occupational field, there are many different factors that can prompt a subject to simulate a disease: to obtain prolongation of a prior disease or its recognition as an occupational affliction, and to attain a higher class of disability pension. The spread of state insurance has certainly increased the number of simulations [1, 51, 52], but although many common cases of self-aggravated spontaneous dermatoses have been reported, only rarely do forms intended to reproduce a picture of professional-type dermatitis seem to be documented.

The first group includes cases of voluntary aggravation of traumatic lesions secondary to accidents at the work site. The wounds do not heal properly, suppurate or eczematize, or else burns appear, that heal but then ulcerate and show a chronic course. Despite occlusive bandaging, which should rapidly resolve such cases, the risk of cunning simulators injecting harmful substances under the bandage should be borne in mind.

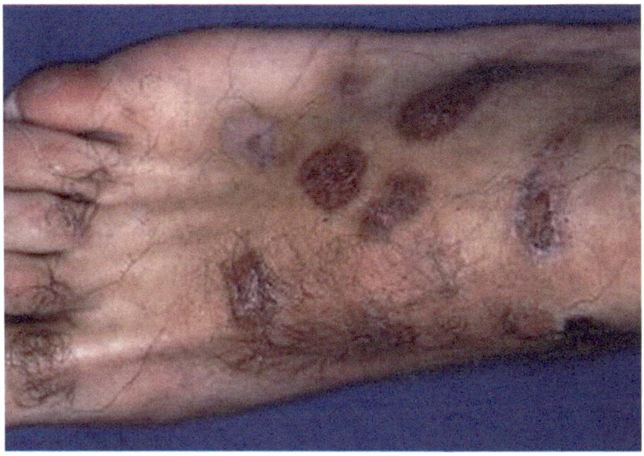

Fig. 5.4 A 22-year-old man with figured pigmented lesions as outcome of dermatitis induced by propane gas from a cigarette lighter. (Reproduced from Angelini and Bonamonte [55]. All rights reserved)

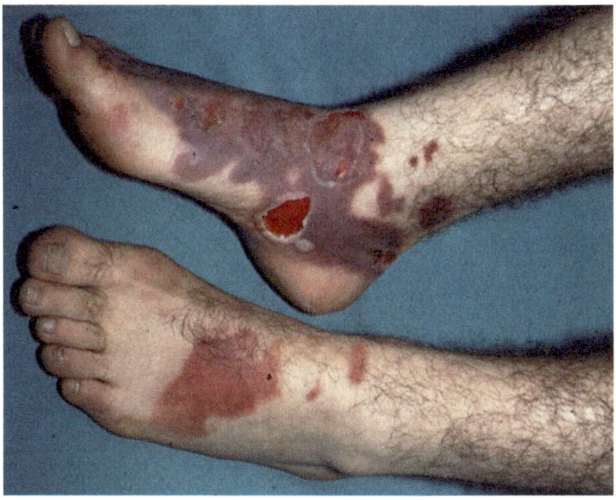

Fig. 5.5 A 22-year-old man with ecchymotic and erosive lesions induced by hot vinegar compresses and physical trauma. (Reproduced with permission by Bonamonte et al. [10])

Occupational dermatitis artefacta of the second type can be provoked directly on healthy skin or can be subsequent to the aggravation of a pre-existing contact dermatitis. The diagnosis can be fairly simple when the simulator attempts to reproduce eczema on healthy skin: in fact, it is difficult to provoke erythematous vesicular spongiotic lesions in different phases of evolution, and so self-inflicted lesions tend to manifest as groups of gross blisters. These criteria do not apply if the subject aggravates a pre-existing spontaneous eczematous dermatitis. The simulator may, in fact, be well aware of what substance provokes the dermatitis and so make use of it.

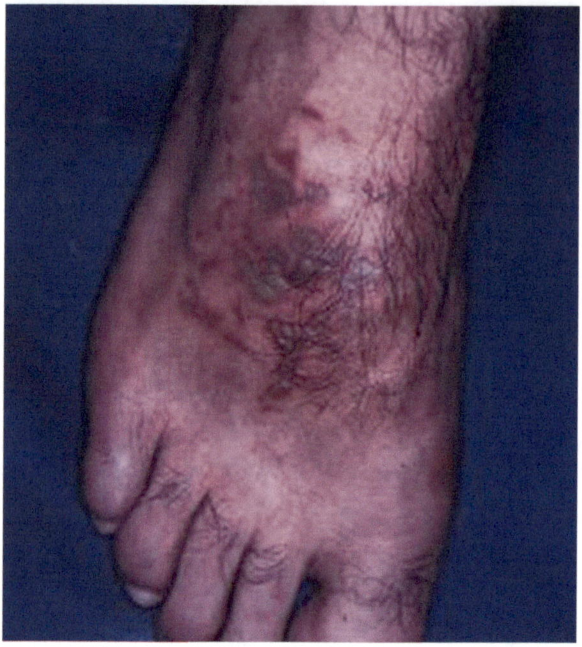

Fig. 5.6 A 23-year-old man with bullous and erosive lesions induced by salted sardines in occlusion. (Reproduced with permission by Bonamonte et al. [10])

In this event, hospitalization and continual supervision of the subject can sometimes enable a precise diagnosis [10, 48, 53–60].

Over the years, we have observed 46 cases of occupational dermatitis artefacta. The suspicion of a true simulation, suggested by the combination of "work problems", the particular morphology of the lesions, and repeated negative findings of all relative tests and clinical dermatological and psychiatric consultations, was then confirmed by confessions obtained from all the patients after repeated confidential and informal discussions [61–63]. The causal agents used included metal objects, incandescent needles, lighted cigarettes, and chrome mixtures (Figs. 5.13, 5.14, 5.15, 5.16, 5.17, 5.18, 5.19, 5.20, 5.21, 5.22, 5.23, 5.24, 5.25, 5.26 and 5.27). Most of the subjects were masons. In 38 cases, the reason for the simulation was to obtain legal recognition of an occupational disease, in 2 to gain a higher class of disability pension, and in 6 to prolong the disease.

Table 5.2 reports some indicative clinical criteria that could be useful for the differential diagnosis between occupational dermatitis artefacta and dermatitis artefacta (aside, of course, from psychiatric problems underlying the latter).

Malingering has to be differentiated from deliberate non-compliance to medical prescriptions, a condition that can lead to the persistence or aggravation of a disease and hence to hospitalization. Many cases of poor compliance need ostensibly to be ignored by physicians that will explore the failed compliance in an empathic way, without making the patient feel guilty [13]. Nevertheless, cases of a hidden

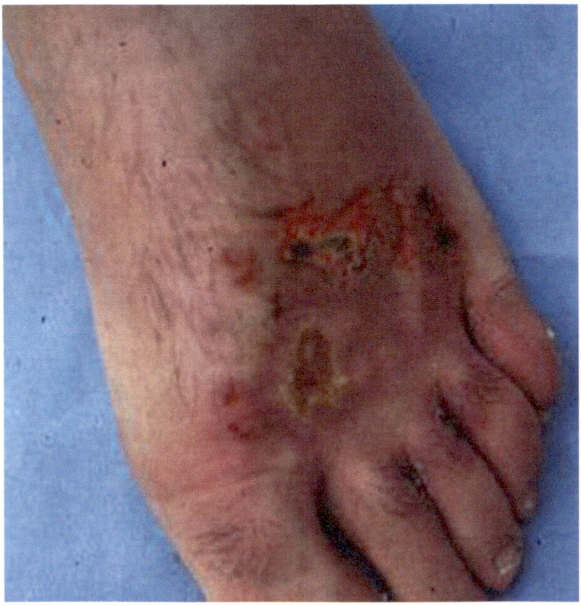

Fig. 5.7 A 22-year-old man with ulcerative lesions induced by salted sardines in occlusion. (Reproduced with permission by Bonamonte et al. [10])

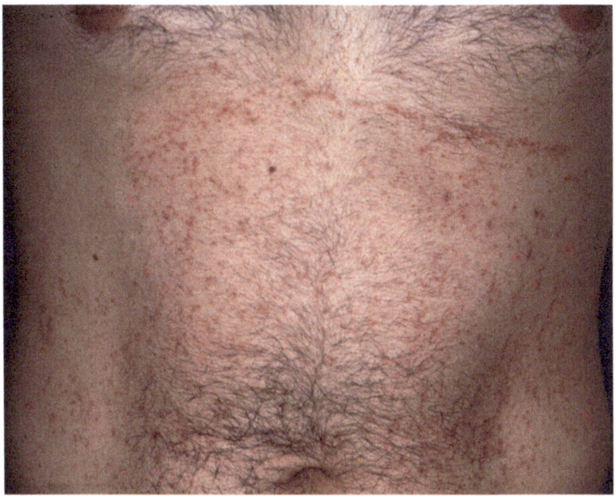

Fig. 5.8 A 23-year-old man with papular dermatitis induced by rubbing a cut leaf of *Agave americana* on abdomen. (Reproduced with permission by Bonamonte et al. [49])

non-compliance can also be supported by a social incentive and so come under the heading of malingering.

Malingering must also be differentiated from dermatological pathomimicry, a condition described in 1984 by Millard in 13 patients who had caused recurrences

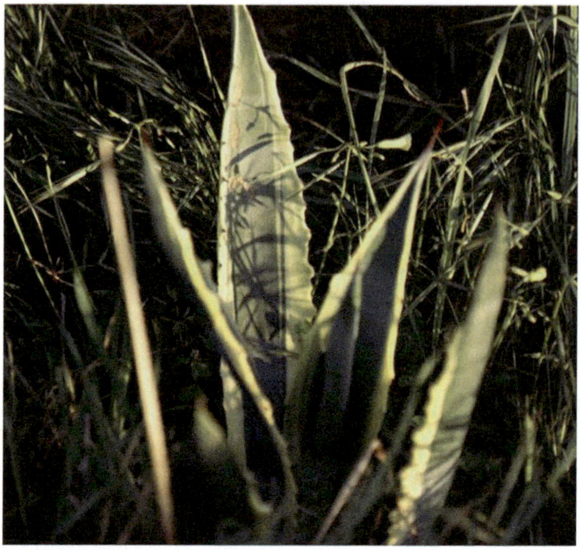

Fig. 5.9 *Agave americana.* (Reproduced with permission by Bonamonte et al. [49])

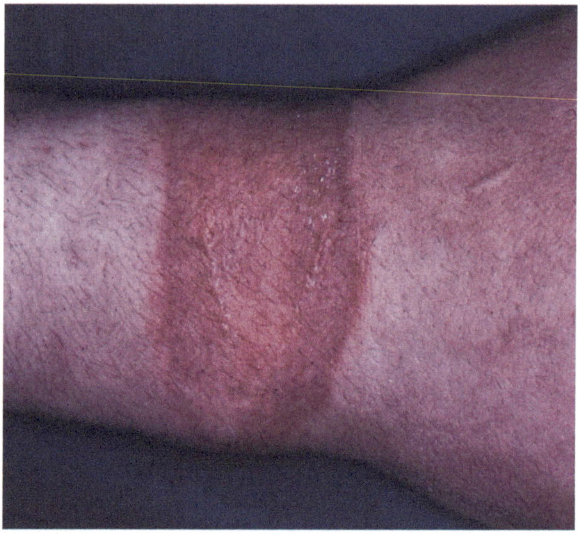

Fig. 5.10 A 22-year-old-man with erythemato-vesicular dermatitis due to wet compresses of leaves of *Urtica dioica.* (Reproduced with permission by Bonamonte et al. [49])

or exacerbations of their existing skin disease [64]. These patients had aggravated their condition by deliberate exposure to the noxae they knew had triggered the complaint. Most of these patients described by Millard were young women, who were trying to gain greater sympathy from their families. The author considers

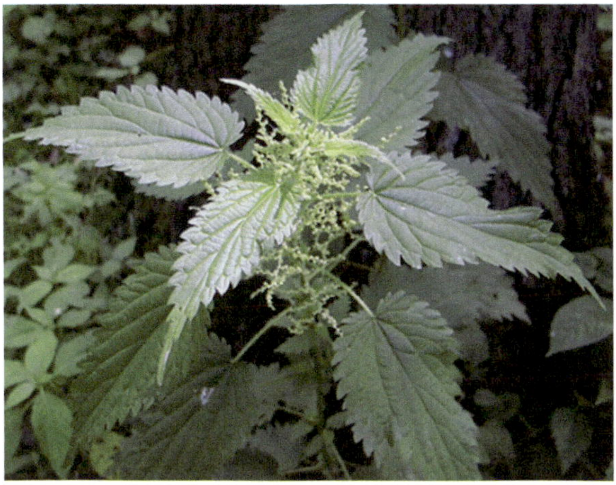

Fig. 5.11 *Urtica dioica.* (Reproduced with permission by Bonamonte et al. [49])

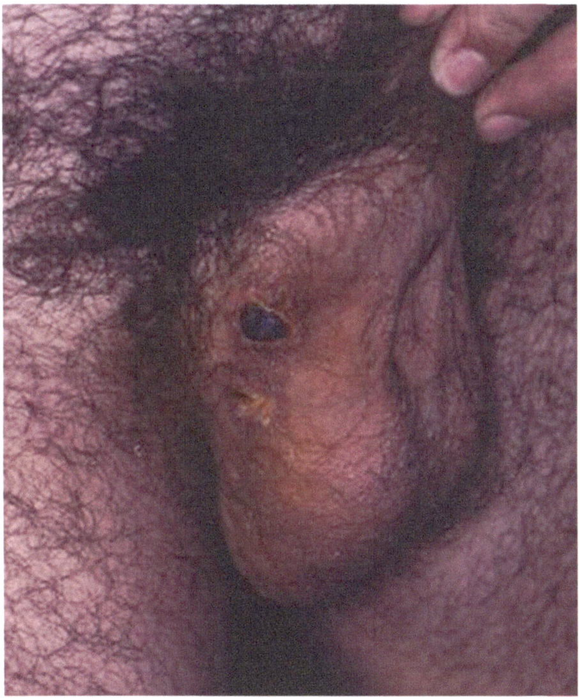

Fig. 5.12 A 21-year-old patient with ulcerative lesions of the scrotum self-induced by incandescent metal object

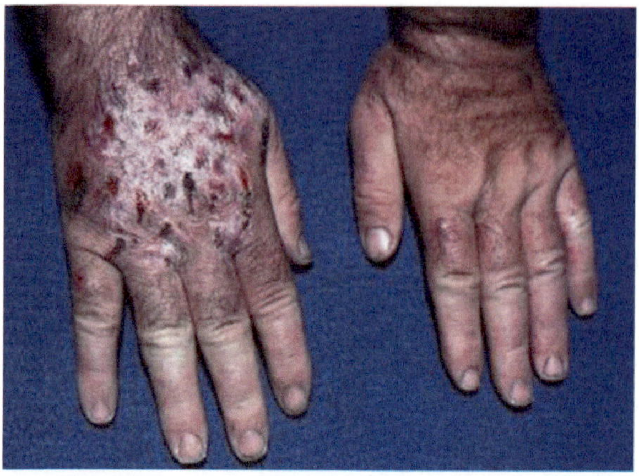

Fig. 5.13 A self-artefact induced by metal object on pre-existing spontaneous contact dermatitis. (Reproduced with permission by Bonamonte et al. [62])

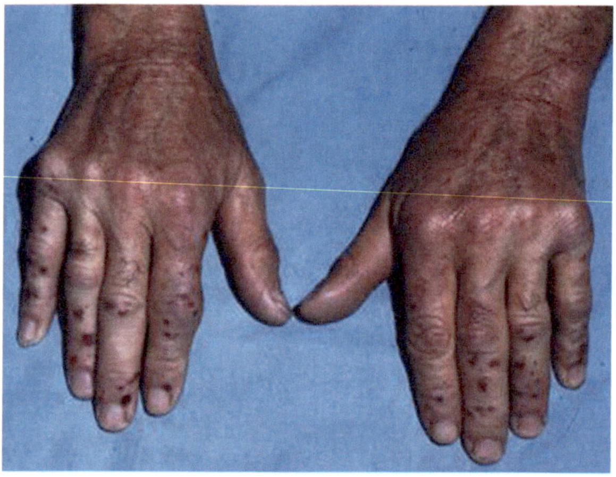

Fig. 5.14 Self-artefact induced by incandescent metal object. (Reproduced with permission by Bonamonte et al. [62])

pathomimicry to differ from dermatitis artefacta, characterized rather by lesions differing from those of true organic skin disease. All the same, it should be remembered that the same behaviour can be observed in conscious simulators with a financial objective, as stated above.

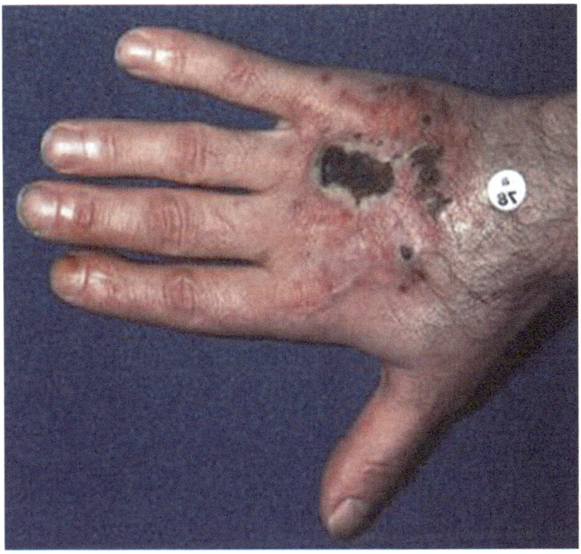

Fig. 5.15 Self-artefact induced by lighted cigarette. (Reproduced with permission by Bonamonte et al. [62])

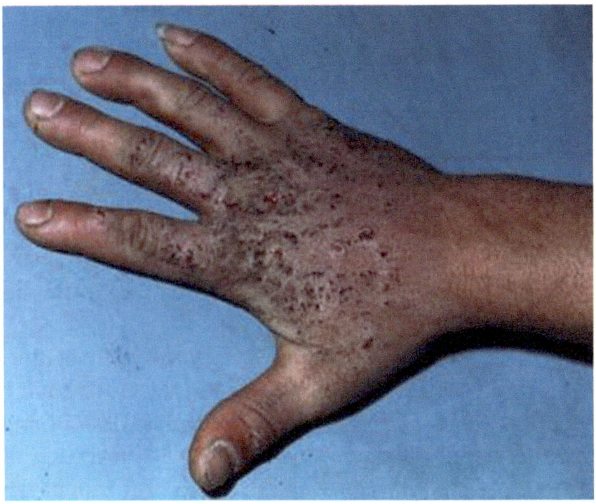

Fig. 5.16 Self-artefact induced by incandescent needles. (Reproduced with permission by Bonamonte et al. [62])

5.3 Dermatitis Artefacta with Patch Test Artefacts

In addition to the above two classical types of occupational dermatitis artefacta, provoked on healthy skin or damaged skin, there is another aspect to the problem.

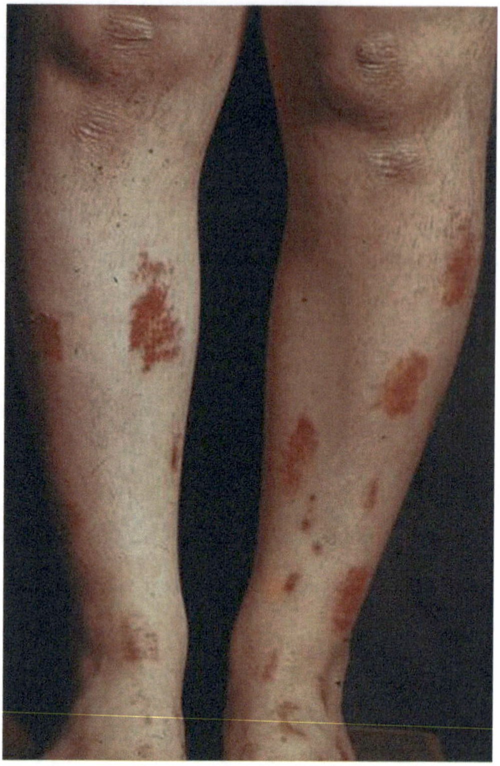

Fig. 5.17 Floor layer (stigmata on the knees) with self-inflicted lesions by metal object. (Reproduced with permission by Bonamonte et al. [62])

This consists of attempts to produce positive results to skin tests which would otherwise give negative results.

As these methods of diagnostic investigation have grown more common, simulators' attention has shifted from the clinical disease picture towards the results of such tests, knowing that recognition of this condition as a professional complaint largely depends on the latter.

The phenomenon had already been reported in 1962 by Meneghini and Rantuccio in two of eight cases of occupational dermatitis artefacta [65] and has since been observed by ourselves [56, 63, 66] (Fig. 5.28). Meigel and Koops reported a case in which the patient attempted to simulate a positive patch test reaction to neomycin by scratching the site [67]. Lyell mentions the case of a patient who was able to produce a chemical burn by applying a caustic liquid on one of her patch test sites [68]. Three cases of dermatitis artefacta with manipulation of patch tests are described by Maurice and Coll. [69]: the subjects were intelligent, single females who produced chemically severe patch tests reactions but denied self-induction.

Clearly, in suspicious cases, the patch tests must be applied without allowing the patient to identify the site of the individual substances and the results must be interpreted with caution. In most such cases, the self-induced reactions are clearly

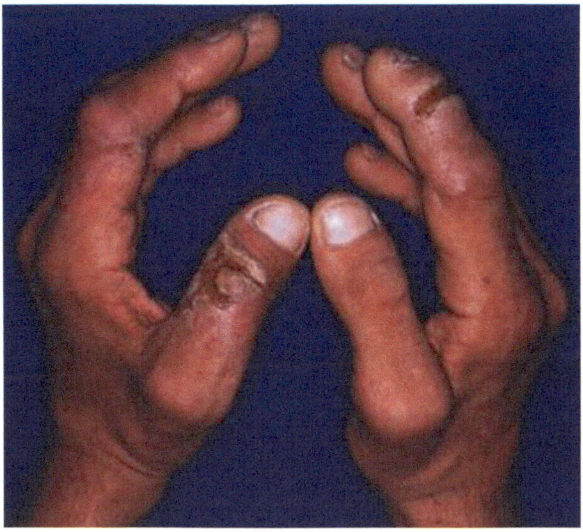

Fig. 5.18 Linear ulcerative lesions self-induced by metal object. (Reproduced with permission by Bonamonte et al. [10])

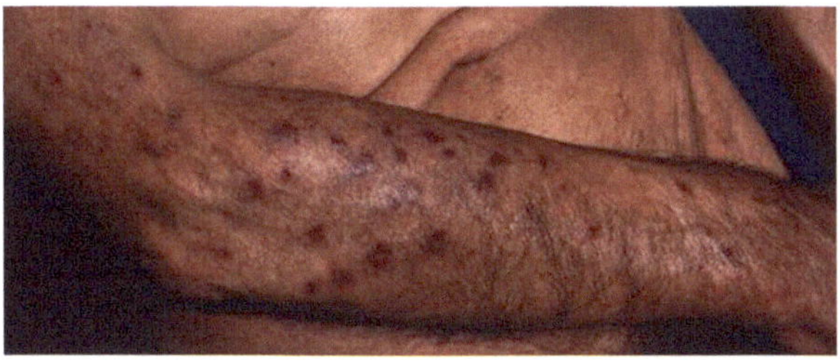

Fig. 5.19 Self-induced lesions by lighted cigarette. (Reproduced with permission by Bonamonte et al. [62])

irritant in nature, but the ingenuity of these patients can be such that even a genuine allergic reaction might be mimicked [69].

5.4 Witchcraft Syndrome

Dermatitis artefacta can even be voluntarily provoked on the skin of unaware subjects by proxy [70, 71]. Various clients of a hairdresser developed urticarial lesions after having been served by the hairdresser's daughter. To revenge herself on her father, she had applied benzyl-ether of nicotinic acid on the clients' skin, inducing local hyperaemia, with some oedema, after about 10 min. The absorption of this

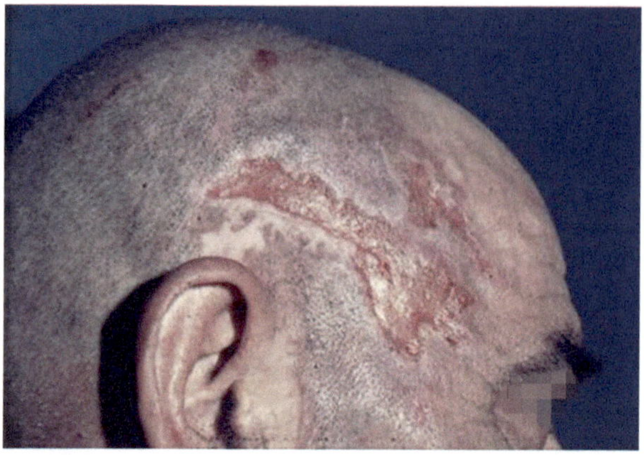

Fig. 5.20 Ulcerative self-induced lesions by chromic mixture. (Reproduced with permission by Bonamonte et al. [62])

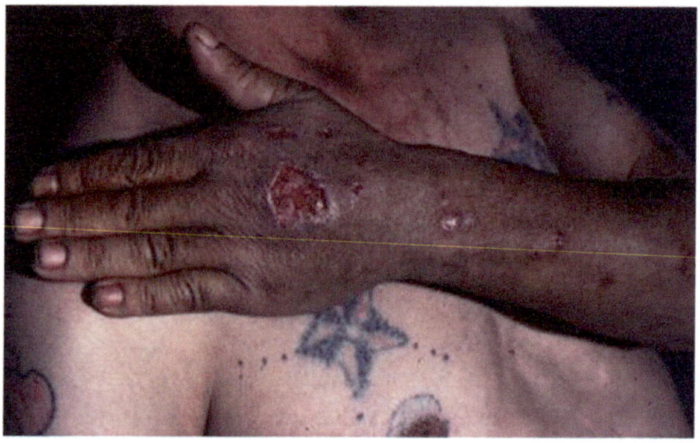

Fig. 5.21 Ulcerative dermatitis artefacta induced by chromic mixture. (Reproduced with permission by Bonamonte et al. [62])

substance on the palms of the hands is very low and so the simulator found it easy to apply it to the customer's skin without harming herself [70].

A 28-year-old man presented a history of several episodes of blisters and intense redness over the cheeks and external ears, associated with a burning sensation. The episodes had a sudden onset and were always associated with a drinking spree the previous night. The peculiar history and the morphology of the lesions, that escaped any classic diagnosis classification, gave rise to the suspicion of simulation. After much persuasion and an assurance of secrecy, the wife of the patient admitted that her husband was an alcoholic and was neglecting his family. When her efforts to prevent his drinking failed, she poured acid, that she used for domestic cleaning, on his cheeks, hoping that the sequelae would frighten him off drinking. The psychiatric evaluation revealed that the patient was an alcoholic with a cyclothymic

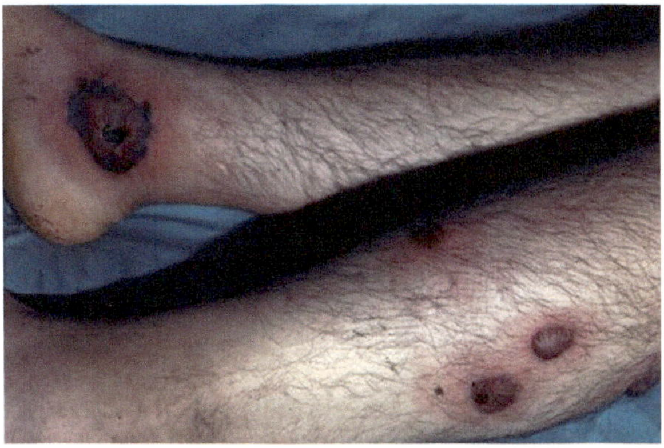

Fig. 5.22 Dermatitis artefacta induced by chromic mixture. (Reproduced with permission by Bonamonte et al. [62])

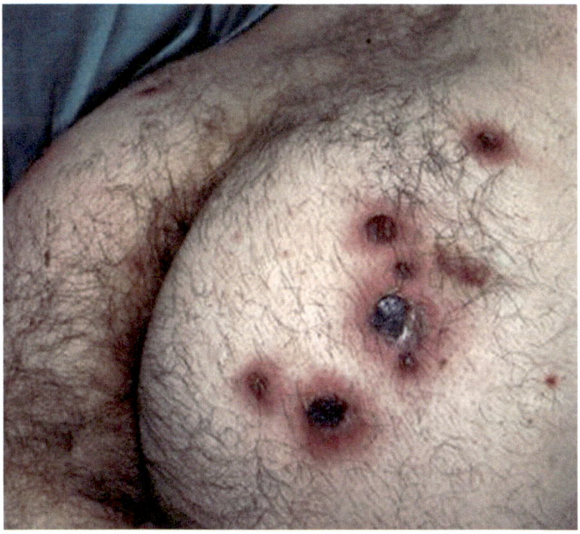

Fig. 5.23 The same patient as in Fig. 5.21. (Reproduced with permission by Bonamonte et al. [62])

personality, whereas his wife showed major depressive symptoms and had a histrionic personality [71].

Both of the above described cases can be considered as forms of dermatitis artefacta imposed on another person, caused by intentional "psychological" malingering without any venal incentive.

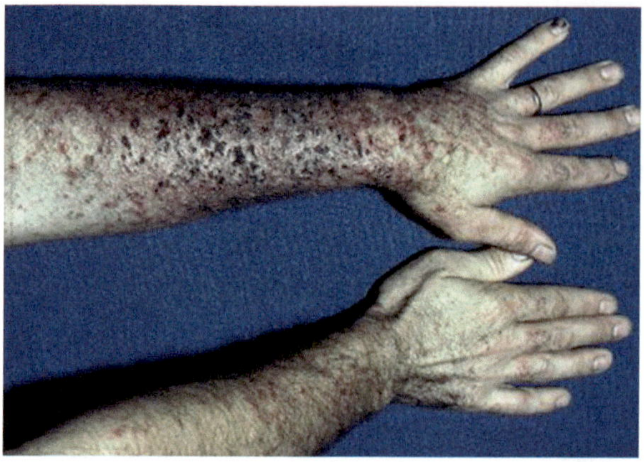

Fig. 5.24 Self-artefact induced by incandescent metal object on pre-existing spontaneous contact dermatitis. (Reproduced with permission by Bonamonte et al. [62])

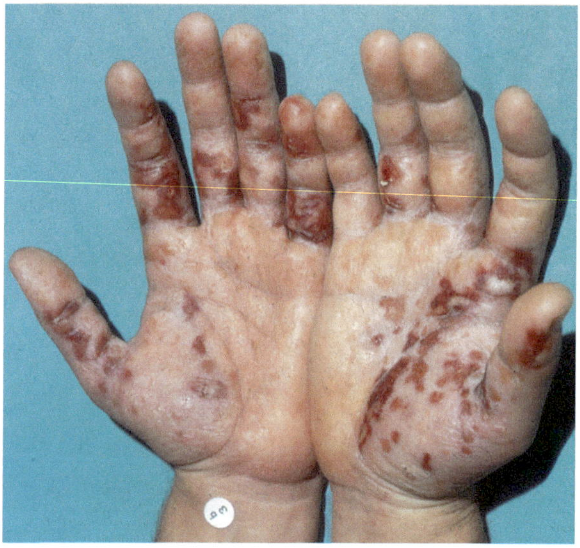

Fig. 5.25 Dermatitis artefacta induced by chromic mixture. (Reproduced with permission by Bonamonte et al. [62])

5.5 Secrétan Syndrome

Secrétan syndrome is characterized by a hard and sometimes cyanotic oedema (Charcot's "edema bleu") on the back of one or both hands and forearms. The affliction can be induced by applying a haemostatic ligature or tight bandaging around the forearms.

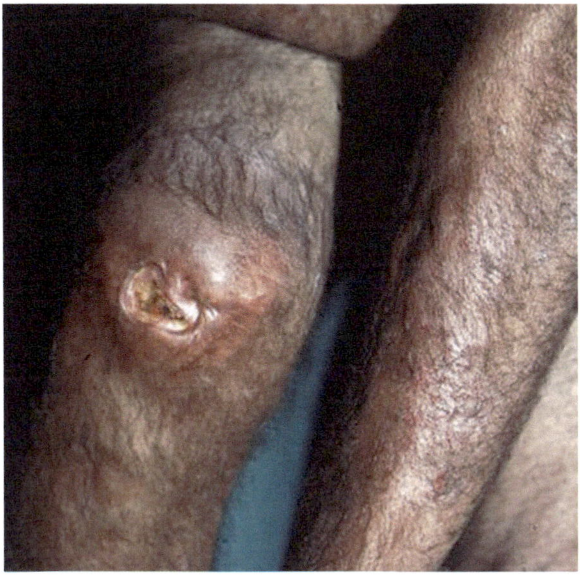

Fig. 5.26 Woody and ulcerative plaque on the right rotular region after 20 years by the subcutaneous injection of liquid paraffin as attempt to obtain a disability pension. (Reproduced with permission by Bonamonte et al. [10])

This picture, first described in 1901 by Henry Secrétan, a Swiss doctor [72], and experimentally reproduced in monkeys by means of repeated injuries [73], has been observed in professional environments in simulators aiming to gain an occupational disease pension. The oedema is likely to be of a lymphatic nature and may be associated with pain and limited flexion of the metacarpal-phalangeal joints. Oedema from a haemostatic ligature can sometimes present, with clear-cut margins and a fairly regular, horizontal, erythematous ring.

The diagnosis of self-inflicted injury was not suggested by Secrétan in his original work, but by authors who reported subsequent, similar cases [74–76]. In all cases the patients were workers who had sustained minor injuries at work and hence were expecting compensation. In all cases, the syndrome was apparently induced either by application of a tourniquet or by repeated self-inflicted contusion of the dorsum of the hand.

Angelini and Coll. observed a case of Secrétan syndrome unrelated to external incentives in a girl aged 16. She had presented six episodes of hard oedema on the dorsum of the left hand that had lasted 10–20 days [77] (Fig. 5.29). The complaint consisted of indurated oedema of the back of the hand, associated with cyanosis, tenderness and limited flexion of the metacarpal-phalangeal joint. A large number of clinical and laboratory investigations were carried out. Examinations by the orthopaedic surgeon and a vascular surgeon proved unhelpful. Repeated X-rays of the left hand and wrist showed no abnormality. Morpho-oscillographic examination of the forearm demonstrated a slowed venous return, an altered vasomotor tone and

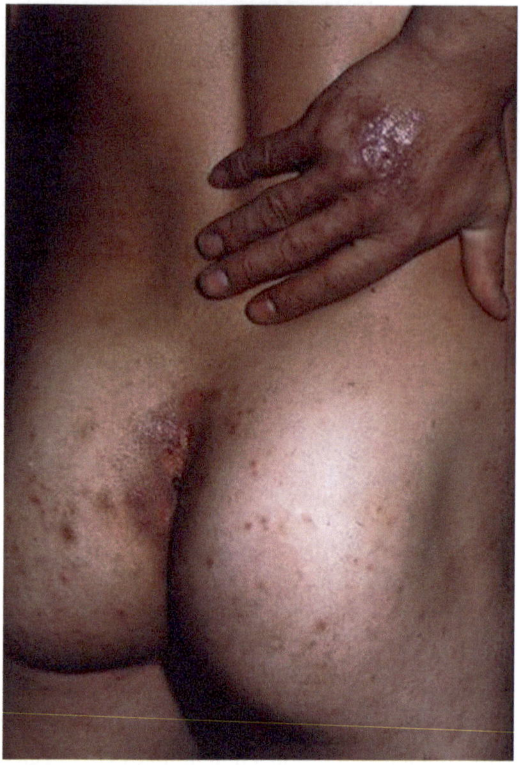

Fig. 5.27 Self-induced ulcerative lesions on dorsal right hand and coccyx. (Reproduced from Meneghini and Angelini [53]. All rights reserved)

Table 5.2 Clinical differential diagnosis between occupational dermatitis artefacta (ODA) and dermatitis artefacta (DA)

Criteria	ODA	DA
Gender	Generally male	Generally female
Age	Young and adult	Young and adult
History	Episodic affliction with acute onset	Chronic history of complaint
Cutaneous sites	Hands, arms, and unusual sites	Generally face and arms
Morphology	More bizarre lesions	Less bizarre lesions
Causal agents	Highly varied, strange and unthinkable	Common mechanical objects or chemical agents

a relative hyposphygmia on the left side. This latter parameter returned to normal after resolution of the oedema. Arteriography and lymphography of the left upper limb showed no abnormality. On the occasion of her last admission to the clinic, the patient presented with atrophic scars on the dorsum of the left hand and excoriated acne on the cheeks (Fig. 5.30). The psychiatric assessment produced evidence of a marked hysterical personality with a "belle indifference" to the primary disease. This led to the suspicion of a self-inflicted aetiology. The patient was enlightened as

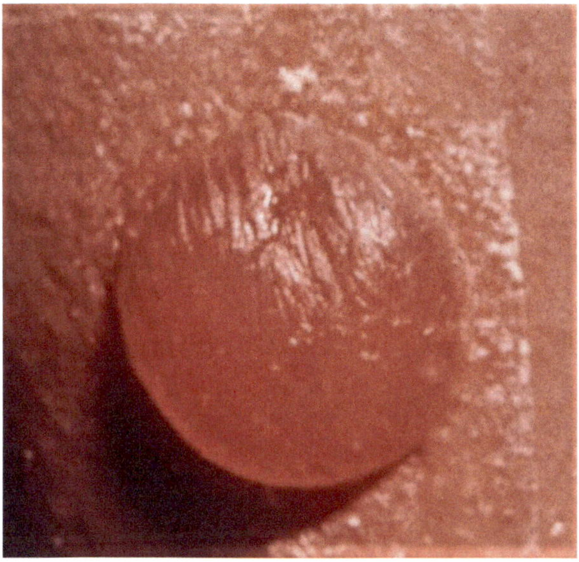

Fig. 5.28 Self-induced irritant bullous patch test. (Reproduced with permission by Foti et al. [66])

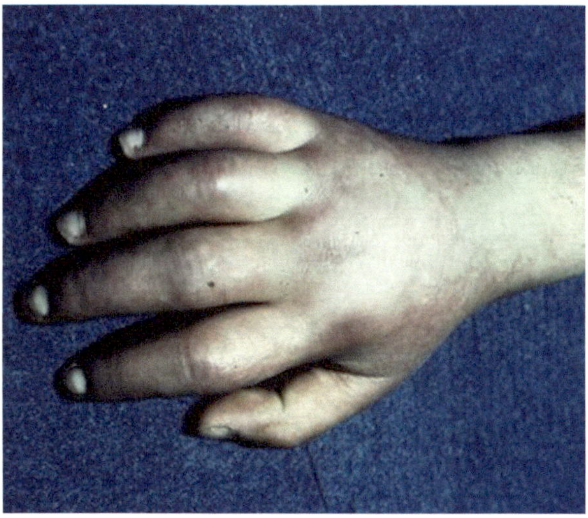

Fig. 5.29 A 16-year-old girl with oedema of the dorsum of the left hand. (Reproduced with permission by Angelini et al. [77])

to the significance of the diagnosis of oedema artefacta and no further lesions were recorded at follow-up examinations. The self-inflicted injury had been induced by repeated contusion of the area using various different hard objects.

Secrétan syndrome must be differentiated from the spontaneous chronic "occupational traumatic lymphoedema of the hands and forearms" described by members

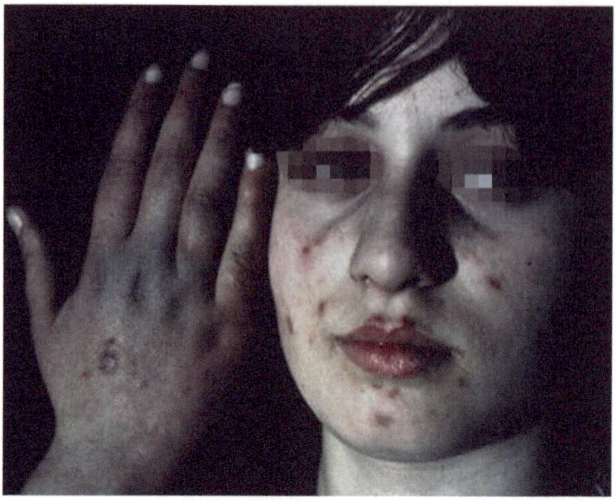

Fig. 5.30 The same patient as in Fig. 5.29. Atrophic scars on the dorsum of the left hand and excoriated acne. (Reproduced with permission by Angelini et al. [77])

of our team in fishermen [78, 79]. This complaint is due to various causes and particularly to repeated trauma from sea urchin spines and the tight cuffs of the wetsuit. In spontaneous, chronic professional cases, lymphography may show alterations of the lymph vessels [79].

Secrétan syndrome must also be differentiated from other types of acute or chronic oedema, such as lymphatic aplasia, recurrent erysipelas, deep thrombophlebitis, angioedema, filariasis, venous obstruction post-surgical disturbances, and carcinoma or other tumours of the breast.

5.6 Religious Stigmata

5.6.1 General Remarks

"Stigma" (the Greek term was originally referred to a wound or sign inflicted on a slave) refers to the reproduction of wounds like those inflicted on Christ during the crucifixion, on the palms of the hands, soles of the feet and head (in lieu of the Crown of Thorns), as well as the chest, the lips (in contact with a vinegar-soaked sponge), and the back (marks of lashing) [80–88]. Over the centuries, stigmata have appeared in saints, priests, nuns, and fraudsters, as well as in subjects suffering from dermatological diseases, such as haematidrosis, and psychiatric disorders [89, 90]. Besides the visible ones, invisible stigmata, such as intense pain affecting the above-mentioned sites, should be considered. The latter could precede the outcome of visible stigmata or be a result of them, but may also be isolated, without any means to ascertain their presence [91, 92]. Whether they are genuine or artefacts, stigmata are still considered a medical enigma; they represent a complex model of interaction between the skin and the psyche.

The wounds can bleed permanently or only just on Fridays or near special Catholic holidays, such as Easter Sunday [85]. They differ in number (from 1 to 10), size and body part affected. Usually, the stigmata are observed on the palms; however, after Barbet reported that contrary to popular belief, nails would have been implanted at the level of the wrists in order to hold the weight of the body on the cross, lesions started also to appear on the wrists [88, 93, 94].

Crucifixion was practised in ancient Rome until the fourth century A.D. as a punishment of criminals. A passage in the Bible (Galatians 6:17) suggests that Saint Paul might have been the first to receive stigmata, since he writes "I bear the marks of the Lord Jesus in my body" [95]. Stigmatization was not then mentioned in the west or east until the beginning of the thirteenth century.

Saint Francis of Assisi (1182–1226) was the first person to receive stigmata during an ecstatic vision in September 1224; these were described 2 years later in his first biography [85, 86, 96]. Saint Francis' stigmata were immediately acknowledged by the papacy, despite minor opposition among the clergy, which accused the Saint of heresy [88, 97].

Kluger and Cribier reported three other cases of self-inflicted stigmata dating back to the thirteenth century [88]. During the following centuries, more than 300 cases of stigmatization were described, most of them in fervent Roman Catholics [88]. In 1908, Imbert-Gourbeyre found that 321 people with stigmata had been described after Saint Francis, 41 were men and 280 were women during their reproductive years [98]. They were mostly from Italy (229 cases) and then France, Spain, Germany, Belgium, Portugal, Switzerland, Holland, Hungary, and Peru.

Among the most famous stigmatized subjects in the nineteenth century, Louise Lateam (1850–1883) stands out, a Belgian girl who bled every Friday from 1868 to 1883, except for two; she was visited by various eminent Belgian doctors [99]. Therese Neumann (1898–1962), a German peasant girl, also developed stigmata in 1926 during an ecstatic vision; her hands and feet bled regularly on Fridays until her death [100]. Finally, in Saint Pius of Petralcina (1887–1968; Apulia, Italy), his hands bled continually from 1918 onwards; however, the lesions faded at the time of his death [85].

As shown by the above-mentioned data, stigmata have been manifesting for centuries in the context of Catholic Europe. In the United States, similar episodes were unheard of until the spread of Catholicism [84]. In the twentieth century, stigmata were reported in other religious contexts (e.g. Muslim ascetics developed lesions in the same sites of injuries suffered by the Prophet in his battles) [84, 101]. Cases in America and Australia were also reported [88].

In 2013, Kluger and Criber compiled a list of the most highly praised stigmatized people [88]. However, few people with stigmata have been beatified or canonized, and the Catholic Church does not allow a mandatory association between stigmata and sanctity, denying the conventional belief that stigmata represent a supernatural event, and are granted by God as a sign of piety. A proclamation by Pope Urban VIII instructs Catholic writers to attribute a purely human nature to this phenomenon [102].

The issue concerning religious stigmata has always been of particular interest, given the complexity of any interpretation and discussion. The question of the etiological interpretation of stigmata remains controversial; indeed, there is no reason to presume that all stigmata should have the same aetiology. Excluding ascertained cases of voluntary self-harm due to malingering, stigmatization is generally referred to as unconscious self-harm during periods of hysteria, autosuggestion, and hypnotism; these are all characteristic factors that can be associated with "mystical delirium" [85, 88, 103].

According to various authors, however, cases of "inexplicable" stigmata with a spontaneous onset and no external triggering factors have been described [85, 88]. Discrete exceptional clinical entities, whose pathogenesis is not fully understood, could possibly constitute the condition underlying some of these cases: for example, autoerythrocyte sensitization syndrome (Gardner-Diamond syndrome or psychogenic purpura), vicarious menstruation (various organs possibly affected), haematidrosis (blood cells in sweat), bloody otorrhea and hemolacria (secondary to ophthalmic conditions) [89, 104–119]. Such conditions usually affect young women; although they often present variable features of a psychosomatic personality, they are considered "natural".

Owing to all the relative debate, the view of religious stigmata is progressively shifting from medieval mysteries to distinct psychiatric and psychosomatic disorders. In studying stigmata, however, we should always consider the possibility that they could be self-inflicted for illegal and/or profit purposes.

5.6.2 Religious Stigmata as Malingering Artefacts

The topic of malingering in the form of religious stigmatization has rarely been treated in the medical literature. Kluger and Cribier treated the subject thoroughly in the light of modern medicine [88].

A case of a 42-year-old Brazilian man with a 5-month history of irregular, nonpainful palmar ulcers at different healing stages has been described [120]. During consultation, the patient theatrically explained how he had been blessed by God with Christ's stigmata. However, the patient's partner revealed that such lesions were self-inflicted using a pocketknife.

The case of a 23-year-old man with stigmata of the hands was reported in a small town in Sicily. He showed some erosions on the dorsal surface of the hands, and small bullous lesions arranged to create the word "pax" on the left palm. Previously, other odd events, promoted as divine, had occurred in the house of the young man (weeping over an effigy depicting the Madonna, weeping and bleeding over a picture of Jesus Christ, lugubrious sounds at night). Accordingly, a prayer hall in the garage of the house had been set up, complete with an altar and iconography of the Stations of the Cross. A flock of people brought gifts and pledges. The patient later turned out to be hysterical, with an easily swayed personality, and easily manipulated by relatives and acquaintances with the aim of making a profit. Intervention by legal authorities stopped the lucrative affair [121]. This case could be considered as a case of malingering stigmatization by proxy.

Fisher and Kollar reported the case of a 23-year-old Mexican-American woman who presented with bleeding on her palms, feet, sides, and head, as well as the oozing of oil from her body. Aside from one video recording, no bloody or oily discharge was directly observed; furthermore, a vial of the said oil, that had a slightly sweet odour, was found. Meanwhile, at the time of the study, the woman's 2-week-old daughter also presented with stigmata [122]. Here, too, the suspicion of a malingering disorder and malingering disorder by proxy is high.

A doubtful case of religious stigmata was reported by Early and Lifschutz [123]. A 10-year-old black Baptist girl experienced religious stigmata periodically over a 3-week period immediately preceding Easter Sunday, 1972. The child, who was intensely religious, came from a large, lower-middle class family in a large city. Her physical examination results were normal. The authors were unable to detect any psychopathology, except within the range of her religious experience, and she showed indifference towards the bleeding and auditory hallucinations of a religious nature.

We observed a case of religious stigmata in a 42-year-old woman, originally from a small town of Calabria (South of Italy) [124]. The patient showed, for the third consecutive year, cutaneous lesions during Easter holidays. Such lesions appeared every year on her forehead and the dorsal surface of hands and feet. The lesions would suddenly manifest on Easter Monday and healed spontaneously within a few weeks. These alleged stigmata were made public, causing a steady flow of devotees and curious onlookers to the patient's house, offering gifts of various kinds. The year before, the local ecclesiastic and police authorities had become interested in the singular event, but legal or religious actions were not undertaken as the stigmata rapidly disappeared some days after Easter. The patient came to our attention on the third day of the clinical manifestation in the third year, accompanied by her general practitioner. At physical examination, a dozen mildly exudative erosions were present on the forehead, along the hairline, measuring 0.5 cm in diameter, regularly spaced at 1 cm from each other (Fig. 5.31). On the dorsal surface of the hands, halfway between the carpus and metacarpus, an irregular, round erythematous-ulcerated lesion, swollen and moderately bleeding, was evident. The left-hand lesion was larger and more infiltrated. Similar erythematous-ulcerated elements (measuring 1.5 × 1 cm) symmetrically involved the central dorsum of the feet (Figs. 5.32 and 5.33). No lesions were present on her wrists, palms, soles, or elsewhere. During consultation, the patient was silent; she gave no specifics about the time and mode of onset of the lesions, and she did not complain of any subjective symptoms. She also showed a wary and absent attitude, occasionally speaking in a detached manner about her religious faith. Psychiatric consultation, which had been refused at the time of the previous episodes, described a hysterical personality with attention-seeking behaviour and an excessive need of approval by her family. Moreover, her general practitioner reported that intervention by the police, the day

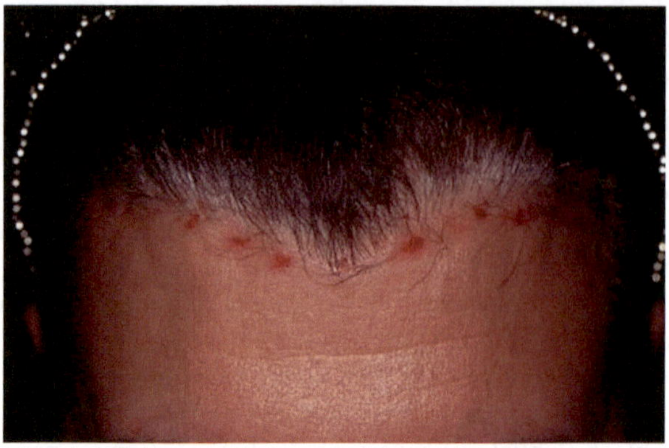

Fig. 5.31 Religious stigmata: multiple erosions following hairline. Notice the consistent diameter and spacing. (Reproduced with permission by Bonamonte et al. [124])

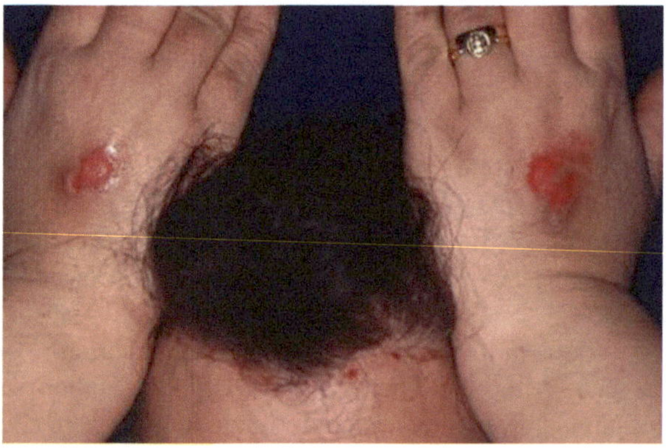

Fig. 5.32 The same patient as in Fig. 5.31. Irregular rounded ulcerative lesions on back of hands. (Reproduced with permission by Bonamonte et al. [10])

before, had stopped people making pilgrimages to the house and had changed the attitude of the patient and her relatives. They showed fear and discretion, diminished the importance of the episode, and argued that most likely it would not occur again. The patient refused hospitalization but promised she would return for follow-up although she never actually showed up. Her general practitioner later reported to us that the lesions were already healing 3 days after our consultation, and there had been complete healing after 3 weeks. Stigmata no longer recurred during the Easter holidays in the following 2 years [124].

This case, because of the affected sites, morphology, acute onset, and duration of the lesions, easily led to the suspicion of an artificially induced disease. As a matter of fact, in this case only the dorsum of the hands and feet were affected, without involvement of the palms and soles. Moreover, in religious texts, the originally described sites of upper limb involvement are the wrists and not the hands. In this

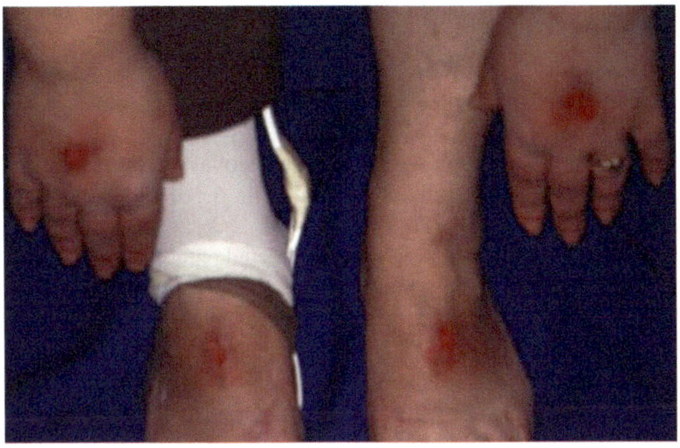

Fig. 5.33 The same patient as in Fig. 5.31. Ulcerative lesions on the back of hands and feet. (Reproduced with permission by Bonamonte et al. [10])

case, moreover, the stigmata had immediately been made public by the patient and her family. Our hypothesis of malingering was indirectly confirmed by the rapid resolution of the lesions and lack of recurrence during the following 2 years. Moreover, the patient's absent attitude, as though she was living inside an inner world, could also underlie a hysterical personality that could be easily exploited by her relatives. This was confirmed by the psychiatric consultation. The skin lesions were probably caused by metal objects, by a mechanism of scraping (on the forehead), or overheating (most likely on the dorsal surface of the hands and feet), although the use of caustic chemicals cannot be excluded [124].

In conclusion, regardless of personal beliefs, the possibility must always be considered that stigmata, as an example of the intricate relationships among medicine, psychology, psychiatry, and spirituality, could be self-inflicted for illegal and/or profit purposes.

References

1. Asher R. Malingering. Talking sense. Bath: Pitman Press; 1973. p. 145–7.
2. Sahoo S, Kumar R, Oomer F. Concepts and controversies of malingering: a re-look. Asian J Psychiatry. 2020;50:101952.
3. Nicholson K, Martelli M. Malingering: overview and basic concepts. In: Young G, Kane A, Nicholson K, editors. Causality of psychological injury: presenting evidence in court. New York: Springer; 2007. p. 375–409.
4. American Psychiatric Association (APA). Diagnostic and statistical manual of mental disorders (DSM-5). 5th ed. Washington, DC: APA; 2013.
5. Udoetuk S, Dongarwar D, Salihu HM. Racial and gender disparities in diagnosis of malingering in clinical settings. J Racial Ethn Health Disparities. 2020;7:1117–23.
6. Park L, Costello S, Li J, et al. Race, health, and socioeconomic disparities associated with malingering in psychiatric patients at an urban emergency department. Gen Hosp Psychiatry. 2021;71:121–7.

7. Zwick T, Sharp C, Severn D, et al. Malingering in the emergency setting. Cureus. 2021;13:e15670–6.
8. Dell NA, Carbone JT, Holzer KJ, et al. Malingering and comorbid psychopathology: evidence from the 2016–2017 nationwide emergency department sample. Gen Hosp Psychiatry. 2021;73:121–2.
9. Sherman EMS, Slick DJ, Iverson GL. Multidimensional malingering criteria for neuropsychological assessment: a 20-year update of the malingered neuropsychological dysfunction criteria. Arch Clin Neuropsychol. 2020;35:735–64.
10. Bonamonte D, Foti C, De Marco A, et al. Self-inflicted pathological cutaneous disorders. Part II. Ital J Dermatol Venereol. 2022;157:480–8.
11. Bonamonte D, Foti C, De Marco A, et al. Self-inflicted pathological cutaneous disorders. Part I. Ital J Dermatol Venereol. 2022;157:389–401.
12. Millard LG, Millard J. Psychocutaneous disorders. In: Burns T, Brethnach S, Cox N, et al. editors. Rook's text book of dermatology. 8th ed. Oxford: Wiley-Blackwell; 2010: chap.64. pp. 1–55.
13. Gieler U, Consoli SG, Tomás-Aragones L, et al. Self-inflicted lesions in dermatology: terminology and classification--a position paper from the European Society for Dermatology and Psychiatry (ESDaP). Acta Derm Venereol. 2013;93:4–12.
14. Mittenberg W, Patton C, Canyock EM, et al. Base rates of malingering and symptom exaggeration. J Clin Exp Neuropsychol. 2002;24:1094–102.
15. Mason AM, Cardell R, Armstrong M. Malingering psychosis: guidelines for assessment and management. Perspect Psychiatry Care. 2014;50:51–7.
16. Chafetz M, Underhill J. Estimated costs of malingered disability. Arch Clin Neuropsychol. 2013;28:633–9.
17. Weiss KJ, Van Dell L. Liability for diagnosing malingering. J Am Acad Psychiatry Law. 2017;45:339–47.
18. Zubera A, Raza M, Holaday E, et al. Screening for malingering in the emergency department. Acad Psychiatry. 2015;39:233–4.
19. Reddy K, Lowenstein EJ. Forensics in dermatology: part I. J Am Acad Dermatol. 2011;64:801–8.
20. Reddy K, Lowenstein EJ. Forensics in dermatology: part II. J Am Acad Dermatol. 2011;64:811–24.
21. Green D, Rosenfeld B. Evaluating the gold standard: a review and meta-analysis of the structured interview of reported symptoms. Psychol Assess. 2011;23:95–107.
22. McCullumsmith CB, Ford CV. Simulated illness: the factitious disorders and malingering. Psychiatr Clin North Am. 2011;34:621–41.
23. Resnick PJ. My favorite tips for detecting malingering and violence risk. Psychiatry Clin North Am. 2007;30:227–32.
24. Lebourgeois HW. Malingering key point in assessment. Psychiatr Times. 2007;24:21.
25. Velsor S, Rogers R. Differentiating factitious psychological presentations from malingering: implications for forensic practice. Behav Sci Law. 2019;37:1–15.
26. Rogers R. Clinical assessment of malingering and deception. New York: Guilford Press; 2008.
27. Overholser JC. Differential diagnosis of malingering and factitious disorder with physical symptoms. Behav Sci Law. 1990;8:55–65.
28. Rogers R, Bender SD. Evaluation of malingering and related response styles. In: Otto RK, editor. Comprehensive handbook of psychology: forensic psychology, vol. 11. 2nd ed. New York: Wiley; 2013. p. 517–9.
29. Rogers R, Sewell KW, Goldstein AM. Explanatory models of malingering: a prototypical analysis. Law Hum Behav. 1994;18:543–52.
30. Vitacco MJ. Syndromes associated with deception. In: Rogers R, Bender SD, editors. Clinical assessment of malingering and deception. 4th ed. New York: Guilford; 2018. p. 83–97.

31. Cumien AJ. Psychiatric and medical syndromes associated with deception. In: Rogers R, editor. Clinical assessment of malingering and deception. 2nd ed. New York: Guilford; 1977. p. 23–46.
32. Deps PD, Aborghetti HP, Zambon TL, et al. Assessing signs of torture: a review of clinical forensic dermatology. J Am Acad Dermatol. 2022;87:375–80.
33. Deps P, Collin SM, Aborghetti HP, et al. Clinical forensic dermatology in cases of torture. Br J Dermatol. 2020;183:773–4.
34. Gargiulo A, Tessitore F, Le Grottaglie F, et al. Self-harming behaviours of asylum seekers and refugees in Europe: a systematic review. Int J Psychol. 2021;56:189–98.
35. Viero A, Amadasi A, Blandino A, et al. Skin lesions and traditional folk practices: a medico-legal perspective. Forensic Sci Med Pathol. 2019;15:580–90.
36. Ravanfar P, Dinulos JG. Cultural practices affecting the skin of children. Curr Opin Pediatr. 2010;22:423–31.
37. Libow JA. Child and adolescent illness falsification. Pediatrics. 2000;105:336–42.
38. Lyell A. Cutaneous artefactual diseases. J Am Acad Dermatol. 1979;1:391–407.
39. Reich P, Gottfried LA. Factitious disorders in a teaching hospital. Ann Intern Med. 1983;99:240–7.
40. Condé-Salazar L, Gomez J, Meza B, et al. Artefactual irritant contact dermatitis. Contact Derm. 1993;28:246–7.
41. Hutchinson GL. Disorders of simulation. Madison: Psychosocial Press; 2001. p. 195–221.
42. Gelmetti G, Bonifazi E. Le patomimie cutanee nel bambino. Pediatric Dermatol News. 1985;4:146–69.
43. Harris MD, Michael R. The malingering of psychotic disorders. Jefferson J Psychiatry. 2000;15:12–24.
44. Fry S. Troy. Salani Editore, s.u.r.l.; 2022. p.139–40.
45. Palmer J. Malingering, shirking, and self-inflicted injuries in the military. In: Halligan PW, Bass C, Oakley DA, editors. Malingering and illness deception. Oxford University Press; 2003. p. 42–53.
46. Palmer J. War based hysteria: the military perspective. In: Halligan PW, Bass C, editors. Contemporary approach to hysteria. New York: Oxford University Press; 2001. p. 12–35.
47. Cohen AD, Vardy DA. Dermatitis artefacta in soldiers. Mil Med. 2006;171:497–9.
48. Petruzzellis V, Angelini G, Vena GA. La dermatite artefatta. Dermatol Allergol Profes. 1988;3:23–40.
49. Bonamonte D, Foti C, Gullo G, et al. Plant contact dermatitis. In: Angelini G, Bonamonte D, Foti C, editors. Clinical contact dermatitis. A practical approach. Berlin: Springer Nature Switzerland AG; 2021. p. 319–52.
50. Crocq MA, Crocq L. From shell shock and war neurosis to posttraumatic stress disorder: a history of psychotraumatology. Dialogues Clin Neurosci. 2000;2:47–55.
51. Mendelson G, Mendelson D. Legal and psychiatric aspect of malingering. J Law Med. 2014;1:28–34.
52. Wessely S. Malingering: historical perspectives. In: Halligan PW, Bass C, Oakley DA, editors. Malingering and illness deception. New York: Oxford University Press; 2003. p. 54–60.
53. Meneghini CL, Angelini G. Occupational dermatitis artefacta. Derm Beruf Umwelt. 1979;27:163–5.
54. Lachapelle JM, Frimat P, Temstealt D, et al. Dermatoses simulées en medicine du travail. In: Dermatologie professionnelle et de l'environnement. Paris: Masson; 1992. p. 263–71.
55. Angelini G. Occupational dermatitis artefacta. In: Kanerva L, Elsner P, Wahlberg JE, et al., editors. Handbook of occupational dermatology. Berlin: Springer; 2000. p. 141–7.
56. Angelini G, Bonamonte D. Occupational dermatitis artefacta. In: Syall-Smith D, Marks R, editors. Dermatology at the millennium. The proceedings of the 19th World Congress of Dermatology. Sidney, 15–20 June, 1998. New York: The Parthenon Publishing Group Inc.; 1999. p. 508–13.

57. Combes FC. Dermatology problems in establishment of workmen's compensation claims. Community Med. 1952;1:5–10.
58. Adams MR. Diagnosis and differential diagnosis. In: Adams MR, editor. Occupational skin diseases. New York/London: Grune and Stratton, Inc.; 1983. p. 110–35.
59. Schwartz L, Tulipan L, Peck SM. Problem or borderline cases: malingering. In: Occupational disease of the skin. London: Henry Kimpton; 1947. p. 87–90.
60. Rietschel RL, Fowler JF. Occupational dermatitis. In: Fisher's contact dermatitis. 5th ed. Philadelphia: Lippincolt Williams and Wilkins; 2001. p. 419–49.
61. Angelini G, Bonamonte D. La dermatite artefatta. G Ital Dermatol Venereol. 1999;134:99–113.
62. Bonamonte D, Foti C, Verni P, et al. Occupational dermatitis artefacta. In: Angelini G, Bonamonte D, Foti C, editors. Clinical contact dermatitis. A practical approach. Berlin: Springer Nature Switzerland AG; 2021. p. 583–95.
63. Angelini G, Vena GA. Dermatosi artefatte. In: Angelini G, Vena GA, editors. Dermatologia professionale e ambientale, vol. 1. Brescia: ISED; 1997. p. 257–68.
64. Millard LG. Dermatological pathomimicry: a form of patient maladjustment. Lancet. 1984;2:969–71.
65. Meneghini CL, Rantuccio F. Patomimia cutanea professionale. G Ital Dermatol. 1962;103:143–55.
66. Foti C, Bonamonte D, Filoni A, et al. Patch testing. In: Angelini G, Bonamonte D, Foti C, editors. Clinical contact dermatitis. A practical approach. Berlin: Springer Nature Switzerland AG; 2021. p. 499–527.
67. Meigel WN, Koops DH. Skarifikationsartefakte der Testreaktion bei einer berufsdermatologischen Begutachtung. Hautarzt. 1976;27:349–51.
68. Lyell A. Dermatitis artefacta in relation to the syndrome of contrived disease. Clin Exp Dermatol. 1976;1:109–26.
69. Maurice PD, Rivers JK, Jones C, et al. Dermatitis artefacta with artefact of patch tests. Clin Exp Dermatol. 1987;12:204–6.
70. Bandmann HJ, Wahl B. Contact urticaria artefacta (witchcraft-syndrome). Contact Derm. 1982;8:145–6.
71. Somani VK. Witchcraft's syndrome: Münchausen's syndrome by proxy. Int J Dermatol. 1998;37:229–30.
72. Secrétan H. Oedema dur et hyperplasie traumatique du metacarpe dorsal. Rev Med Swiss Romande. 1901;21:409–15.
73. Omer GE Jr, Riordan DC, Conran PB, et al. Peritendinous fibrosis of the dorsum of the hand in monkeys. An experimental approach. Clin Orthop Relat Res. 1969;62:251–9.
74. Reading G. Secrétan's syndrome: hard edema of the dorsum of the hand. Plast Reconstr Surg. 1980;65:182–7.
75. Smith RJ. Factitious lymphedema of the hand. J Bone Joint Surg Am. 1975;57:89–94.
76. Saferin EH, Posch JL. Secrétan's disease: post-traumatic hard edema of the dorsum of the hand. Plast Reconstr Surg. 1976;58:703–7.
77. Angelini G, Meneghini CL, Vena GA. Secrétan's syndrome: an artefact oedema of the hand. Contact Derm. 1982;8:345–6.
78. Angelini G, Vena GA, Meneghini CL. Occupational traumatic lymphedema of the hands. Dermatol Clin. 1990;8:205–8.
79. Bonamonte D, Angelini G, editors. Aquatic dermatology. Biotic, chemical and physical agents. Berlin: Springer; 2016. p. 240–4.
80. Goffman E. Stigma notes on the management of spoiled identity. Englewood Cliffs: Prentice Hall; 1963.
81. Kent G. Stigmatization and skin conditions. In: Walker C, Papadopoulos L, editors. Psychodermatology. Cambridge: Cambridge University Press; 2005. p. 44–52.
82. Klauder J. Stigmatization. Arch Derm Syphilol. 1938;37:650–9.
83. Whitlock FA, Hynes JV. Religious stigmatization: an historical and psychophysiological enquiry. Psychol Med. 1978;8:185–202.

84. Harrison T. Stigmata: a medical mystery in the modern age. New York: Penguin Books; 1994.
85. Simpson CJ. The stigmata: pathology or miracle? Br Med J. 1984;289:1746–8.
86. Kechichian E, Khoury E, Richa S, et al. Religious stigmata: a dermato-psychiatric approach and differential diagnosis. Int J Dermatol. 2018;57:885–93.
87. Kluger N. Devotional dermatoses. Ann Dermatol Venereol. 2012;139:309–20.
88. Kluger N, Cribier B. Les stigmates: de Saint-François d'Assise à l'hématidrose idiopathique. Ann Dermatol Venereol. 2013;140:771–7.
89. Manonukul J, Wisuthsarewong W, Chantorn R, et al. Hematidrosis: a pathologic process or stigmata. A case report with comprehensive histopathologic and immunoperoxidase studies. Am J Dermatopathol. 2008;30:135–9.
90. Techasatian L, Waraasawapati S, Jetsrisuparb C, et al. Hematidrosis: a report with histological and biochemical documents. Int J Dermatol. 2016;55:916–8.
91. Mucci C. Il fenomeno delle stigmate. La Civiltà Cattolica. 1993;144:217–26.
92. Glaz S. Characteristics of extraordinary religious phenomena accompanying the Christian religious experience. Reflection-Religious. 2014;5:1146–60.
93. Barbet P. Les cinq plaies du Christ. 2nd ed. Paris: Procure du Carmel de l'Action de Graces; 1937.
94. Barbet P. A doctor at Calvary. In: Image books. New York: Kennedy PJ and Sons; 1995.
95. Lussiez B. Anatomy of crucifixion. Chir Main. 2005;24:132–47.
96. Thurston H. The physical phenomena of mysticism. London: Burns and Oates; 1952.
97. Vanchez A. Les stigmates di Saint François et leur détracteurs dans les derniers siècle du moyen âge. Melanges Archeol Histoire. 1968;80:595–625.
98. Imber-Gourbeyre A. La stigmatization. Clermont: Bellet; 1894-.
99. Bion R. The riddle of the stigmata. London: Burnes and Oates; 1962.
100. Shimberg AP. The story of Therese Neumann. New York: All Saints Press; 1962.
101. Ramesh V, Al Aboud K. Cutaneous signs of piety. Cutis. 2014;94:e13–8.
102. Tocquet R. L'ombra svelata. Torino: Dellavalle; 1971.
103. Maroldi V. La scienza moderna e i miracoli. Torino: SAIE; 1955.
104. Boussault P, Doutre MS, Beylot-Barry M, et al. Painful bruising syndrome: a psychogenic disease. Rev Med Interne. 2005;26:744–7.
105. Ivanov OL, Lvov AN, Michenko AV, et al. Autoerythrocyte sensitization syndrome (Gardner-Diamond syndrome): review of the literature. J Eur Acad Dermatol Venereol. 2009;23:499–504.
106. Gauba V, Cooper M, Liu C. Vicarious menstruation in primary localized conjunctival amyloidosis. Arch Ophthalmol. 2006;124:1361–2.
107. Carvalho AC, Machado-Pinto J, Nogueira GC, et al. Hematidrosis: a case report and review of the literature. Int J Dermatol. 2008;47:1058–9.
108. Wang Z, Yu Z, Su J, et al. A case of hematidrosis successfully treated with propranolol. Am J Clin Dermatol. 2010;11:440–3.
109. Praveen BK, Vincent J. Hematidrosis and hemolacria: a case report. Indian J Pediatr. 2012;79:109–11.
110. Latorre Martinez N, Betlloch Mas I, Monteagudo Paz AF, et al. Recurrent bleeding in an 18-year-old girl. Arch Dermatol. 2012;148(8):960–1.
111. Ho JZ, de Silva J, Olver J. A very rare case of bloody tears with enigmatic epistaxis and haematuria. Orbit. 2011;30:116–7.
112. Holoubek JE, Holoubek AB. Blood, sweat and fear. A classification of hematidrosis. J Med. 1996;27:115–33.
113. Mishra KL. Bloody tears and hematohidrosis in a patient of PF3 dysfunction: a case report. Cases J. 2009;2:9029.
114. Jerajani HR, Jaju B, Phiske MM, et al. Hematohidrosis—a rare clinical phenomenon. Indian J Dermatol. 2009;54:290–2.
115. Bhagwat PV, Tophakhane RS, Rathod RM, et al. Hematohidrosis. Indian J Dermatol Venereol Leprol. 2009;75:317–8.

116. Uber M, Rohl R, Abagge K, et al. Hematidrosis: insights in the pathophysiology. Int J Dermatol. 2015;54:e542–61.
117. Ho VH, Wilson MW, Linder JS, et al. Bloody tears of unknown cause: case series and review of the literature. Ophthalmic Plast Reconstr Surg. 2004;20:442–7.
118. Aberer E, Riedl A. (Stigmatization. Consideration from a theological-dermatologic perspective). Hautarzt 2004;55:1168–1171.
119. Agle DP, Ratnoff OD. Purpura as a psychosomatic entity. A psychiatric study of autoerythrocyte sensitization. Arch Intern Med. 1962;109:685–94.
120. Hissa-Elian A, Valera CF, Pires GJT et al. Dermatitis artefacta. Stigmata Christ as a self-inflicted disorders. In: 21st World Congress of Dermatology, Buenos Aires, Argentina, 2007: P4937.
121. Randazzo SD. Quando la pelle è testimone d'accusa. Med Psicosom. 1995;4:299–308.
122. Fisher JG, Kollar EJ. Investigation of a stigmatic. South Med J. 1980;73:1461–6.
123. Early LF, Lifschutz JE. A case of stigmata. Arch Gen Psychiatry. 1974;30:197–200.
124. Bonamonte D, Vestita M, Filoni A, et al. Religious stigmata as malingering artifact: report of a case and review of the literature. Medicine (Baltimore). 2016;95:e5354–7.

Chapter 6
Psychocutaneous Diseases in Children: A Clinical Dermatological Approach

Marco Adriano Chessa, Annalucia Virdi, and Iria Neri

Psychodermatology is a medical specialty concerning the biological mechanisms and the clinical expression of the connection between skin and psyche and is gaining a growing interest. The skin and the brain originate from ectoderma and share many neurotransmitters and hormones. In the clinical practice, we can observe a greater prevalence of psychiatric disorders among dermatologic diseases and vice versa. The prevalence of psychiatric comorbidity in outpatient dermatology has been estimated at 30% [1].

Self-inflicted cutaneous disorders (SICD), or factitious (from the Latin factitious: artificial, not natural or self-induced) diseases, can be caused on almost all the organ systems by the use of exogenous or endogenous methods. Skin artifacts provoked intentionally by subjects with a psychological disorder, without any venal interest, are described as "pathomimic." Instead, artifact skin disorders caused with illicit intent, aiming to gain various advantages, are true simulations and are called "malingering." In both cases, affected subjects reject or purposely hide their pathological conduct [2].

In children, factitious skin disorders are observed inapproximately 1 in 23,000 pediatric consultations [3]. Considering all pediatric cases of factitious skin disorders, the most common lesions reported are: excoriations, purpura, trichotillomania, contact dermatitis, and miscellaneous lesions (edema, panniculitis, bullae, eschars). Head, neck, and arms are the most affected cutaneous sites [4, 5].

For dermatologists, it is very important to be aware of SICD, their clinical symptoms, and the basic principles of treatment, especially in children.

M. A. Chessa (✉) · A. Virdi · I. Neri
Dermatology Unit, Department of Experimental, Diagnostic and Specialty Medicine, University of Bologna, Bologna, Italy

Dermatology Unit, IRCCS Azienda Ospedaliero-Universitaria di Bologna, Bologna, Italy
e-mail: marcoadriano.chessa2@unibo.it; annalucia.virdi@aosp.bo.it; iria.neri@aosp.bo.it

G. Angelini et al. (eds.), *Psychocutaneous Diseases*,
https://doi.org/10.1007/978-3-031-70296-9_6

The clinical symptoms and basic treatment principles of SICD, particularly in children, require dermatologists to be aware of their importance as a disease.

Several SICD with "pathological" clinical manifestations according to Statistical Manual of Mental Disorders [6] (DSM-5) and the classifications reported in the position paper drawn up by the European Society for Dermatology and Psychiatry and Diagnostic [7] will be discussed focusing on children such as: (1) factitious disorder imposed on self or another, (2) excoriation disorders, (3) trichotillomania, (4) body-focused repetitive behavior disorder. Skin damage may be self-induced in delusional parasitosis (5) by scratching and pricking to eliminate imagined parasites. In addition, the following psychiatric disorders with cutaneous involvement will be debated in order to define skin signs to achieve the diagnosis: (6) body dysmorphic disorder or dysmorphophobia, (7) eating disorders, and (8) olfactory reference syndrome.

No account will here be taken of psychiatric disorders with no significant dermatological disease.

6.1 Factitious Disorder Imposed on Self or Another

Factitious disorder imposed on self or another is a term that should replace the following dermatological uses in literature: dermatitis artefacta, factitious dermatitis, self-induced factitial dermatitis, dermatitis factitial, artifactual skin disease, factitious illness, illness falsification, dermatology pathomimicry, cutaneous artifactual disease, dermatitis simulates, and factitious skin disease [6, 7]. Dermatitis artefacta (DA) is the term the most reported by dermatologist in literature. In this condition, the patient may not be fully aware of this and usually denies any responsibility; the true extent of this disorder, especially in children, is currently unknown [8].

Clinically, the most common lesions reported in DA in childhood are excoriations and ulcers followed by blisters, burns, irritant contact dermatitis, hematomas, panniculitis, cheilitis, and hyperpigmentation [4, 9, 10].

Lesions are monomorphic, generally well-demarcated, with sharp edges and geometric shapes [11] (Fig. 6.1). In several studies and in our experience, the most commonly affected areas in children are the face and extremities [5, 12].

A rare psychodermatological condition occurring most frequently in children and in young adult females is Gardner-Diamond syndrome [13] (GDS). GDS is characterized by the formation of spontaneous, painful skin lesions that develop into ecchymosis following episodes of severe psychological stress (Fig. 6.2). Self-injury can serve to relieve tension or may be a self-punitive function exerted to mitigate guilt feelings.

In DA and GDS, the diagnosis is of exclusion after other primary dermatologic disease, coagulopathies, purpura, child abuse should be ruled out.

Management's role is to prevent self-harm self-mutilation with occlusive dressings and the treatment of the skin lesions. In addition, psychotherapy for

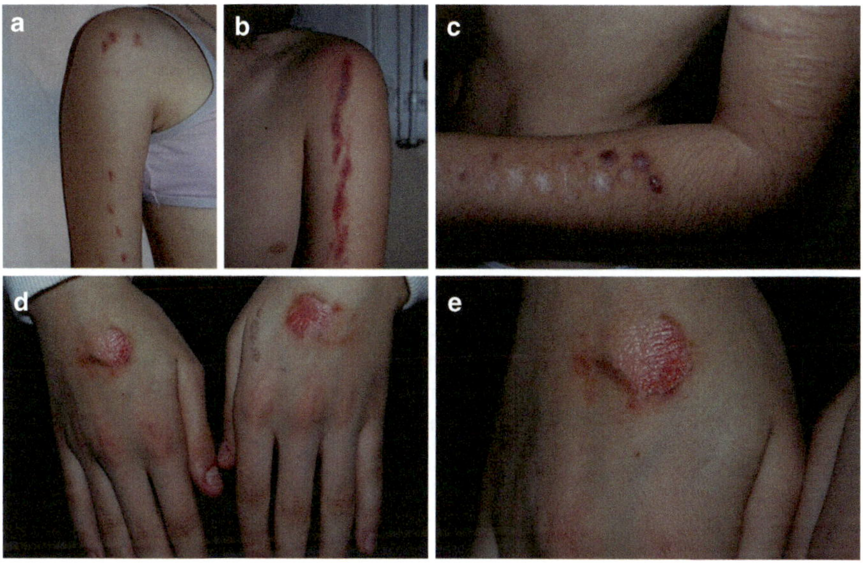

Fig. 6.1 (**a**) A 9-year-old girl presented with row of painful linear purpura on the flexor surface of the upper limbs; (**b**) a 10-year-old girl presented with round atrophic scars and painless purple streaks on the arms of 2 months' duration diagnosed as factitial purpura; (**c**) well-demarcated, dusky-red oval scars on the left dorsal surface of the left forearm and linear cutting scars on the arm; (**d**) geometric shapes excoriations on the dorsum of the hands of a 13-year-old girl; (**e**) higher magnification of geometrical erosion and crusting on the left hand of a 13-year-old girl

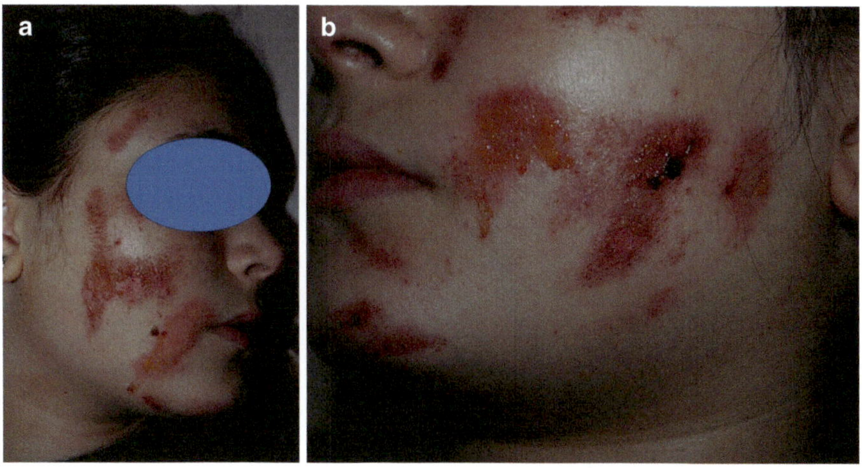

Fig. 6.2 (**a**) Geometric excoriations on the face of a 16-year-old girl; (**b**) higher magnification of multiple exudating excoriations

restructuring the patient's personality and sometimes pharmacologic therapy for the psychiatric condition could be effective [5, 14].

The prognosis for recovery is poor and the disease tends to vary according to the patient's life circumstances [14].

6.2 Excoriation Disorders

Excoriation disorder is the term that should be used in place of the following dermatological uses: dermatillomania, psychogenic excoriation, compulsive skin picking, pathological skin picking disorder, dermatitis para-artefacta, self-injurious skin picking, repetitive skin picking, emotional excoriation, nervous scratching artefacta, para-artificial excoriation, epidermatillomania, neurotic excoriation, neurodermatitis [2].

These disorders describe the repetitive rubbing of the skin that provokes visible tissue damage. The most common onset is during childhood or adolescence [15].

In literature, several types of compulsive skin picking have been described but the most common in pediatric age are stereotypical linear purpura of the upper limbs (Fig. 6.3), acne excoriate, knuckle pads, and pachydermodactyly [16, 17].

In children, knuckle pads are often benign idiopathic subcutaneous nodules that appear most frequently on the extensor surfaces of the proximal interphalangeal joints [18]. On the contrary, the name pseudo-knuckle pads may be considered as a

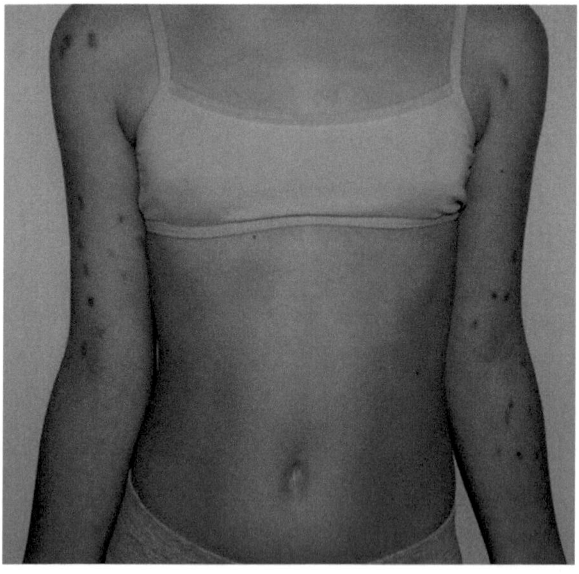

Fig. 6.3 Bilaterally symmetrical, multiple oval or square purpuric macules, forming a discontinuous linear purpuric streaks over arms and forearms

form of callosity that appears after repeated trauma. In children exhibiting obsessive behaviors has been described also as chewing pads [19].

In addition, pachydermodactyly is a benign fibromatosis described in children characterized by asymptomatic, progressive, fusiform swelling over the dorsal and lateral aspects of the proximal interphalangeal joint with no loss of joint function. In some cases, this clinical manifestation is associated to systemic disease, whereas obsessive-compulsive behavior is probably the main cause [20, 21].

In these patients, psychiatric comorbidities such as body dysmorphic disorder (BDD), trait anxiety, and borderline personality disorder could be investigated [22]. Occlusive dressings could be considered as treatment of the skin lesions.

6.3 Trichotillomania (Hair-Pulling Disorder)

The term trichotillomania (TTM) should be used instead of trichotemnomania, trichoteiromania, and trichodaganomania (hair-biting habit). Biting hair without pulling it falls under body-focused repetitive behaviors.

Hair disorders are very stressful in pediatric population. Both physicians and families are often unsatisfied leading to non-compliance [23]. There is evidence for a bimodal onset of trichotillomania, with peaks in the pre-school years and in early adolescence, predominantly in females, with poorer prognosis as it persists into adulthood [24].

This disease commonly affects the scalp, followed by the eyebrows and eyelashes. The extent of hair loss is determined by the individual's hand. In severe cases involving the vertex (tonsure pattern) or occipital area (Fig. 6.4a), hair at the

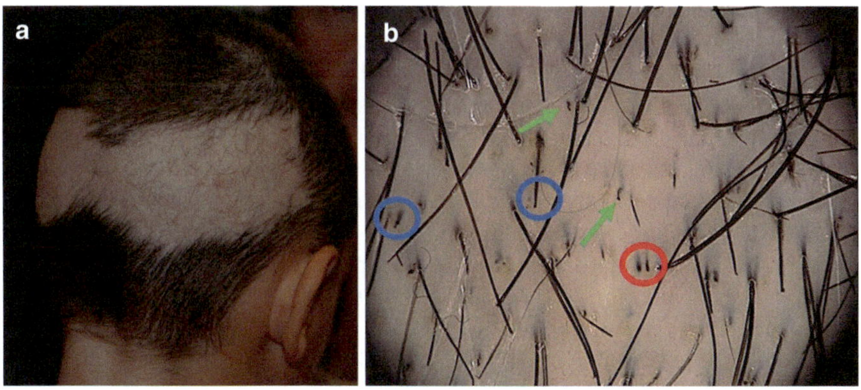

Fig. 6.4 (**a**) Alopecic area with geometrical borders and varying hair lengths located in the occipital region; (**b**) trichoscopic examination showing signs of trichotillomania. Red circles: black dots with high variability in diameter and shape; blue circles: broken hairs or tulip hair (short hairs with darker shaped ends); green arrow: hook hairs (partially coiled hairs). The images were obtained by computerized polarized-light videomicroscopy (FotoFinder Dermoscope, Teachscreen Software, Bad Birnbach, Germany) at 20-fold magnification

periphery is typically spared (Friar Tuck sign) [25]. Dermoscopy evaluation of scalp and hair disorders improves diagnostic capability beyond simple clinical inspection also in diagnosis of TTM. At dermoscopy alopecic lesions show broken hairs of different lengths with three important dermoscopic signs: (i) V sign 2 hairs broken at equal lengths from 1 follicular opening: (ii) coiled hairs and (iii) tulip hairs [26–30] (Fig. 6.4b).

Histopathologic findings can help in diagnosis, like increased catagenic hairs, traumatized hair bulbs, pigmentary casts, and trichomalacia.

Differential diagnoses include tinea capitis, alopecia areata, traction alopecia, androgenetic alopecia, and trichotemnomania [29].

Several studies reported cognitive-behavioral therapy, pharmacological management, or combination therapies for management of TTM. Dermatologists should be encouraged to develop relationships with community psychologists and psychiatrists experienced in behavioral intervention. In pediatric population, pharmacological options are not well understood still today [31]. Whereas N-acetylcysteine is effective in adults, there are little data on efficacy in the pediatric age. Serotonin reuptake inhibitors (SSRI), tricyclic antidepressants (TCA), and antipsychotics have limited efficacy data in pediatric patients [32].

6.4 Delusional Disorder Somatic Type

Delusional disorders somatic type is defined in the Diagnostic and Statistical Manual of Mental Disorders (DSM-5) as the presence of one or more delusions that persist for 1 month or longer [6].

The term delusional disorder somatic type includes all of the following terms that have been reported in the literature: delusions of parasitosis, delusional parasitosis, Ekbom syndrome, psychogenic parasitosis, delusional infestation.

Delusional infestation (DI), also known as delusions of parasitosis, is the most common monosymptomatic, hypochondriacal psychosis in dermatology [33]. There is a peak prevalence in patients in their 20s and 30s and over 50 years of age; 2:1 ratio of women to men has been reported [33].

Children affected usually refer that they are infested with parasites or have foreign objects extruding from their skin and try to remove the organisms with nails or tools, producing self-imposed erosions, ulcers, prurigo nodules, and lichenification [34, 35]. Usually, the patients describe skin dysesthesias attributed to the infestation, such as crawling, biting, and stinging [34]. Typically, the patients or their parents require the prescription of disinfectants and pesticides to achieve eradication.

The diagnosis of DI can be established on the basis of clinical features and history, and after excluding other etiologies. Primary formication (without conviction of infestation), often caused by underlying neurologic disease or substance abuse, should be ruled out [32]. Two criteria are essential for diagnosis of delusions of parasitosis: (i) individuals have a conviction of being infested despite evidence to the contrary and (ii) abnormal cutaneous sensations are attributed to this belief [36].

A rare form of this disease is known as delusions of parasitosis by proxy, which encompasses a delusional belief projected onto another person that lacks capacity to hold the same belief [37]. Delusions of parasitosis by proxy is most frequently reported in vulnerable individuals such as children [37, 38].

Patients known to lack insight and often refuse psychiatric care so the goal of the visit is to improve the patient's condition; it is by no means to convince the child or the parents of being delusional [39, 40].

In this point of view perform initial laboratory tests, obtain skin biopsy specimens and cultures, rule out the organic causes of formication, could represent an ideal approach to build a relationship with the patient [7].

6.5 Body-Focused Repetitive Behavior Disorder (BFRB)

This disorder manifests with repetitive and intentional acts of habitual grooming behaviors causing physical injuries and social avoidance for incapacity to control them [41] BFRB disorders pertain to 20% of adults but subclinical forms are higher common, involving up to 60% of undergraduated students. The subjects are unable to control these behaviors due to emotional tension or to more severe disease or unconscious self-punishment or autoerotic maneuvers [42]. BFRBs may be categorized as focused and automatic characterized respectively by awareness of behavior with high emotional tension (excoriation disorder, onychophagia) and unawareness of it (trichotillomania). According to previous study, trichotillomania, onychophagia, and skin-picking behavior are often associated with attention-deficit hyperactivity disorder, obsessive-compulsive disorder, and Tourette syndrome [41]. People suffering from BFRB may have problems with physical functioning and emotional well-being. Impulsivity and mood and anxiety disorders are the main underlying factors in these subjects. Triggering factors may be various and in a recent pediatric study were sensorial, emotional (anxiety, distress, anger), cognitive (related to appearance), or calming activities (watching TV, reading book) [41].

Although the patients do not deny the self-infliction, they hardly accept medical or psychiatric help.

BFRBs are quite frequent in children and adolescents with intellectual disability [41].

The clinical features are very variable. Automatic and focused behaviors characterized different entities such as trichotillomania, dermatillomania, dermatophagia, onychophagia, onychotillomania, morsicatio labiorum, linguarum, and buccarum (chewing of the lips, tongue, cheek), and cheilitis. In addition, severe nail biting, defined as biting past the nail bed, can cause also paronychia and gingival lesions.

- Pica is persistent, compulsive ingestion of substances considered inedible, beyond the normal developmental phase of occasional indiscriminate and experimental mouthing and swallowing over a period of at least 1 month. The prevalence is greatest in children aged 18 months to 6 years. It is commonly seen in

children who suffer from developmental delay, in lower socioeconomic classes or emotionally deprived, and it is an important cause of anemia. It includes trichophagia, onychophagia, eating scabs after skin picking [43].
- Onychophagia (i.e., biting on the nail with teeth) begins during childhood, after the age of 3–4 years, and adolescence with the fingernails and toenails. Usually, the nails are not swallowed, but are thrown out. Epidemiological data are limited because it is not considered a disorder. Thumb sucking and onychophagia are manifestations of difficulty in the evolution of oral stage of child's psychological development [44]. The rate of prevalence is 50% in childhood, with a slight female preponderance, reaches a peak during adolescence and decreases thereafter, until 4.5% in late adulthood [41]. It is a most common BFRB disorder in a recent retrospective cohort study on 67 children [41]. At physical examination, nails appear short and uneven, with erythematous folds, hang nails, splinter hemorrhages, ragged or absent cuticles. Rubbing of the proximal nail fold and cuticle may cause nail matrix damage and deformity. A significant distress due to behavior and the failure of attempts to stop it are required as diagnostic criteria of BFRB according to DSM-5 [6].

No treatment is necessary for mild disease beyond proper nail hygiene, trimming. Covering the nails with bandages, regular manicure, or applying a bitter substance to the nails may discourage nail biting. N-acetylcysteine 800 mg/day promotes nail and hair growth after 1 month, but efficacy is limited in onychophagia. The pharmacological treatment should be individualized depending on the severity of tic and the underlying psychiatric condition. The first-line use of behavioral therapy has level 2 of evidence [44].

- Onychotillomania is a recurrent trauma of the paronychium or manipulation and removal of the cuticle and/or nail that led to onychodystrophy, and sometimes to chronic paronychia and anonychia. Clinical and dermoscopic examination shows the absence of nail plate and the presence of scales, wavy lines, crusts, linear or pinpoint hemorrhages, and melanonychia due to melanocyte activation [42]. It is less common than onychophagia but is more often associated with underlying neuropsychiatric comorbidities (fixed hypochondriacal delusions, depression, obsessive-compulsive disorder) [44].
- Trichophagia may involve up to 50% of patients affected by trichotillomania and consists of chewing and swallowing hairs. A trichobezoar may develop in stomach or intestinal tract (Rapunzel syndrome) causing pain, nausea, vomiting, failure to thrive, and intestinal obstruction. Trichobezoar is reported almost exclusively in young female, up to 90% between 13 and 20 years of age with trichotillomania and trichophagia, and often it is associated to psychiatric illness, intellectually disabled or young children. The clinical findings of non-scarring alopecia of the scalp (occasionally of other body regions) with broken hair of varying lengths, trichophagia, and abdominal pain are important to suspect trichobezoar [45].
- Rhinotillexomania is the pathological habit of nose picking (e.g., squeezing comedones) and the compulsive extraction of dried nasal mucus with fingers. It

is more common in children and young adults. It may rarely cause bacterial infections, nasal bleeds, serious self-inflicted lesions such as perforation of the nasal septum and destruction of facial bone structures (ethmoidal sinuses and orbit wall). It may be associated to onychotillomania, onychophagia, neurotic excoriation, and other obsessive-compulsive behaviors [46].

- Morsicatio buccarum, labiorum, linguarum: compulsive sucking and biting of oral mucosa that causes irregular leukodermic lesions with rough surface and symmetric localization. The most frequent sites are: the pericommissural part of the lips, the mucosal cheek at the level of occlusive plane, the lateral edges of the tongue [42].
- Cheilitis factitial (or self-inflicted cheilitis): repetitive lip-licking, sucking, biting, or picking that causes cyclical peeling of keratinaceous scale involving the vermilion lip [42, 47], painful skin fissures, and sometimes superinfection and development of "lip-eczema." The diagnosis is one of exclusion and may be suggested by resistance to therapy. The condition is more prevalent in adolescent and young women and is associated to an underlying behavioral health condition [47]. Differential diagnosis includes other type of cheilitis associated with lip-licking dermatitis, especially: (i) eczematous cheilitis: erythema and scaling of vermilion and cutaneous lips, with possible fissuring, frequent association with allergens; (ii) exfoliative cheilitis: thick desquamative scale, most often along the vermilion border and involving the lower lip; possible association with actinic damage, lip-licking, nutritional deficiencies, and body-focused repetitive behaviors [47].

Diagnosis of BFRB is often of exclusion. The initial question to patient with suspected BFRB disorder may be "Do you find yourself making this behavior when you fill stressed or bored?" If the answer is yes, the patient may be screened fitting existing screening tools for trichotillomania and excoriation disorder (no validated screening tools exist for other BFRBs) [48].

There is no defined treatment algorithm for children and adolescents with BFRB disorder. Habit reverse training is the first-line treatment but a limited evidence is reported. Other psychotherapeutic treatments seem effective, including comprehensive behavioral treatment, acceptance and commitment therapy, and dialectical behavioral therapy [48]. In addition, the most commonly used pharmacological agents are atypical antipsychotics and SSRIs [41].

6.6 Body Dysmorphic Disorder (BDD) or Dysmorphophobia

It belongs to obsessive-compulsive and related disorders, and if BDD symptoms are related to actual flaws with an excessive concern it is also defined as other specified obsessive-compulsive and related disorders with body dysmorphic-like disorder with actual flaws [6]. BDD is an excessive worry about an imagined or a slight defect in appearance, causing clinical significant distress and limitation in social life and work and leading to time-consuming repetitive behaviors. Some patients have moderate insight into their disease, but many others especially adolescents have poor insight or delusional thoughts. Whenever patients are completely convinced that their view of the defect is undistorted the disorder is called "monosymptomatic hypochondriasis and delusions of dysmorphosis" or "delusional form of BDD."

Up to 6.7% of general dermatology patients and 14% of cosmetic dermatology patients could be affected by BDD. The onset is during adolescence or childhood (even at 4 years of age), the course is chronic but prognosis is favorable with appropriate psychiatric treatment. It affects 1.9% of adults, 3.3% of college-aged students, and 1.7% of adolescents [49].

The face or head including hair is often the cause of the concern, but any part of the body can be involved. Nonexistent or minimal defects such as acne, marks, scarring, thinning hair, excessive body hair, too large or misshapen nose are considered very unattractive by patient and cause uncontrolled preoccupation. Most patients think that other people notice and talk about the supposed defect and mock them for it (ideas or delusion of reference).

One third of patients compulsively pick at their skin with fingers, needles, pins, etc. in order to clear or perfect their skin, exacerbating mild acne and causing cutaneous damage.

These behaviors led to concentration impairment and large amount of time consumption, avoidance of works, social relationship, psychiatric recovery, and risk of suicide.

The diagnosis in pediatric age is difficult because the symptoms are considered typical adolescent body image issues. Dermatologist should ask the patient appearance-specific and open-ended questions in sensitive manner, including questions about social media use. This latter and photo manipulation are associated to negative body image mainly in adolescent girls.

Red flags in the history are: (1) the excessive concern or a number of secondary excoriative lesions out of proportion of primary visible lesions; (2) excessive camouflaging behavior or time spent for skin care out of proportion to the visible skin problem; (3) previous multiple visits by other doctors who do not satisfactorily explain or cure perceived problem [49].

The attempt to convince him that the defect is not real can lead to distress and mistrust, whereas it is better to reassure him that the other people do not notice what we notice when we are looking at ourselves. The correction of patient's unhealthy skincare regimen should be made by dermatologist. A referral to mental health should be considering according to clinical and emotional status of the patient after establishing a therapeutic relationship. This should be presented to the patient and parents as an opportunity to discuss the emotional distress [11].

Its management necessitates an empathetic, non-dismissive approach. Although most BDD patients resort to cosmetic treatments, interventions rarely improve symptoms. The first-line therapy is cognitive-behavioral therapy with deliberate exposure and response prevention, and whether it fails or is rejected, SSRIs may be considered [11].

6.7 Eating Disorder (ED)

Examination of the skin is a helpful tool for the diagnosis of eating disorders, considering the customary of patients to deny the problem. Higher prevalence is among adolescent and young adults of high-income Western population. More than 90% of patients affected by ED are women; in fact, the prevalence of anorexia nervosa (AN) and bulimia nervosa (BN) is, respectively, 1.4% and 1.9% in women and 0.2% and 0.6% in men. Amenorrhea is a key diagnostic feature in AN, whereas BN has been linked to polycystic ovary syndrome.

DSM-5 classified feeding and EDs into:

- anorexia nervosa (AN): restricted type and binge-eating/purging type
- bulimia nervosa (BN): purging and nonpurging
- binge-eating disorders (BED), pica, rumination disorder, avoidant/restrictive food intake disorder, other specified and unspecified feeding or eating disorder.

Skin manifestations are various and frequent with a body mass index (BMI) $\leq$ 16 kg/m^2. According to literature cutaneous manifestations could be classified into five main groups [50] (Table 6.1).

Among these there are some more typical signs helping to make ED diagnosis: Russell's sign, self-induced dermatitis, perimylolysis, and lanugo like hair (Fig. 6.5). These signs may be absent in males because self-induced vomiting and laxative abuse are less common, and they prefer to make excessive fasting and exercise [50]. Fine lanugo hair is a specific marker of AN and permits to distinguish it from other

Table 6.1 Cutaneous manifestations in eating disorders

Cutaneous Manifestations in Eating Disorders	
Skin Signs of Self-Purging	*Russel's sign* (knuckle calluses on the dorsal aspect of dominant hand due to friction against teeth during introduction of it into the mouth to induce vomiting), *self-phlebotomy, perimylolysis* (severe chemical erosion of tooth enamel by exposure to gastric acid from chronic vomiting)
Skin Signs of Starvation (due to nutritional deficiency)	Xerosis, lanugo-like hair, nail changes, telogen effluvium, mucosal signs (dry mouth, cheilitis, angular cheilitis, gingivitis, geographic tongue, aphthae), striae distensae, pellagra, acrodermatitis enteropathica, scurvy, carotenoderma
Skin Signs Related to Drug Abuse	Xerosis, drug reactions (urticaria.), photosensitivity (thiazides), retention edema, myopathy with dermatomyositis-like skin findings (ipecac syrup)
Skin Signs of Psychiatric Comorbidity	*Self-inflicted injuries*, interdigital intertrigo, erythema ab igne, trichotillomania, acne excorie, dissatisfaction with the appearance of the skin
Miscellaneous Signs	Delayed wound healing, manifestations due to nutritional deficiencies (pellagra, acrodermatitis enteropathica, scurvy), seborrheic dermatitis, folliculitis, prurigo pigmentosa, evident blood vessels due to decreased subcutaneous tissue, pili torti, linear erythema craquelé, acute edema/cutaneous distension syndrome with refeeding

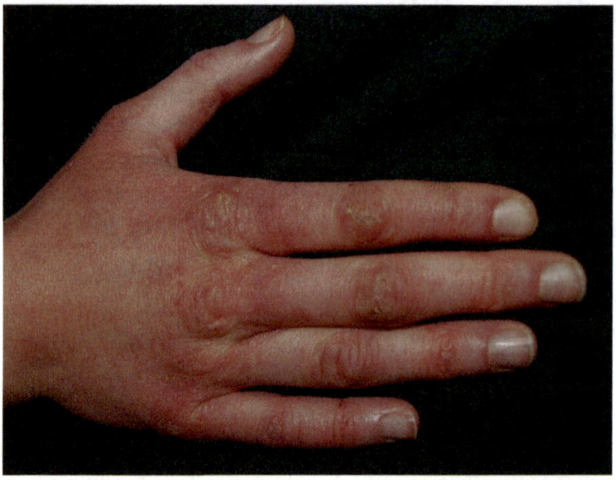

Fig. 6.5 Calluses and abrasions on the dorsal aspects of the dominant hand induced by the patient's repeated introduction of the hand into the mouth. This sign predominates in BN rather than AN

types of malnutrition. It develops mainly on the back, arms, and sometimes on the face and neck as an attempt to keep the body warm. A modest improvement is likely with re-nutrition.

Principal nail changes reported are: koilonychia due to iron deficiency, Terry nails, Muehrcke's lines, color changes seen in B12 deficiency (blue nails, wavy longitudinal dark streaks and brownish pigmentation), splinter hemorrhages, nail dystrophy, longitudinal ungual striae, onychocryptosis, and periungual erythema.

Acquired pili torti (hair shaft flattened at irregular intervals and twisted 180° along its long axis; increased fragility) is reported in AN and seems to be related to excessive vitamin A due to intake of yellow vegetable and vitamin supplements containing carotenes. Clinically patients have fragile, brittle, dry, and coarse hair, especially in temporal and occipital areas.

Dermatological manifestations usually resolve with weight gain. Dermatologic therapies include emollients, including those containing urea 10–30% for Russel's sign, avoidance of topical and systemic retinoids for acne (risk of hypervitaminosis A in AN) [50].

In addition, in ED disorders is recommended a referral to a multidisciplinary center in order to perform psychotherapy (cognitive-behavioral therapy), psychopharmacotherapy, and management of medical complications.

6.8 Olfactory Reference Syndrome (ORS)

ORS is a psychiatric condition more common than generally recognized. It is concern about a false belief that one emits a malodorous body smell, which others notice but is not really perceived by others. ORS is classified under "other specified OCDs and Related Disorders" in DSM-5 [6]. The etiology and exact prevalence is unknown; it is more predominant in single males and develops in the early adulthood, with a mean age of onset 21.1 year [51], but it may begin in the teenage years in many instances [52]. Recently, Sejdiu A et al. reported 14-year-old male with a history of high functioning autism and attention-deficit/hyperactivity disorder (ADHD) presenting with a new onset of obsessive-compulsive disorder with symptoms similar to olfactory hallucinations and olfactory reference syndrome in the setting of the COVID-19 pandemic [53].

The symptoms of ORS overlap with several other psychiatric disorders, including OCD, delusional disorder, social anxiety disorder, body dysmorphic disorder, depression, and hypochondriasis.

Three diagnostic criteria could be considered to achieve diagnosis: (i) a persistent false belief that one emits a malodorous smell; may encompass a range of insight (i.e., symptoms can be nondelusional); (ii) The belief causes clinically significant distress, is time-consuming (i.e., preoccupies the individual for ≥1 h/day) or results in significant impairment in social, occupational, or other important areas of functioning; (iii) The belief is not better accounted for by another mental disorder or a general medication condition.

The patients misinterpret behavior of other people around them, believing their gesture and remarks are a response to smell (ideas of reference). They spend a lot of time with rituals to rid of the smell, wash repeatedly, use perfumes and deodorants excessively, change frequently their clothes, limit travel and social life, avoid intimacy, and physical activity. Depression, anxiety, substance abuse, social phobia, OCD, BDD, personality disorders (obsessional, dependent, and avoidant) may coexist.

Regarding treatment SSRIs are the first line of treatment for pediatric OCD, but clomipramine is resulted more effective in a meta-analysis study [53]. Psychotherapy and exposure therapy may be helpful [51].

References

1. Jafferany M, Ferreira BR, Abdelmaksoud A, Mkhoyan R. Management of psychocutaneous disorders: a practical approach for dermatologists. Dermatol Ther. 2020;33:e13969.
2. Bonamonte D, Foti C, De Marco A, Hansel K, Cecchini E, Filoni A, De Prezzo S, Ambrogio F, Angelini G, Stingeni L. Self-inflicted pathological cutaneous disorders. Part I. Ital J Dermatol Venerol. 2022;157(5):389–401.
3. Sneddon I, Sneddon J. Self-inflicted injury: a follow-up study of 43 patients. BMJ. 1975;3:527–30.

4. Alcántara Luna S, García Bravo B, Rodríguez Pichardo A, Camacho Martínez FM. Dermatitis artefacta in childhood: a retrospective analysis of 44 patients, 1976–2006. Pediatr Dermatol. 2015;32(5):604–8.
5. Saez-de-Ocariz M, Orozco-Covarrubias L, Mora-Magaña I, Duran-McKinster C, Tamayo-Sanchez L, Gutierrez-Castrellon P, Ruiz-Maldonado R. Dermatitis artefacta in pediatric patients: experience at the national institute of pediatrics. Pediatr Dermatol. 2004;21(3):205–11.
6. American Psychiatric Association. DSM-5 task force. Diagnostic and statistical manual of mental disorders: DSM-5. 5th ed. Arlington: American Psychiatric Association; 2013.
7. Gieler U, Consoli SG, Tomás-Aragones L, Linder DM, Jemec GB, Poot F, et al. Self-inflicted lesions in dermatology: terminology and classification—a position paper from the European Society for Dermatology and Psychiatry (ESDaP). Acta Derm Venereol. 2013;93:4–12.
8. Rodrıguez Pichardo A, Garcıa BB. Dermatitis artefacta: revision. Actas Dermosifiliogr. 2013;104:854–66.
9. Persad L, Salim S, Motaparthi K. Factitious dermatitis due to thermal burn with histologic features simulating fixed drug eruption. Am J Dermatopathol. 2017 Aug;39(8):622–4.
10. Alexander T, Cohen B. Painless purple streaks on the arms and chest. Cutis. 2019 Jul;104(1):E8–9.
11. Yamada K, Sakurai Y, Shibata M, Miyagawa S, Yoshioka A. Factitious purpura in a 10-year-old girl. Pediatr Dermatol. 2009;26(5):597–600.
12. Zack JM, Fults M, Saxena H, Green B. Factitial dermatitis due to the "salt and ice challenge". Pediatr Dermatol. 2014;31(2):252–4.
13. Block ME, Sitenga JL, Lehrer M, Silberstein PT. Gardner-Diamond syndrome: a systematic review of treatment options for a rare psychodermatological disorder. Int J Dermatol. 2019 Jul;58(7):782–7.
14. Koblenzer C. Dermatitis artefacta: clinical features and approaches to treatment. Am J Clin Dermatol. 2000;1:47–55.
15. Odlaug BL, Grant JE. Clinical characteristics and medical complications of pathologic skin picking. Gen Hosp Psychiatry. 2008;30:61–6.
16. Shah KN, Fried RG. Factitial dermatoses in children. Curr Opin Pediatr. 2006;18(4):403–9.
17. Sarkar S, Ghosh SK, Sil A. Stereotypical linear purpura of the upper limbs: a report of three cases of a rare psychocutaneous disorder and review of the literature. Indian J Psychiatry. 2020;62(2):212–6. Erratum in: Indian J Psychiatry. 2020 Nov-Dec;62(6):752.
18. Nenoff P, Woitek G. Images in clinical medicine. Knuckle pads. N Engl J Med. 2011;364(25):2451.
19. Calikoðlu E. Pseudo-knuckle pads: an unusual cutaneous sign of obsessive-compulsive disorder in an adolescent patient. Turk J Pediatr. 2003;45(4):348–9.
20. Bardazzi F, Neri I, Fanti PA, Patrizi A. Pachydermodactyly in two young girls. Pediatr Dermatol. 1996;13(4):288–91.
21. Bardazzi F, Neri I, Raone B, Patrizi A. Pachydermodactylie: 7 nouveaux cas [Pachydermodactyly: seven new cases]. Ann Dermatol Venereol. 1998 Apr;125(4):247–50.
22. Nemeh MN, Hogeling M. Pediatric skin picking disorder: a review of management. Pediatr Dermatol. 2022;39(3):363–8.
23. Chandran NS, Novak J, Iorizzo M, Grimalt R, Oranje AP. Trichotillomania in children. Skin Appendage Disord. 2015;1(1):18–24.
24. Bruce TO, Barwick LW, Wright HH. Diagnosis and management of trichotillomania in children and adolescents. Paediatr Drugs. 2005;7(6):365–76.
25. Woods DW, Flessner CA, Franklin ME, et al. The trichotillomania impact project (TIP): exploring phenomenology, functional impairment, and treatment utilization. J Clin Psychiatry. 2006;67:1877–88.
26. Rakowska A, Slowinska M, Olszewska M, et al. New trichoscopy findings in trichotillomania: flame hairs, V-sign, hook hairs, hair powder, tulip hairs. Acta Derm Venereol. 2014;94:303–6.

27. Martín JM, Montesinos E, Cordero P, Gonzalez V, Ramon D. Trichoscopy features of trichotillomania. Pediatr Dermatol. 2019;36(2):265–267. https://doi.org/10.1111/pde.13756. Epub 2019 Feb 11. PMID: 30746759.
28. Lee DY, Lee JH, Yang JM, Lee ES. The use of dermoscopy for the diagnosis of trichotillomania. J Eur Acad Dermatol Venereol. 2009 Jun;23(6):731–2.
29. Kaczorowska A, Rudnicka L, Stefanato CM, Waskiel-Burnat A, Warszawik-Hendzel O, Olszewska M, Rakowska A. Diagnostic accuracy of trichoscopy in trichotillomania: a systematic review. Acta Derm Venereol. 2021;101(10):adv00565. https://doi.org/10.2340/00015555-3859. PMID: 34184065; PMCID: PMC9425589.
30. Happle R. Trichotemnomania: obsessive-compulsive habit of cutting or shaving the hair. J Am Acad Dermatol. 2005;52:157–9.
31. Henkel ED, Jaquez SD, Diaz LZ. Pediatric trichotillomania: review of management. Pediatr Dermatol. 2019;36(6):803–7. https://doi.org/10.1111/pde.13954. Epub 2019 Oct 6.
32. Mosca M, Martin K, Hadeler E, Hong J, Brownstone N, Koo J. Review of the diagnosis and management of pediatric psychodermatologic conditions: part I. Pediatr Dermatol. 2022;39:17–21.
33. Heller MM, Wong JW, Lee ES, Ladizinski B, Grau M, Howard JL, Berger TG, Koo JY, Murase JE. Delusional infestations: clinical presentation, diagnosis and treatment. Int J Dermatol. 2013;52(7):775–83.
34. Fisher JD. Emergency department presentation of 'delusional parasitosis by proxy'. Delusional parent, injured child. Am J Emerg Med. 2019;37(9):1806.e1–2.
35. Foster A, Hylwa S, Bury J, et al. Delusional infestation: clinical presentation in 147 patients seen at Mayo Clinic. J Am Acad Dermatol. 2012;67:673.e1–673.e10.
36. Mosca M, Martin K, Hong J, Hadeler E, Brownstone N, Koo J. A review of the diagnosis and management of pediatric psychodermatologic conditions: part II. Pediatr Dermatol. 2022 Jan;39(1):12–6.
37. Moriarty N, Alam M, Kalus A, O'Connor K. Current understanding and approach to delusional infestation. Am J Med. 2019;132(12):1401–9.
38. Kalra K, Whittington CP, Sevey W, Hunt E, Metz JB. Delusions of parasitosis and delusions of parasitosis by proxy in a mother and her children. Pediatr Dermatol. 2023;40(3):544–6.
39. Ahmed H, Blakeway EA, Taylor RE, Bewley AP. Children with a mother with delusional infestation--implications for child protection and management. Pediatr Dermatol. 2015;32(3):397–400.
40. Friedmann AC, Ekeowa-Anderson A, Taylor R, Bewley A. Delusional parasitosis presenting as folie à trois: successful treatment with risperidone. Br J Dermatol. 2006;155(4):841–2.
41. Hangül Z, Tuman TC, Altunay-Tuman B, Saygılı GY, Tufan AE. Body-focused repetitive behaviors in children and adolescents, clinical characteristics, and the effects of treatment choices on symptoms: a single-center retrospective cohort study. Acta Dermatovenerol Alp Pannonica Adriat. 2022;31(4):141–6.
42. Bonamonte D, Foti C, De Marco A. Self-inflicted pathological cutaneous disorders. Part II. Ital J Dermatol Venereol. 2022;157(6):480–8.
43. Leung AKC, Hon KL. Pica: a common condition that is commonly missed—an update review. Curr Pediatr Rev. 2019;15(3):164–9.
44. Singal A, Daulatabad D. Nail tic disorders: manifestations, pathogenesis and management. Indian J Dermatol Venereol Leprol. 2017;83:19–26.
45. Ahmed MM, Tahir KS, Gubari MIM, Rasul RHK, Rashid MJ, Abdul Aziz JM. Large trichobezoar associated with misdiagnosis, a rare case report with a brief literature review. Int J Surg Case Rep. 2021;88:106551.
46. Martin-Callizo C, Sacristà M, Fortuno Y, Penin RM, Tribò MJ. Rhinotillexomania. Actas Dermosifilogr. 2018;109:370–1.
47. Fonseca A, Jacob SE, Sindle A. Art of prevention: practical interventions in lip-licking dermatitis. Int J Women's Dermatol. 2020;6:377–80.

48. Najera DB. Body-focused repetitive behaviors: beyond bad habits. JAAPA. 2022;35(2):28–33.
49. Dennin MH, Lee MS. Body dysmorphic disorder in pediatric dermatology. Pediatr Dermatol. 2018;35:868–74.
50. Stamu-O'Brien C, Shivakumar S, Messas T, Kroumpouzos G. Through the looking glass: skin signs that help diagnose eating disorders. Clin Dermatol. 2023;41(1):67–74.
51. Kuhn H, Mennella C, Magid M, Stamu-O'Brien C, Kroumpouzos G. Psychocutaneous disease: clinical perspectives. J Am Acad Dermatol. 2017;76(5):779–91.
52. Begum M, McKenna PJ. Olfactory reference syndrome: a systematic review of the world literature. Psychol Med. 2011;41:453–61.
53. Sejdiu A, Basith SA, Ayala V, et al. The emergence of new-onset obsessive and compulsive disorder in an adolescent during COVID-19 pandemic. Cureus. 2021;13(9):e17907.

Chapter 7
Compulsive Skin Disorders

Anna Belloni Fortina and Francesca Caroppo

7.1 Introduction

Skin is intimately related with emotional and psychological aspects, with various skin disorders caused by or resulting in psychiatric disturbances.

In fact, psychological stress conditions can induce or manifest themselves in the form of several types of skin disorders and dermatoses. On the other hand, psychological symptoms can be induced by several dermatological diseases. Furthermore, most of patients with pre-existing dermatological diseases often additionally develop psychological symptoms, which can negatively affect the primary skin disease.

The current DSM-5 includes several psycho-dermatological disorders in the category of obsessive–compulsive and related disorders, such as body dysmorphic disorder, neurotic excoriation, trichotillomania, and body-focused repetitive behavior disorder.

The percentage of patients with obsessive–compulsive disorders associated with skin diseases, referred to dermatologist, ranges between 9% and 35% [1–5].

However, there are several disorders which can be defined as "compulsive skin disorders" that include several dermatological diseases having the characteristics of compulsiveness and obsessive thoughts. Patients with these compulsive skin disorders cannot prevent themselves from performing a certain action in a repetitive and purposeless way [1–9].

Although these conditions do not perfectly match the criteria for the obsessive–compulsive and related disorders identified in DSM-5, they represent disorders with

A. Belloni Fortina · F. Caroppo (✉)
Pediatric Dermatology Regional Center, Department of Medicine (DIMED) and Department of Women's and Children's Health (SDB), University of Padua, Padua, Italy
e-mail: anna.bellonifortina@unipd.it; francesca.caroppo@unipd.it

G. Angelini et al. (eds.), *Psychocutaneous Diseases*,
https://doi.org/10.1007/978-3-031-70296-9_7

the characteristics of compulsiveness and obsessiveness which request a psychological and/or psychiatric evaluation.

The main types of compulsive skin disorders are summarized in Table 7.1.

Considering that patients with compulsive skin disorders usually have a diagnosis and enter into psychiatric follow-up and treatment only 8–10 years after the onset of initial signs and symptoms, it is very important to early recognize these disorders and to recommend to these patients an adequate psychiatric and psychological follow-up and treatment.

7.1.1 Psychogenic Pruritus

Psychogenic pruritus is defined as itch not related to dermatologic or systemic causes.

In particular, psychogenic itch is defined by the French Psycho-Dermatology Group (FPDG) as "an itch disorder where itch is at the center of the symptomatology and where psychological factors play an evident role in the triggering, intensity, aggravation, or persistence of the pruritus," also suggesting to call it "functional itch disorder" (FID).

It should be considered that pruritus, one of the most reported symptoms of skin diseases, is closely influenced by psychological and emotional factors, as it can represent the root cause or reason for maintenance of itching. Furthermore, data currently available support the hypothesis that psychogenic and emotional factors increase the perception of pruritus.

It is not a surprise that a high percentage (25–60%) of patients with skin diseases have a high incidence of psychiatric comorbidities and that 70% of patients with chronic pruritus are affected by psychiatric disorders [10–13].

Table 7.1 Main types of compulsive skin disorders

Compulsive skin disorders
Psychogenic pruritus
Prurigo nodularis
Lichen simplex
Acne excoriée
Trichotillomania
Trichotemnomania
Trichoteiromania
Onychophagia
Onychotillomania
Factitious cheilitis
Morsicatio buccarum
Pseudo-knuckle pads

However, there is a lack of consensus on how to classify the condition of "psychogenic pruritus," in part due to the overlap between the fields of psychiatry and dermatology.

When a patient presents with pruritus, regardless of the presumed cause, the standard work-up should include a thorough history, dermatologic examination, and laboratory examinations or biopsies as needed.

The physician should build a relationship with the patient, as is often difficult to convince many patients that their condition could have a psychiatric component.

7.1.2 Diagnosis

Investigating the possible diagnosis of psychogenic pruritus, it is important to rule out medical, dermatologic, and neuropathic causes.

In case of psychogenic pruritus, dermatitis is not generally present, but a great range of secondary skin manifestations can be seen. Skin lesions are generally found on areas accessible by the patient sparing other body areas such as the midback.

In patients with pruritus, a complete physical examination and a complete medical history collection is essential in order to exclude acariasis of the skin.

In patients with pruritus and no specific skin signs, dermatologists and physicians should exclude any potential organic cause of pruritus and, finally, psychogenic pruritus can be considered a diagnosis of exclusion.

Physicians should investigate for potential alcohol and drug abuse, as many substances can contribute to the sensation of pruritus.

A thorough medical history should be collected and appropriate labwork should be drawn.

Blood exams should consider Complete Blood Count, Erythrocyte Sedimentation Rate, liver, renal and thyroid panel, considering that abnormalities in these fields can contribute to pruritus.

Patients with pruritus should be screened for hepatic and renal disease such as alcoholic liver disease, cholestasis, primary biliary cholangitis, hepatitis B and C, and chronic kidney disease.

If no systemic diseases were detected, the diagnosis of psychogenic pruritus is made.

There are also several signs that indicate that the patient has a psychogenic itch: the disability out of proportion to symptoms, the presence of psychiatric comorbidities (anxiety, depression), often correlating with itch intensity, dysfunctional coping behaviors (helplessness), high number of doctor visits, lack of cutaneous findings, and pruritus of face more likely.

However, the physicians should also consider that a pre-existing skin condition can have triggered the psychiatric issue related to anxiety and pruritus [11–15].

7.2 Treatment

In case of patient with a pre-existing skin condition, dermatologists should focus on the improvement of the skin disease, considering topical and/or systemic medications. Among topical medications, topical corticosteroids and emollients can be considered. Among systemic medications, antihistamines or corticosteroids can be considered.

Dermatologists must remember that, in these cases, the psychiatric consequences of the skin disease (related to anxiety and pruritus) cannot be proportionate to the extent of the disorder.

In the majority of case, dermatologists treat patients with known skin diseases with a worsened pruritus with related psychiatric stress.

The treatment of pruritus with no pre-existing skin disease should include topical therapies, injections, or anticonvulsants.

For patients with an obsessive–compulsive component, cognitive behavior therapy has been shown effective.

Therefore, physicians should investigate the presence of obsessive thoughts and compulsive habits in the patients with pruritus: obsessions are recurrent and persistent thoughts, images, or impulses that are experienced as intrusive or inappropriate and cause marked distress and anxiety. Compulsions are negative behaviors that a subject needs to perform according to rules that must be rigidly applied or reacting to an obsession [11–15].

7.2.1 Prurigo Nodularis

Prurigo nodularis is an uncommon compulsive skin disorder characterized by intense pruritus associated with the habit of compulsive and repetitive manipulation of the skin, leading to pruritic papulo-nodular skin lesions with similar characteristics if compared with classic excoriation disorders.

In patients with prurigo nodularis, we can identify the classic characteristics of compulsive habits: compulsions are negative behaviors that a subject needs to perform according to rules that must be rigidly applied or reacting to an obsession.

The habit of the patient to the repetitive, compulsive, and recurrent manipulation of the skin induces the onset of multiple erythematous, hyperkeratotic papules and nodules, involving typically the legs and arms with symmetric distribution. The body areas where the patient cannot reach are usually spared [16–18].

7.3 Diagnosis and Pathophysiology

The diagnosis of prurigo nodularis is essentially clinic, based on the observation of typical nodular lesions induced by the repetitive scratching. Skin biopsy is not routinely necessary.

Patients with prurigo nodularis have intense pruritus present from at least 6 weeks, sometimes associated with burning or stinging sensations.

An accurate collection of dermatological history of the patient, including pre-existing or previous skin dermatoses, such as atopic dermatitis, can be useful in the diagnostic process.

A complete medical history about previous or concomitant diagnosed psychiatric comorbidities can also be helpful.

The pathophysiology of prurigo nodularis is not well understood. However, factors related to immune and neural dysregulation seem to be implicated in the pathogenesis of prurigo nodularis: immune cells and neuropeptides are involved in the pathogenesis of skin inflammation, while altered neural circuits are involved in the pathogenesis of pruritus.

The result of these complex interactions is a vicious cycles of chronic pruritus followed by repeated scratching.

Sometimes, patients with prurigo nodularis can have a pre-existing primary pruritic skin disease, in most of cases atopic dermatitis. Patients with atopic dermatitis are at greater risk to develop prurigo nodularis and have an early onset of prurigo nodularis if compared to patients without atopic dermatitis.

Furthermore, patients with prurigo nodularis seem to have a greater risk to develop psychiatric comorbidities, such as anxiety and depression, especially in female patients.

Furthermore, prurigo nodularis is a severe and generally chronic disease with a great impact on the quality of life, with patients having the third worst self-reported health among other skin disorders.

The lack of efficacious treatments and the common association with psychiatric comorbidities made this disease a challenging condition for dermatologists [16–18].

7.4 Treatment and Management

In patients with prurigo nodularis, the diagnostic workup should include a complete blood cell count with differential liver and renal function exams.

The management and treatment of patients with prurigo nodularis is very challenging, also considering the importance of psychological and/or psychiatric evaluation.

Dermatological therapy for prurigo nodularis is essentially based on topical, intralesional, and systemic neuroimmune modulatory treatments, with the aim to break a short-circuited itch-scratch cycle.

There are currently no approved topical therapies for prurigo nodularis; topical corticosteroids, pimecrolimus, and calcipotriol showed limited evidence of efficacy.

About systemic treatments, dupilumab (a human monoclonal antibody against IL-4 receptor alpha inhibiting IL-4 and IL-13 signaling), was recently approved by the Food and Drug Administration as the first and unique drug specifically indicated for prurigo nodularis in adult patients [16–18].

7.4.1 Lichen Simplex

Lichen simplex is a common form of chronic neurodermatitis, presenting as dry, patchy areas of skin which are thick and scaly, with a hypertrophic epidermis resulting of repetitive rubbing or scratching of a specific skin area. The etiology of lichen simplex is usually related to psychological factors or, in some cases, could be secondary to other cutaneous diseases such as eczema or psoriasis. The common development of skin plaques is the result of the itching dermatoses that typically result from the psychological stressors.

Clinical evidence reported a link between lichen simplex and emotional factors, which often results in repeated and cyclic itching. The most common involved areas are self-accessible areas of the body, including the scalp, neck, head, arms, and hands.

The irritation and the need to constantly scratch induced by the emotional stress, is often cyclic, inducing plaques, chronic itching, alterations of skin pigmentations.

The perception of itch and changes involved in lichen simplex is related to central and peripheral neural tissue and to several inflammatory mediators.

Furthermore, it should be considered that itching could be related to several psychiatric and psychological conditions, such as anxiety, obsessive–compulsive disorder, and depression.

Managing patients with lichen simplex, dermatologists should also consider that these patients have high risk of the aforementioned psychiatric comorbidities.

The treatment of lichen simplex can include several topical therapies: occlusion of the area, anti-inflammatory drugs (essentially corticosteroids), but also topical inhibitors of calcineurin (tacrolimus or pimecrolimus) and/or emollients with specific anti-pruritus properties. In the most severe cases, systemic medications can be used (essentially antihistamines).

Not less important is to consider the role of psychological treatment, such as psychotherapy as well as correlate systemic drugs, such as anti-anxiety treatments, which can help the patient, considering the etiological nature of the disorder. Surgical therapeutic options may include cryosurgery.

However, the outcomes of lichen simplex depend on the primary cause; if the patient has a mental health disorder and it is not managed, the disorder can become chronic, leading to a very poor quality of life [19–23].

7.4.2 *Acne excoriée*

Acne excoriée is an acne variant and excoriation disorder, characterized by the repetitive and uncontrollable scratching, picking, and squeezing of the inflammatory skin lesions by patients. The lesions of acne excoriée commonly evolve in skin erosions, ulcerations, and scarring in the long-term period. The term "Acne excoriee" was first described by Brock in 1898 as "acne excoriee des jeunes filles," which means "excoriated acne of young females." The age onset may vary between 11 and 40.4 years. Even the condition is more common among female adolescents, and it can also be seen in males.

It is not clear yet the question of why in some patients with acne the disease evolves into the form of acne excoriée. However, several evidence suggest an underlying impulsive behavior, as most of these patients show psychiatric comorbidities which seem to play a central role in the etiology of acne excoriée, such as obsessive–compulsive disorder, anxiety disorder, and body dysmorphic disorder.

Furthermore, an association between acne picking and the non-planning facet of impulsivity in patients with acne excoriée was demonstrated. Therefore, it could be helpful to investigate in terms of impulsivity the acne patients in order to predict the course of the disease and to consider treatments that affect impulse control in patients.

In clinical practice, managing patients with acne excoriée is very challenging, considering the common overlapping with associated psychiatric component [24, 25].

7.4.3 *Trichotillomania*

Trichotillomania (also called "hair-pulling disorder") is a compulsive disorder characterized by a recurrent, repetitive, impulsive, and irresistible urges to pull out hair from the scalp, eyebrows, or other areas of the body.

Hair pulling from the scalp often leaves patchy bald spots, inducing significant distress, also interfering with social life or work functioning of the patient.

The prevalence of trichotillomania ranges between 0.6% and 4%, with the highest incidence in females and in children and adolescents.

Trichotillomania is usually preceded by an increase in inner tension and anxiety, which is reduced by pulling out hair. The increase in tension and the neutralization through compulsive–obsessive behaviors is similar to the symptoms and emotional feelings of patients with trichotillomania. However, some patients even experience feelings of guilt and shame after pulling their hair. Patients affected by trichotillomania attempt to hide the body areas with hair loss implementing several habits, such as inappropriately wearing sunglasses, wigs, or excessive makeup. In this way, the patient attracts even more attention, exposing him to ridicule by others, often resulting in social withdrawal and symptoms of depression.

Furthermore, patients affected by trichotillomania for several months or years could develop several physical complications, such as carpal tunnel syndrome due to overuse of the wrists or, in patients with trichophagia, gastrointestinal diseases caused by ingested hair [26, 27].

7.5 Risk Factors

Several risk factors related to trichotillomania have been detected.

- Age: this disorder usually onset before or during adolescence, most often between 10 and 13 years.
- Sex: females seem at higher risk compared with males.
- Family history: genetic factors can play a role in the development of trichotillomania. Patients with a close relative affected by this disorder can be at higher risk to develop it.
- Psychiatric disorders: people who have trichotillomania may have psychiatric comorbidities, such as anxiety, depression, anxiety, or obsessive–compulsive disorders.
- Stress: severely stressful or traumatic situations or events may act as a trigger factor for the onset of trichotillomania.

7.6 Diagnosis

Patients with trichotillomania commonly come to the attention of dermatologist for the evaluation and treatment of alopecia in the involved body area. Alopecia in these patients is usually characterized by round patches of incomplete and irregular hair loss. The scalp usually does not show inflammation signs. Potentially, trichotillomania could induce alopecia in all body areas (lashes, eyebrows, and pubic hair).

In case of suspected trichotillomania, dermoscopic examination of the involved area could be very useful for dermatologists, showing hair broken at different heights.

The diagnostic process in patients with suspected trichotillomania is often complicated by the overlap between trichotillomania and other psychiatric and psychological disorders (obsessive–compulsive disorders and severe structural personality disorders).

Trichotillomania represents a multifactorial disorder, in which evolutionary biology, neurobiology, genetic and psychodynamic factors play a role.

Most of patients with trichotillomania can also show deficits in regulating emotions and in perceiving and express emotions (alexithymia).

An early detection and diagnosis of trichotillomania is essentially in order to early identify possible psychiatric comorbidities; in fact, an adequate and early treatment of the underlying psychiatric disease lead to an improvement of the skin condition.

Psychopharmacological and psychotherapeutic treatments should be used first line according to the diagnosis, depending on the presence of a comorbid DSM-IV disorder or a personality disorder. In this context, a psychiatric evaluation is essential as there is no standard pharmacological treatment for factitious disorder [26, 27].

7.6.1 Trichotemnomania

Trichotemnomania (term derived from Greek—"temnein"—to cut) is an obsessive–compulsive disorder characterized by the habit of the patient to cut the hair with scissors or to shave hair with a razor, in the context of an obsessive–compulsive disorder.

Obsessions are recurrent and persistent thoughts, images, or impulses that are experienced as intrusive or inappropriate and cause marked distress and anxiety. Compulsions are negative behaviors that a subject needs to perform according to rules that must be rigidly applied or reacting to an obsession.

Trichotemnomania should not be confused with trichotillomania, which is characterized by tonsural patterns of hairlessness and irregular length of hair shafts.

Very few cases of trichotemnomania are described and reported in literature although this disorder is probably under-diagnosed.

Trichotemnomania shares with trichotillomania the characteristic that the patients are very resistant to admitting their habit and often the patients had a history of multiple dermatologic and other medical consultations without reaching the diagnosis.

Trichotemnomania clinically is characterized by a loss of scalp hair, but can also occur in other locations (such as the eyebrows, axilla, or pubis). The hair is usually cut with scissors or shaved, and the diagnostic key is the evidence of follicle openings with filled hair shafts with a healthy scalp.

In contrast to trichotillomania, trichotemnomania has no diagnostic histopathological features and has a normal trichogram.

Psychopharmacological and psychotherapeutic treatments should be used first line according to the diagnosis, depending on the presence of a comorbid DSM-IV disorder or a personality disorder. In this context, a psychiatric evaluation is essential as there is no standard pharmacological treatment for factitious disorder [27–29].

7.6.2 Trichoteiromania

Trichoteiromania is an obsessive–compulsive disorder ("teiro," of Greek derivation meaning "I rub"), characterized by hair loss subsequent to rubbing of the hairs, causing splitting and breakage of the hairs. Clinically, the result is bald spots with hair of different length, which may be similar to hair cutting with scissors. At the end of the hair shafts are evident white tips and brush-like ends of the hair, which are the hallmark of trichoteiromania. Light microscopy of the hair shafts revealed brush-like cracking of the ends.

Hair loss in patients with trichoteiromania is the consequence of chronic rubbing of the scalp hairs resulting in brush-like splitting of the ends.

In contrast to trichotillomania, trichoteiromania has no diagnostic histopathological features and has a normal trichogram.

Psychopharmacological and psychotherapeutic treatments should be used first line according to the diagnosis, depending on the presence of a comorbid DSM-IV disorder or a personality disorder. In this context, a psychiatric evaluation is essential as there is no standard pharmacological treatment for factitious disorder [29, 30].

7.6.3 Onychophagia

Onychophagia is a chronic habitual nail-biting behavior. The onset of onychophagia is usually during childhood or adolescence, and this condition affects approximately 20–30% of the general population. Its prevalence is assumed to be low and underestimated, as many patients are ashamed or socially inclined to admit nail biting.

Physicians in several fields, such as dermatology, pediatrics, and psychiatry may be faced with this condition.

Onychophagia could be associated with disorder of nail unit and orodental complications, which may significantly have an impact on the quality of life.

Onychophagia cannot be considered as a cosmetic problem or an innocuous behavior. In fact, it was demonstrated that chronic nail biting may cause significant dental alterations, such as malocclusion, gingival recession, or incisor rotation. Onychophagia may also cause severe local complications, such as infections of the tissue around the nails, irreversible fingernail shortening, or formation of epidermoid cysts.

Nail biting can also have negative psychological and social effects on patients, especially considering that in most of cases the disorder has the onset during the adolescence [31–39].

7.6.4 Onychotillomania

Onychotillomania (named by Jan Alkiewicz, a Polish dermatologist) is a condition characterized by compulsive behaviors inducing the person to picks constantly at the nails or tries to tear them off.

It should be clearly distinguished from onychophagia, where the nails are chewed or bitten.

Onychotillomania can be categorized in the DSM-5 as a body-focused repetitive behavior in the DSM-5 in the category of excoriation disorder.

Onychotillomania is clinically characterized by alterations of the nail bed, with onychodystrophy, paronychia, and darkening of the nail.

Some cases have been treated successfully with antipsychotics.

A cheap solution suggested by some authors is to cover the proximal nail fold with a cyanoacrylate glue, realizing a physic obstacle to picking [40–44].

7.6.5 *Factitious Cheilitis*

Factitious cheilitis is a compulsive disorder characterized by lip crusting, localized crusting, or artifactual and exfoliative cheilitis, often associated with crusts and ulcerative lesions.

This condition is based on a self-induced trauma related to compulsive and repetitive picking, biting, or licking of the lips.

Compulsions are negative behaviors that a subject needs to perform according to rules that must be rigidly applied or reacting to an obsession.

The prevalence is higher in young women, but factitious cheilitis could be observed in any age group in males and females.

The etiopathogenesis of factitious cheilitis is unknown and the underlying motivations of the behaviors are unconscious.

Psychological and psychiatric factors involved in the pathogenesis of factitious cheilitis were proposed, suggesting that these patients could show a nervous instability, status of anxiety or depression, or borderline personality disorders.

However, patients often have immature coping skills, not matching any effective category of personality disorder. On the other hand, poor coping may be part of several personality disorders, such as borderline personality or dependent and narcissistic personality traits.

In the differential diagnosis of crusted and ulcerated lesions of the lips area, several conditions should be considered, such as atopic dermatitis, cheilitis, actinic damage, contact dermatitis, photosensitivity reactions, and neoplasia.

Psychopharmacological and psychotherapeutic treatments should be used first line according to the diagnosis, depending on the presence of a comorbid DSM-IV disorder or a personality disorder. In this context, is essential a psychiatric evaluation, as there is no standard pharmacological treatment for factitious disorder [45–48].

7.6.6 Morsicatio Buccarum

Morsicatio buccarum is a type of frictional keratosis. It is a condition characterized by repetitive chewing, biting, or nibbling inducing chronic irritation or injury to the buccal mucosa (the lining of the inside of the cheek within the mouth).

The involved areas are usually mucosa, bilaterally in the central part of the anterior buccal mucosa and along the level of the occlusal plane. In some cases, the labial mucosa tongue or the labial mucosa is affected by similar lesions, called "morsicatio linguarum" and "morsicatio labiorum," respectively.

The lesions are white with shredding and thickening of mucosa, usually combined with areas characterize by erythema or ulceration.

Morsicatio buccarum is a disorder related to a chronic parafunctional activity of the masticatory system, which induces crushing, frictional and incisive damage to the mucosal surface and over time the characteristic mucosal lesions.

In some cases, poorly constructed prosthetic teeth could be the cause if the original bite is altered. Similar or more severe damage may be caused by self-mutilation in people with learning disabilities or psychiatric disorders.

The diagnosis of morsicatio buccarum is usually based on the clinical evidence and on the observation of the lesions; the biopsy is not generally necessary. The histologic characteristics of lesions involved in morsicatio buccarum are marked hyperparakeratosis, vacuolated cells in the upper portion of the prickle cell layer and superficial colonization by bacteria [45–49].

7.6.7 Pseudo-Knuckle Pads

Knuckle pads have been described for the first time by Garrod in 1893. Knuckle pads are also known as athlete's nodules, discrete keratoderma, subcutaneous fibroma, keratosis supracapitularis, and tylositas articuli.

Knuckle pad is a condition characterized by discrete fibromatosis with well-defined, mobile, dome-shaped plaque-like or nodule lesions. These lesions usually seem flesh-colored or hyperpigmented and commonly involve the proximal interphalangeal joints over the dorsal surface of fingers more than toes. The metacarpophalangeal or distal interphalangeal joints could be involved by knuckle pads.

Skin lesions are usually asymptomatic and not associated with rheumatology symptoms.

Knuckle pads can be differentiated in two categories: inherited (primary) knuckle pads or secondary (acquired) knuckle pads (pseudo knuckle pads). Most of the inherited cases of knuckle pads are idiopathic; however, in some cases knuckle pads could be associated with several fibromatosis disorders (such as palmar Dupuytren contracture, plantar Ledderhose disease). Secondary knuckle pads are usually called "pseudo knuckle pads" and should be recognized separately, considering that clinical and management approaches are different.

Pseudo knuckle pads usually appear in childhood and adolescence. Skin lesions of pseudo knuckle pads are hyperkeratotic and appear secondary to chronic friction or repeated trauma, but they could also be associated with several psychiatric disorders (such as chewing or sucking fingers, bulimia nervosa) or with particular occupational or athletic/sport activities, such as surfing or boxing. The diagnosis of knuckle pads is essentially clinic, based on the observation of clinical features of lesions. However, some further investigations could be considered to rule out differential diagnosis. Ultrasound shows a subcutaneous hypoechoic nodule without vascularization on color Doppler. Histologic examination of knuckle pads shows acanthosis, hyperkeratosis, and proliferation of myofibroblasts with a decrease of elastic filaments in the deep dermis [50, 51].

References

1. Zhu TH, Nakamura M, Farahnik B, et al. Obsessive-compulsive skin disorders: a novel classification based on degree of insight. J Dermatolog Treat. 2017;28(4):342–6.
2. Mavrogiorgou P, Bader A, Stockfleth E, Juckel G. Obsessive-compulsive disorder in dermatology. J Dtsch Dermatol Ges. 2015;13(10):991–9.
3. Leon A, Levin EC, Koo YM. Psychodermatology: an overview. Semin Cutan Med Surg. 2013;32:64–7.
4. Sheikhmoonesi F, Hajheidari Z, Masoudzadeh A, et al. Prevalence and severity of obsessive-compulsive disorder and their relationships with dermatological diseases. Acta Med Iran. 2014;52:511–4.
5. Garcia-Soriano G, Rufer M, Delsignore A, et al. Factors associated with non-treatment or delayed treatment seeking in OCD sufferers: a review of the literature. Psychiatry Res. 2014;220(1–2):1–10.
6. Buteau A, Reichenberg J. Psychogenic pruritus and its management. Dermatol Clin. 2018;36(3):309–14.
7. Misery L, Dutray S, Chastaing M, Schollhammer M, Consoli SG, Consoli SM. Psychogenic itch. Transl Psychiatry. 2018;8(1):52.
8. Dalgard F, Lien L, Dalen I. Itch in the community: associations with psychosocial factor among adults. J Eur Acad Dermatol Venereol. 2007;21:1215–9.
9. Picardi A, Abeni D, Melchi CF, et al. Psychiatric morbidity in dermatological outpatients: an issue to be recognized. Br J Dermatol. 2000;143:983–91.
10. Radmanesh M, Shafiei S. Underlying psychopathologies of psychogenic pruritic disorder. Dermatol Psychosom. 2001;2:130–3.
11. Schneider G, Driesch G, Heuft G, et al. Psychosomatic cofactors and psychiatric comorbidity in patients with chronic itch. Clin Exp Dermatol. 2006;31:762–7.
12. Swarna SS, Aziz K, Zubair T, Qadir N, Khan M. Pruritus associated with chronic kidney disease: a comprehensive literature review. Cureus. 2019;11(7):e5256.
13. Suh KN, Keystone JS. 153 - Delusional parasitosis. In: Magill AJ, Hill DR, Solomon T, Ryan ET, editors. Hunter's tropical medicine and emerging infectious disease. 9th ed. London: W.B. Saunders; 2013. p. 1074–8.
14. Savas JA, Pichardo RO. Female genital itch. Dermatol Clin. 2018;36(3):225–43.
15. Lee HG, Stull C, Yosipovitch G. Psychiatric disorders and pruritus. Clin Dermatol. 2017;35(3):273–80.
16. Tan WS, Tey HL. Extensive prurigo nodularis: characterization and etiology. Dermatology. 2014;228:276–80.

17. Schneider G, Hockmann J, Stumpf A. Psychosomatic aspects of prurigo nodularis. Hautarzt. 2014;65:704–8.
18. Williams KA, Huang AH, Belzberg M, Kwatra SG. Prurigo nodularis: pathogenesis and management. J Am Acad Dermatol. 2020;83(6):1567–75.
19. Muylaert BPB, Borges MT, Michalany AO, Scuotto CRC. Lichen simplex chronicus on the scalp: exuberant clinical, dermoscopic, and histopathological findings. An Bras Dermatol. 2018;93(1):108–10.
20. Voicu C, Tebeica T, Zanardelli M, Mangarov H, Lotti T, Wollina U, Lotti J, França K, Batashki A, Tchernev G. Lichen simplex chronicus as an essential part of the dermatologic masquerade. Open Access Maced J Med Sci. 2017;5(4):556–7.
21. Fruchter R, Melnick L, Pomeranz MK. Lichenoid vulvar disease: a review. Int J Women's Dermatol. 2017;3(1):58–64.
22. Day T, Bohl TG, Scurry J. Perianal lichen dermatoses: a review of 60 cases. Australas J Dermatol. 2016;57(3):210–5.
23. Liao YH, Lin CC, Tsai PP, Shen WC, Sung FC, Kao CH. Increased risk of lichen simplex chronicus in people with anxiety disorder: a nationwide population-based retrospective cohort study. Br J Dermatol. 2014;170(4):890–4.
24. Öğüt Ç, Öğüt ND. Impulsivity in patients with acne excoriee. J Cosmet Dermatol. 2023;22(3):1099–104.
25. Zaenglein A, Thiboutot D. Acne vulgaris. In: Bolognia J, Jorizzo L, Schaffer J, et al., editors. Dermatology. Elsevier; 2012. p. 549.
26. Huynh M, Gavino AC, Magid M. Trichotillomania. Semin Cutan Med Surg. 2013;32:88–94.
27. Happle R. Trichotemnomania: obsessive-compulsive habit of cutting or shaving the hair. J Am Acad Dermatol. 2005;52(1):157–9.
28. Orgaz-Molina J, Husein-Elahmed H, Soriano-Hernández MI, Arias-Santiago S. Trichotemnomania: hair loss mediated by a compulsive habit not admitted by patients. Acta Derm Venereol. 2012;92(2):183–4.
29. Obsessive-compulsive disorder. In: American Psychiatric Association: Diagnostic and statistical manual of mental disorders. 4th ed, text revision. Washington, DC: American Psychiatric Association, 2000. p. 457.
30. Banky JP, Sheridan AT, Dawber RP. Weathering of hair in trichoteiromania. Australas J Dermatol. 2004;45(3):186–8.
31. Shin JO, Roh D, Son JH, et al. Onychophagia: detailed clinical characteristics. Int J Dermatol. 2022;61(3):331–6.
32. de Berker D. Childhood nail diseases. Dermatol Clin. 2006;24:355–63.
33. Pacan P, Reich A, Grzesiak M, Szepietowski JC. Onychophagia is associated with impairment of quality of life. Acta Dermato-Venereologica. 2014;94:703–6.
34. Ghanizadeh A, Shekoohi H. Prevalence of nail biting and its association with mental health in a community sample of children. BMC Res Notes. 2011;4:116.
35. Halteh P, Scher RK, Lipner SR. Onychophagia: a nail-biting conundrum for physicians. J Dermatol Treat. 2017;28:166–72.
36. Alessandri Bonetti G, Incerti Parenti S, Zucchelli G. Onychophagia and postorthodontic isolated gingival recession: diagnosis and treatment. Am J Orthod Dentofacial Orthop. 2012;142:872–8.
37. Sachan A, Chaturvedi TP. Onychophagia (nail biting), anxiety, and malocclusion. Indian J Dent Res. 2012;23:680–2.
38. Van Tongel A, De Paepe P, Berghs B. Epidermoid cyst of the phalanx of the finger caused by nail biting. J Plast Surg Hand Surg. 2012;46:450–1.
39. Ghanizadeh A. Nail biting; etiology, consequences and management. Iran J Med Sci. 2011;36:73–9. 22. Lee DY. Chronic nail biting and irreversible shortening of the fingernails. J Eur Acad Dermatol Venereol 2009;23:185.
40. Ameen Sait M, Reddy BS, Garg BR. Onychotillomania. 2 case reports. Dermatologica. 1985;171(3):200–2.

41. Kim MH, Park HJ, Lee JY, Cho BK. Two cases of Onychotillomania. Korean J Dermatol (in Korean). 2006;44(7):855–7.
42. Harth W, Gieler U, Kusnir D, Tausk F. Clinical management of psychodermatology. Berlin: Springer; 2009. p. 21.
43. Baran R. Nail biting and picking as a possible cause of longitudinal melanonychia. A study of 6 cases. Dermatologica. 1990;181(2):126–8.
44. Ring DS. Inexpensive solution for habit-tic deformity. Arch Dermatol. 2010;146(11):1222–3.
45. Aydin E, Gokoglu O, Ozcurumez G, Aydin H. Factitious cheilitis: a case report. J Med Case Rep. 2008;2:29.
46. Rogers RS 3rd, Bekic M. Diseases of the lips. Semin Cutan Med Surg. 1997;16:328–36. https://doi.org/10.1016/S1085-5629(97)80025-9.
47. Calobrisi SD, Baselga E, Miller ES, Esterly NB. Factitial cheilitis in an adolescent. Pediatr Dermatol. 1999;16:12–5.
48. Daley TD, Gupta AK. Exfoliative cheilitis. J Oral Pathol Med. 1995;24:177–9.
49. Bouquot JE, Neville BW, Damm DD, Allen CM. Oral & maxillofacial pathology. 2nd ed. Philadelphia: W.B. Saunders; 2002. p. 253–4.
50. Cunliffe T. Knuckle pads. Primary Care Dermatology Society (PCDS) website. 2020.
51. Line M, Farah E, Mariame M, Karima S. Pseudo-knuckle pads a bridge to psychodermatology. J Clin Case Rep Stud. 2022;4(2):120.

Chapter 8
Cutaneous Diseases Precipitated or Perpetuated by Emotional Factors

Luca Stingeni, Katharina Hansel, and Elisa Cecchini

8.1 Atopic Dermatitis

Atopic dermatitis (AD) is a chronic-relapsing inflammatory skin disease characterized by the presence of eczema in multiple areas of the body with erythema, edema, crusting, excoriation, lichenification, and diffuse xerosis as main clinical features and characterized by severe itch and often sleep loss.

Recent data about the estimated prevalence of AD differs according to age groups with higher rates in children which are affected between 10–20% and lower in adults with 2–8% [1, 2] and geriatric patients with 1–3% [3]. Most typical and frequent onset is in early childhood (<2 years) and in adult patients (20–60 years); childhood (2–12 years) and adolescent (12–18 years) onset are a little less common, and a late-onset in patients with more than 60 years is rare. Given the chronic nature of the dermatosis, patients with AD will experience phases of relapses and remission throughout their lives but sometimes, when atopic dermatitis appears in early childhood, patients can experience complete remission in a few years [4, 5].

Eczemas can develop in every part of the body but in AD mainly occur in the flexural areas of the limbs, like the antecubital/popliteal fossae, and on the face and neck area. Usually, eczemas have a round or ovalar shape of centimetric size, which can merge into wider areas in severe cases, and they can have an acute or chronic course. Acute eczema is characterized by erythematous-edematous areas that are sometimes exuding and crusty as a result of scratching, while chronic eczema presents with intense lichenification, desquamation and hypo-hyperchromic scarring. During flares, coexistence of acute and chronic eczema is possible [4]. When atopic dermatitis

L. Stingeni · K. Hansel · E. Cecchini (✉)
Department of Medicine and Surgery, Dermatology Section, University of Perugia, Perugia, Italy
e-mail: luca.stingeni@unipg.it; katharina.hansel@unipg.it; elisa.cecchini@specializzandi.unipg.it;

G. Angelini et al. (eds.), *Psychocutaneous Diseases*,
https://doi.org/10.1007/978-3-031-70296-9_8

involves the face, the most frequent findings are erythema and xerosis of the periocular/perioral regions and fissurative cheilitis although in infants <1 year also checks and scalp can be involved [4]. Other suggestive facial signs of atopic dermatitis are paleness of the face, the presence of Dennie-Morgan folds (several linear wrinkles beneath the lower eyelids), the Hertoghe sign (thinning or loss of the outer third of the eyebrows), and periorbital darkening [1]. Nipple eczemas and hand and foot involvement are other possible, sometimes isolated, localizations of atopic eczema. However, in some patients, especially adults, elementary lesions of AD can differ from the classic eczema and mimic other dermatosis: these morphological variants are known as nummular, psoriasis, seborrheic, prurigo-like, lichenified, and follicular ones. Lastly, when almost the entire skin surface is involved, atopic dermatits is called erythrodermic.

AD pathogenesis is complex: genetic disorders, defects in the epidermal barrier, imbalance of the skin's bacterial flora, and an altered immune response are the most important factors. Mutations of gene encoding for filaggrin, a structural protein of epidermis, or other genes that codes for epidermal barrier elements, can impair skin integrity leading to increased transepidermal water loss, skin dryness, penetration of allergens, higher pH of surface and favouring imbalance of skin microbiota. Reduction of normal bacteria of skin (*Streptococcus, Corynebacterium, Cutibacterium*) with an increase of staphylococcal colonization has been associated with AD development. Moreover, an excessive differentiation of CD4 lymphocytes in Th2 way, which leads to high production of IL-4, IL-5, IL-13, IgE, and eosinophils, plays a key role in AD pathogenesis [6]. Research of last decades indicates that glucocorticoids released in stressful situations may promote Th2 differentiation, suggesting how psychological stress can influence disease trend and relapses. In fact, AD patients may have an acute response to stress in terms of T-cell and mast cell activation, hypothalamic-pituitary-adrenal (HPA) axis dysregulation and neurogenic inflammatory mediator release [7]. Excessive cytokine production may activate brain microglia, a mechanism supposedly underlying depression and anxiety which are frequent comorbidities in patients with chronic diseases, including AD [8].

Allergic asthma, rhino-conjunctivitis with sensitization to pollen and house dust, and allergy to metals or foods are the most frequent comorbidities in patients with atopic dermatitis. Sometimes high levels of IgE in serum can be found, but this finding does not seem to correlate with disease severity neither to predict response to therapies. Patients with atopic dermatitis are more prone to develop skin bacterial, viral, and fungal infections than healthy people due to impaired skin barrier. An increased cardiovascular risk is discussed. AD is associated with higher rates of anxiety, depression, and sometimes suicide that all directly correlate with severity of AD [9]. The emotional burden of AD can be evaluated through many questionnaires like Dermatology Life Quality Index (DLQI), SCORAD, or Patient Oriented Eczema Measure (POEM) that allows physicians to monitor changes and impact of disease in patient life. Signs and symptoms of AD like red inflamed skin, scaling, oozing, itch, skin pain, and sleep disturbance are the most burdensome problems that limit patients activities and relationships with consequences depending on the age of dermatitis onset and evolution. In children and adolescents, sleep disturbances can reduce school performance and the presence of eczema, especially on visible areas, can lead to episodes of bullying, isolation, and problems in sexual sphere. In young patients also caregivers can experience the burden of the disease with low sleep quality and deteriorated psycho-emotional state due to unpredictable recurrent flares despite therapies. Occupational problems and low quality of life are more common in adults [10–12]. Presence of anxiety and depressive symptoms may suggest a more aggressive treatment to achieve better AD control and impairment of mental health.

The diagnosis of atopic dermatitis is mostly clinical since there are no specific tests or pathognomonic signs; without an appropriate clinical contest not even histological examination is decisive because it usually shows nonspecific features like spongiosis, perivascular dermal infiltration, and acanthosis. Differential diagnosis between atopic dermatitis and other skin diseases is influenced by morphology of the lesions, history, comorbidities, triggers, and the presence of atopy in first-degree relatives of the patient. Scabies, tinea, psoriasis, pityriasis rosea, seborrheic dermatitis, adverse drug reaction, T cell lymphomas (especially in erythrodermic forms), and Paget disease for nipple localization are some examples. Allergic and irritant contact dermatitis also need to be investigated through patch testing when atopic dermatitis is suspected because they can mimic this dermatosis and often coexist/overlap with it. In fact, frequent use of topical medication, emollients and impaired skin barrier enhances risk of contact sensitization [1]. Depending on each patient, blood examinations, microbiological, allergological testing, and eventually biopsies may be necessary.

Choice of therapy is guided by multiple factors: disease severity, patient's age, daily habits, and local legislations. All patients with AD must follow some daily precautions like the use of emollients, especially after the shower to help reduce the epidermic water loss, oil baths, and the avoidance of products that contain common allergens to prevent sensitizations. Based on severity, that can be mild, moderate, or severe and which is mainly evaluated with the EASI score, BSA calculation (body surface area) and quality of life questionnaires listed above, therapy will range from topical to systemic drugs. Topical steroids and topical inhibitor of calcineurin are the first-line medications and are followed by phototherapy, oral steroids, just recommended for the management of severe flares in short periods, oral immunosuppressants like cyclosporin A (methotrexate, azathioprine, and mycophenolate mofetil are used off-label), and eventually to biological therapies that target IL-4/IL-13 (dupilumab, tralokinumab and lebrikizumab) or JAK-inhibitors (upadacitinib, abrocitinib, baricitinib). In patients with high disease burden, psychotherapy can be helpful, along with pharmacological treatment, to improve quality of life [12, 13].

8.2 Psoriasis

Psoriasis is a chronic immune-mediated inflammatory disorder that affects the skin, joints, and that has strong association with some systemic diseases. It is characterized by well-circumscribed, erythematous papules and plaques covered with silvery scales and predominantly affect the extensor surfaces of the limbs.

Approximately 125 million people are affected worldwide with variable prevalence across countries. Psoriasis has a bimodal age distribution with the first peak between 18 and 39 years and the second between 50 and 69 years [14].

Clinically, psoriasis can manifest in plaque, flexural, guttate, pustular, or erythrodermic form. These main presentations differ among them for the aspect of the elementary lesion, for the triggers and clinical course. Sometimes, in the same patients, two or more types of psoriasis can coexist. In 80% of patients, psoriasis manifests itself with the classic well-demarcated pink plaques covered with silvery-white scales whose removal cause bleeding point spots (Auspitz sign). Plaque psoriasis, also known as psoriasis vulgaris, has a typical symmetrical distribution mainly affecting extensor surfaces like elbows and knees, trunk, and scalp. However, psoriatic lesions can appear at any site and when they appear in an area of skin where previous trauma has occurred this is called Koebner's phenomenon [15]. Flexural psoriasis involves inguinal and inframammary folds, axillae, retroauricular, perianal area, umbilicus and sometimes interdigital spaces, antecubital and popliteal fossae: scales are minimal or absent with the surface of lesions looking moist, smooth, shiny often fissured [16]. The guttate form (GP) has different epidemiological, clinical, and histological characteristics. GP is characterized by several small "drop-like" scaly plaques on trunk and limbs that frequently appears 1–3 weeks after an acute infection like streptococcal tonsillitis. It is more frequent in children and adolescents than in adults and has a good prognosis because sometimes can resolve even without treatment after weeks or months following its appearance [17]. Pustular psoriasis is characterized by 2–3 mm sterile pustules overlying erythematous skin often accompanied by systemic symptoms and malaise. Pustules occur especially at the edges of expanding erythematous plaques and can coalesce into wider areas finally resolving with desquamation; when nail bed and matrix are affected, onychodystrophy may occur. Pustular psoriasis can be limited or generalized: palmoplantar forms and acrodermatitis continua of Hallopeau are peculiar localizations. In annular pustular psoriasis, lesions have a polycyclic distribution. Impetigo herpetiformis is a GPP (generalised pustular psoriasis) in pregnant women, a dangerous condition because of its both maternal and fetal morbidity [18]. Lastly, erythrodermic psoriasis is defined as prominent erythema and scaling affecting 75–90% of body surface area: the extensive cutaneous involvement impairs the homeostatic function of skin and can lead to dehydration, electrolytes imbalances, pruritus, fever, asthenia, and lymphadenopathy. Triggers of EP can be infections, withdrawal of systemic corticosteroids, and severe emotional stress [19]. Nail alterations can be observed in almost 80% of patients with psoriasis, sometimes preceding skin and joint involvement, and are associated with more severe disease, earlier onset, and a higher risk of psoriatic arthritis. In the 6% of cases, nail psoriasis can be the only manifestation of disease. Pitting, leukonychia, dystrophy, splinter hemorrhages, onycholysis, oil-salmon patches, and subungual hyperkeratosis reflect matrix and bed nail affection by psoriasis [20]. Regarding changes in the oral cavity, psoriasis's patient shows a higher prevalence of benign migratory glossitis and fissured tongue [21]. Due to its joint involvement, psoriasis is an inflammatory condition that often requires rheumatological evaluation: in 15–10% of patients, arthritis can precede skin psoriasis. Psoriatic arthritis is a seronegative spondyloarthritis with possible associated enthesitis, dactylitis, and axial involvement that has a similar impact on rheumatoid arthritis on quality of life and functional ability: early diagnosis and treatment are the key to reduce its consequences [22].

Children psoriasis resemble the adult's disease but some features are more characteristics: plaque are smaller and finer, neonatal diaper rash (napkin psoriasis) is relatively specific; guttate psoriasis is more common than in adults and severe scalp psoriasis can present with thick fixed, silver scales called pityriasis amiantacea. Frequency of arthritis increases with age and is exceptional in infants [23].

Psoriasis is a multifactorial disease where genetic, environmental, and behavioral factors interact, being the genetic predisposition probably the most determinant one: in genetically susceptible individuals, skin trauma, infections, smoking, medications such as lithium and interferon, and stress can exacerbate the disease. In psoriasis's pathophysiology, an excessive feed-forward activation of the adaptive immune system determines a high production of cytokines and chemokines like IL-12, and IL-23 that stimulates differentiation and survival of TH1, TH17, and TH22 T helpers that secrete IL-17, IL-22, and TNF α [14]. These cytokines are responsible for the typical histological changes in skin like hyperkeratosis, parakeratosis, acanthosis, and neovascularization that eventually cause the clinical appearance of psoriatic lesions [24].

Psoriasis has a strong association whit metabolic syndrome, obesity, non-alcoholic fatty liver disease, and vascular accident. It is postulated that psoriasis is responsible for different degree of systemic inflammation leading to increased insulin resistance, vascular endothelial damage, atherosclerosis, and myocardial infarction: patients with severe psoriasis have higher risk of cerebral and cardiovascular accidents [25]. Patients with psoriasis have an increased risk of psychological and psychiatric disorderse like depression, anxiety, and suicidal ideation: difficult to treat lesions, especially in visible areas, pruritus, articular pain, and everyday life limitations can reduce quality of life of these patients. On the other side, depression and emotional stress can exacerbate psoriasis through HPA axes resulting in a vicious cycle [26, 27]. DLQI, as for the atopic dermatitis and other skin disease, can help monitoring the impact of psoriasis on patients' mental health.

Diagnosis is mostly clinical, requires an appropriate anamnesis looking for familiarity with psoriasis, triggers and eventually blood tests to evaluate systemic alterations. Biopsies may help when other diseases are suspected: pityriasis lichenoides chronica, pityriasis rosea, secondary syphilis, mycotic infections, acute generalized exanthematous pustulosis, cutaneous lymphomas, allergic contact dermatitis can mimic some psoriasis spectra. In flexural and nail psoriasis, superinfection by bacteria and fungi is frequent [28].

Severity of psoriasis can be evaluated clinically and with the help of IGA, PASI, and BSA score. Topical steroids, alone or in combination with Vitamin D analogs and keratolytics are first-line treatment in mild cases. Topical inhibitor of calcineurin and phototherapy (NB-UVB and PUVA) are other effective options with the latter being used for both localized and extensive areas to treat. Oral treatment for moderate to severe cases comprehends traditional agents such as methotrexate, acitretin, cyclosporine, and apremilast, a phosphodiesterase 4 inhibitor. Biologics for psoriasis treatment represent an effective and safe option: TNFα inhibitors, IL-12/23 inhibitor, IL-17 inhibitors, IL-23 inhibitors and JAK-inhibitors are the main classes used nowadays; most of them are also effective on arthritis [14–22].

8.3 Seborrheic Dermatitis

Seborrheic dermatitis (SD) is a common chronic skin disorder characterized by erythematous plaques with greasy scales on body areas with higher density of sebaceous glands.

SD has a bimodal epidemiological distribution: the first peak is during infancy, in the first months of life and before puberty, while the second one is in early adulthood.

When presenting in infancy, it usually involves symmetrically the diaper and scalp areas, the latter known as cradle cap, but also face, retroauricular area, body folds, and trunk can be affected. In adult patients, the most affected areas are the scalp, nasolabial folds, ears, eyebrows, chest, and presternal region. Itching can be present and sometimes, in severe cases, scales and inflammation can determine a transient hair loss. Seborrheic dermatitis of babies tends to be self-limited, while in adults is more often a chronic condition [29]. Unlike general population which is affected between 1 and 3% with male predilection, immunosuppressed patients have higher rates of SD: HIV/AIDS, previous organ transplant, chronic alcoholic pancreatitis, hepatitis C, and various malignancies can be considered as risk factors. Also patients with neurologic and psychiatric diseases like Parkinson and depression, or patients with genetic disorders such as Down syndrome, Hailey–Hailey disease, and cardio-facio-cutaneous syndrome have higher risk of suffering from SD [30].

Many factors contribute to the development of this skin disorder: interaction between hormonal, immunological, nutritional, environmental, and genetic factors is complex [31]. Malassezia yeasts, normal human skin commensals, may have a causative role in SD inducing an immunologic response in predisposed subjects. Good response to antifungals and higher rates of other fungal diseases such as tinea pedis, onychomycosis, and pityriasis versicolor in patients with SD supports this theory [32]. Furthermore, stress is often reported as a trigger factor [33].

SD is diagnosed clinically: further investigations like biopsies or serologies can help differentiate this condition from others that can present with similar features like atopic dermatitis, lupus, rosacea, acne, tinea, psoriasis, Langerhans cell histiocytosis in children [29] and, anecdotally with leukemia cutis [31].

Several over-the-counter products are available to treat SD containing keratolytic or antifungal agents. Topical or oral antifungal drugs like azoles, ciclopiroxolamina, and allylamine are effective. Corticosteroids can be used alone or in combination with antifungals for short periods and sometimes also topical inhibitors of calcineurin can help reduce associated inflammation [34].

8.4 Alopecia Areata

Alopecia areata (AA) is a common non-scarring hair loss disorder with an unpredictable chronic-relapsing course. Since any body site with pilifer annexes can be affected, AA has an heterogeneous clinical presentation.

Lifetime incidence of AA is approximately 2% with no clear difference between men and women. The age of onset is usually between 20 and 40 years, but an earlier onset is possible and it often correlates with a most severe disease [35].

Clinically, patients with AA presents hairless patches of round or oval shape with a normal skin color and texture on the involved area. The scalp is the most affected site [35]. Dysesthesia, tingling, or itching can precede the hair loss, but normally patients are asymptomatic. Nearly 75% patients present a *patchy* AA pattern that is characterized by the presence of one single or more areas of alopecia. Sometimes patches can be in different phases, some can be active, and thus hair-less, while others can be in remission showing initial re-growth: this clinical presentation is called *alopecia reticularis*. When patient lost the totality of hair alopecia is *totalis* (AT) and if all scalp and body hairs are affected alopecia is *universalis* (AU). Other clinical presentations are the ophiasis (occipital alopecia) and sisaipho (temporal and occipital alopecia) type, the band-like, the perinevoid, the sudden hair whitening and a diffuse pattern of hair loss that mimic androgenic alopecia and telogen effluvium known as alopecia incognita. Isolated involvement of the beard, eyelashes, and eyebrows can occur. Lastly, acute diffuse and total alopecia is a rare form of alopecia characterized by rapid progression and extensive hair loss, but with a favorable prognosis [36]. Nail changes can appear in almost 30% of patients with alopecia, especially in severe cases and in children. Pitting, trachyonychia, red spotted lunulae, onycholysis, Beau's lines and punctate leukonychia are the main findings and can determine functional impairment or disfigurement. Moreover, AA nail alterations can coexist with other diseases such onychomycosis, psoriasis, or lichen planus; thus, fungal cultures or biopsies may be necessary to achieve a right diagnosis [37].

AA is an autoimmune phenomenon resulting from loss of the hair follicle immune privilege (IP) normally maintained through INFγ expression and modulation of MHC presentations. Causes of IP collapse are discussed [38], but stressful emotional events and some lifestyle factors can be a pathogenetic trigger [39, 40]. As a consequence of hair loss, patient with AA can manifest social anxiety, low self-esteem, and major depression [41].

Diagnosis of AA is clinical and can be supported by dermoscopic evaluation: exclamation point hairs (broken hair that is thicker at the distal end relative to the base), dystrophic, broken hairs, yellow and black dots, empty hair bulbs, and vellus regrowing hairs are common findings. Pull test can be positive at the periphery of patches. As for nail involvement, biopsies, fungal culture, and serology may be required to exclude diseases that can mimic AA as for example trichotillomania, tinea, temporal triangular alopecia, telogen effluvium, an early scarring alopecia, secondary syphilis, and systemic lupus erythematous. Multiple autoimmune disorders including thyroid and celiac disease, psoriasis, and vitiligo have a high association with AA. Some studies report a higher risk of AA also in patients with atopic dermatitis, asthma, and allergic rhinitis [42, 43].

Most patients, between 30 to 50%, will recover spontaneously in the first year after diagnosis although relapses can occur. Severe cases like AT (alopecia totalis) and AU (alopecia universalis), ophsiasis phenotype and cases with an early onset have a worse prognosis instead. Topical, intralesional, and systemic steroids, the latter also with a pulse scheme administration, are effective but side effects need to be considered, especially in children. Topical immunotherapy with contact allergens (diphenylcyclopropenone and squaric acid dibutyl ester) and topical anthralin are other options. Methotrexate and azathioprine can be used in severe non-steroid-responsive cases. JAK-inhibitors as baricitinib or ritlecitinib appear to be effective. Psychological support is recommended [44].

8.5 Flushing and Rosacea

Flushing is defined as a sudden and transient reddening of the skin often accompanied by warmth or burning sensation. It usually occurs in visible areas like face, neck, ears, and chest but, depending on the cause, can also have a different localization or be generalized.

Emotional, thermoregulatory, or climacteric are physiologic and common forms of flushing that appear as a consequence of cutaneous vasodilation mediated by vasoactive substances and nervous stimulation. Flushing can also be caused by several medications, food, alcohol, or can be a sign of an underlying disease. Several neurological and endocrinological dysfunctions, tumors like pheochromocytoma, the Dumping syndrome, or the superior vena cava obstruction can be associated with flushing phenomena [45].

Rosacea is a common benign inflammatory chronic skin disease often presenting with flushing. Subjects with fair skin are the most affected, typical onset is after 30 years, but it can appear at any age and with different clinical patterns. Erythema and telangiectasia of the centrofacial area, papulo-pustular lesions, phymatous changes, and ocular involvement are the most common features of rosacea along with flushing, burning sensation, sometimes localized facial edema and dry skin. Ocular manifestations can range from dryness and foreign body sensation to photophobia, conjunctivitis, blepharitis, and keratitis. Diagnosis is clinical and is made when one or more of the diagnostic signs are present or if two or more of the major phenotypes are observed [46]. Differential diagnosis includes acne, seborrehic dermatitis, erysipelas, perioral dermatitis, polymorphous light eruption, angiosarcoma, and many more [47]. Also lupus and facial granulomas can mimic a rare variety of rosacea, the lupoid or granulomatous form which distinguishes herself for the presence, along with the typical features of rosacea, of monomorphic yellow-brown, red papules, and nodules on the cheeks and periorificial areas that histologically correspond with non-caseating epithelioid cell granulomas [48]. In classic presentation of rosacea, skin biopsy findings are usually nonspecific, they reflect the clinically observed lesions like dilated vessels, perifollicular inflammation, or pustules and do not show granulomas [49]. Lastly, in a few number of cases rosacea can appear abruptly with numerous pustules, nodules, and cysts with severe erythema and edema: this form is known as rosacea fulminans [50].

Pathogenesis is unclear, but a dysregulation of immune system and of neurocutaneous mechanisms are supposed to have a central role inducing inflammation, vascular, lymphatic, glandular, and fibrotic processes seen in rosacea [51]. Bacterial and mites colonization of skin, especially by *Demodex* spp., might contribute to trigger innate and adaptive immune response in these patients [52].

Some cardiovascular, gastrointestinal, neurologic disorders can be more frequent in patients with rosacea, probably because of an associated systemic inflammation [53]. Chronic redness and involvement of the face can lead to embarrassment, low self-esteem, anxiety, and depression: these psychiatric disorders are higher in rosacea patients and determine low quality of life [54].

Sun exposure, emotional stress, hot or cold weather, wind, exercise, alcohol consumption, spicy foods, and some drugs often trigger flushing and flares in rosacea, interfering with patients' daily life. Topical therapies with azelaic acid, ivermectin, or metronidazole are the most used along with specific moisturizers and sun filters [55]. Systemic treatment with tetracyclines or retinoids is reserved to severe cases. Topical antibiotics, steroids, and immunosuppressants can be used in ocular rosacea and ablative laser or surgerical treatments helps reducing the sebaceous hypertrophy in phymatous cases. Alpha-adrenergic agonist like topical brimonidine reduces temporarily facial redness inducing vasoconstriction [47].

8.6 Hyperhidrosis

Hyperhidrosis (HH) is a medical condition characterized by an increased sweating that largely exceeds the quantity of secretions needed for body thermoregulation. The excess of secretion itself does not determine an unpleasant odor in HH; when this happens it is called bromhidrosis, caused by the bacterial breakdown of substances on the skin surface, and when sweat became colored we have a rare condition called chromhidrosis.

HH usually affects males and females equally, although females seem to look for medical help more frequently, with higher prevalence between the age of 18 and 39 and an early onset before 18 and years. Sometimes, patients have a positive family history for same condition suggesting the possibility of a genetic predisposition and inheritance [57, 58].

Primary HH is a condition *per se* and needs to be distinguished from secondary HH which can be physiologic (heat, fever, menopause) or caused by an underlying disease of neurological, oncological, cardiovascular, endocrine, or infectious nature. In primary HH, the most frequent areas involved are axillae, palmoplantar regions and face, often with a simultaneous and bilateral involvement of more areas. Trunk, inguinal folds, and genitalia are less commonly affected [59].

Principal mechanisms hypothesized for focal primary HH are a dysregulated activity of sympathetic nerves, a localized higher density of the eccrine glands or an abnormal central control of emotions. This latter theory postulates that the sweat center in hypothalamus, in HH patients, is exclusively under control of the cortex and emotions and does not receive any input from thermoregulatory components [59]. Human sweat glands are subdivided into three types (eccrine, apocrine, and apoeccrine). HH usually occurs in areas where there is a prevalence of eccrine glands that produce a watery secretion, while the apocrine glands have not been shown to contribute to excessive sweat. In fact, apocrine glands are found in limited areas over the body (axillary region, perineum, nipples, ears, eyelids) and are not present in palmoplantar regions which represent common involved areas in HH [56–59].

In HH, oversecretion tends to be independent from environmental factors but can also be triggered by physiological stimuli like heat and emotions. Stressful situations induce higher sweat production in HH patients than in healthy people [60]. Excessive sweating, especially in public situations, can lead to embarrassment and shame because of its association with lacking of hygiene resulting in a vicious circle of stress-sweating and social anxiety. The chronic stress caused by fear of over-sweating, particularly in visible areas like axillae, can lead to anxiety and depression with an impairment of the quality of life, isolation, and low self-esteem [61]. Eventually, these patients show a higher risk of cutaneous infections in affected body sites: pitted keratolysis, warts, dermatophytosis, and eczematous dermatitis can appear more easily on macerated skin [62].

Diagnostic criteria are excessive sweating for at least 6 months with four or more of the following features: primary involvement of eccrine-dense sites (axillae/palms/soles/craniofacial), bilateral and symmetric distribution, absence of signs at night, episodes at least weekly, onset at 25 years of age or younger, positive family history, and impairment of daily activities [56]. Qualitative and quantitative tests for sweat evaluation are available but not frequently used in clinical practice. When criteria are not satisfied or if patient complaints other symptoms, further investigations to exclude secondary causes are recommended.

HH therapy should follow a step-by-step approach. Topical medications are first-line treatment: aluminum salt solutions are the most used because of their antiperspirant effect, especially the aluminum-chloride one with concentration between 10% and 20%. Aluminum ions precipitate mucopolysaccharides damaging the epithelial cells of the duct and so plugging the lumen mechanically temporary. Other available topical compounds are the anticholinergic ones like glycopyrrolate, glycopyrronium, and oxybutynin which reduce the sympathetic nerves effects on glands and their secretions. Local repeated injections of botulinum toxin A are effective, and also iontophoresis, laser and microwave therapies show good results. Systemic therapies with anticholinergic drugs are used but adverse effects often determine treatment discontinuation. Finally, sympathectomy of thoracic ganglion or local surgical approach with excision, liposuction, and curettage are possible [63].

8.7 Urticaria and Angioedema

Urticaria is a common, mast cell-driven disease presenting with wheals, angioedema, or both.

The prevalence in the general population is 0.7%, with higher rates in children [64].

Wheals are circumscribed edematous skin lesions often surrounded by erythema that appear abruptly and last less than 24 h often associated with intense itching or burning sensation. Angioedema is a well-demarcated edema of the deep dermis, subcutis, or mucous membranes that can persist for several days, sometimes accompanied by burning or pain; when angioedema affects upper airways (pharynx or larynx), risk of asphyxiation may occur. Recurrent wheals with or without angioedema lasting less than 6 weeks are defined as acute urticaria whereas if clinical manifestations persists for a longer time, even if with periods of remission, urticaria is considered chronic [65].

Clinical manifestations are mainly determined by mast cell degranulation with consequent release of histamine, PAF (platelet activating factor), and cytokines but mechanisms of mast cells activation are often unclear: sometimes the presence of IgE autoantibodies to self-antigens or mast cell-directed activating autoantibodies [66] is responsible for degranulation. Moreover, when urticaria is the manifestation of an acute allergic reaction, mast-cell activation is determined by the presence of specific IgE mainly directed to drugs [67] and foods [68]. Food, drugs, thyroid disease, infections, inflammatory processes [66], and stress [69] may both be the cause or an aggravating factor of urticaria. Some patients report a stressful event before the onset or appearance of urticaria: the complex interaction between stress, skin, and the nervous system, including the HPA axis, may in fact play a role in the degranulation of mast cells [70]. Urticaria can also be induced by specific factors: dermographic, cold, heat, delayed pressure, vibratory, cholinergic, aquagenic, contact, and solar urticaria are triggered by physical and environmental stimuli. Anyway, in most patients, causes remain unknown so both acute and chronic urticaria can be spontaneous.

Diagnosis is clinical and needs a detailed anamnesis to investigate the presence of eliciting/worsening factors or the presence of systemic symptoms. Blood tests looking for infections, inflammation, atopy, autoimmune diseases are recommended in chronic urticaria or if patient history requires further investigations. Allergologic workup is necessary when urticaria has a suspected allergic genesis. Histological examination is not pathognomonic but can help with differential diagnosis [66]. Urticaria vasculitis, mast cell-activating syndrome, mastocytosis, Still disease, cryopyrin-associated syndromes, Schnitzler's syndrome, prebullous stage of bullous pemphigoid or PUPP in pregnant women can present with urticaria or mimic her. When patient presents isolated angioedema without urticaria, bradykinin-mediated angioedema (ACE, HAE, AAE), Gleich and Melkersson-Rosenthal syndromes need to be investigated [71].

First-line treatment of urticaria are antihistamines drugs, second generation's one are preferred due to their less sedative effect. Systemic steroids are not recommended in the long term for chronic urticaria treatment, while a short course of rescue oral steroids in patients with an acute exacerbation urticaria may be considered. Omalizumab, an anti-IgE antibody has been shown to be very effective and safe in the treatment of CU not responsive to antihistamines. Cyclosporine is used in patients with CU resistant to the previous drugs. In induced and allergic urticaria, triggers need to be avoided. Some foods, containing high levels of histamine, and NSAIDs should be avoided or taken with caution [66].

8.8 Vesicular Eczema of Palms and Soles

Vesicular eczema of palms and soles is a medical condition also known as dyshidrotic eczema or pompholyx.

Dyshidrosis is a relatively common dermatitis with no clear predilection for sex or age.

It is characterized by the transient and recurrent appearance of vesicular lesions on palms, soles, and lateral areas of fingers on non-inflamed skin. Vesicles are small, between 1 and 2 mm, deep-seated, and their development may be preceded by intense itching: lesions tend to persist for 2 to 3 weeks and then resolve leaving desquamation. Sometimes patients can present a more severe abrupt eruption with large bullae and surrounding inflamed skin: in these cases, the term pompholyx is preferred. Itching and pain, the latter caused by fissures and tightening of skin due to relapses, along with impairment of hand functions and social stigma can significantly reduce quality of life and increase psychological distress. Ulcerations, infections, and lymphedema may also occur [72].

The pathomechanism of dyshidrosis is unknown but several causes can determine this vesicular dermatitis: allergic or irritant contact dermatitis, especially to metals like nickel, chromium, and cobaltum, fungal infections, drugs, and foods are the most frequent etiological agents [73, 74]. As previously said, dyshidrosis can also be a peculiar phenotype of atopic dermatitis [4]. Stress, smoking, irritants, hyperhidrosis, and prolonged use of gloves are considered potentials aggravating factors of dyshidrosis, and rarely, if most of relapses occur during summer, it can also be a photoaggravated condition [75]. Cases of pompholyx are also reported after IVG administration [76] and during IL-17 inhibitors therapy in patients with psoriasis [77].

Diagnosis is clinical and needs a detailed anamnesis: patch tests, fungal cultures, serologies, and biopsies may be necessary, especially when other diseases are suspected. Many other conditions like palmoplantar pustulosis, infantile acropustulosis, bullous pemphigoid and linear IgA dermatitis can debut with vesico-bullous lesions of palms and soles [73].

Avoidance of precipitating factors and topical steroids are the cornerstone of treatment. Topical calcineurin inhibitors, bexarotene, PUVA, and high-dose UVA-1 seem to be effective; iontophoresis and botulinum toxin can help in patient that complaints relapses due to hyperhidrosis. Systemic steroids, immunosuppressants (azathioprine, methotrexate, cyclosporine) or oral retinoids (alitretinoin) can be used in severe and difficult-to-treat cases [78]. A few cases of severe dyshidrosis resistant to classic treatments showed a successful outcome with dupilumab, an anti-IL4/IL13 frequently used in patients with atopic dermatitis [79].

8.9 Aphthosis

Aphthosis is a medical condition characterized by the presence of multiple spherical or oval painful ulcers on mucous membranes. Lesions can vary in size, from a few millimeters to centimeters, and have a yellowish-grey floor surrounded by an erythematous halo. Aphthae mainly appear on the oral mucosa, but also genital area can be involved.

Developed countries have the highest prevalence of aphthous oral ulceration with general population affected between 20 and 25% [80]. The onset of the idiopathic and recurrent form is in early adolescence, while it is variable when determined by an underlying cause. Patients with a family history for recurrent oral aphthosis seem to have a higher risk of suffering of same condition [81].

Idiopathic form is also known as recurrent aphthous stomatitis (RAS), a chronic inflammatory disease that presents with three different clinical spectra: minor, major, and herpetiform. The minor form, the most common, is characterized by the presence of multiple aphthous lesions with a diameter <10 mm mainly located on the non-keratinized mucosa of the lip, cheeks, floor of mouth, and ventral/lateral surface of tongue that cure spontaneously in 4–14 days. In major form, lesions larger than 10 mm and deeper tend to affect the posterior part of the mouth, like soft palate, tonsillar fauces, and pharynges persisting for more than 6 weeks and sometimes leaving a scarring area. Lastly, in the herpetiform one we observe a large number of millimetric ulcers, from 10 to 100, that tend to coalesce and disappear in less than 30 days [82].

Etiology of RAS is unknown; autoimmune or hypersensitivity mechanisms are considered possible causes [82], oral bacteria and virus are sometimes associated with aphthous ulcers [80] and also stressful events can trigger RAS episodes [83]. Pain, recurrences, difficulty in eating, and sometimes in swallowing food lead to higher rates of stress and anxiety in this patients, thus may be contributing to aphthae development [84].

Diagnosis of RAS is clinical and needs a detailed collection of patient history and physical exploration to exclude an underlying disease. As said, oral aphthous lesions can appear in chronic inflammatory or autoimmune context like IBD, celiac disease, pemphigus, Behçet or can be caused by infections, nutritional deficiencies, repetitive traumas or drugs. Blood tests to evaluate blood count, autoantibodies, vitamins, and iron levels are generally recommended while microbiological tests or biopsies should be performed when ulcers do not cure even if treated or if suggested by clinical history, especially to exclude oral cancer [85].

Local therapies with antimicrobial agents to prevent/treat infections and topical corticosteroids to suppress local immune response helps reduce pain and duration of flares but are not curative. Severe cases of RAS can be treated with systemic steroids, colchicine, thalidomide, anti-TNF agents. Treatment of specific underlying disease usually improves general conditions of patient and ulcerative lesions [86, 87].

References

1. Patruno C, Amerio P, Chiricozzi A, Costanzo A, Cristaudo A, Cusano F, Foti C, Girolomoni G, Guarneri F, Naldi L, Offidani A, Pigatto P, Prignano F, Stingeni L, Calzavara-Pinton P. Optimizing a clinical guidance for diagnosis of atopic dermatitis in adults: joint recommendations of the Italian Society of Dermatology and Venereology (SIDeMaST), Italian Association of Hospital Dermatologists (ADOI), and Italian Society of Allergological, Occupational and Environmental Dermatology (SIDAPA). G Ital Dermatol Venereol. 2020;155(1):1–7. https://doi.org/10.23736/S0392-0488.19.06522-2. Epub 2019 Dec 16.
2. Costanzo A, Amerio P, Asero R, Chiricozzi A, Corazza M, Cristaudo A, Cusano F, Ferrucci SM, Nettis E, Patrizi A, Patruno C, Peris K, Picozza M, Stingeni L, Girolomoni G, Italian AD Study Group. Long-term management of moderate-to-severe adult atopic dermatitis: a consensus by the Italian Society of Dermatology and Venereology (SIDeMaST), the Association of Italian Territorial and Hospital Allergists and Immunologists (AAIITO), the Italian Association of Hospital Dermatologists (ADOI), the Italian Society of Allergological, Environmental and Occupational Dermatology (SIDAPA), and the Italian Society of Allergy, Asthma and Clinical Immunology (SIAAIC). Ital J Dermatol Venerol. 2022;157(1):1–12. https://doi.org/10.23736/S2784-8671.21.07129-2. Epub 2021 Dec 21.
3. Chatrath S, Silverberg JI. Phenotypic differences of atopic dermatitis stratified by age. JAAD Int. 2022;11:1–7. https://doi.org/10.1016/j.jdin.2022.08.026. PMID: 36818679; PMCID: PMC9932465.
4. Girolomoni G, de Bruin-Weller M, Aoki V, Kabashima K, Deleuran M, Puig L, Bansal A, Rossi AB. Nomenclature and clinical phenotypes of atopic dermatitis. Ther Adv Chronic Dis. 2021;26(12):20406223211002979. https://doi.org/10.1177/20406223211002979. PMID: 33854747; PMCID: PMC8010850.
5. Bieber T, D'Erme AM, Akdis CA, Traidl-Hoffmann C, Lauener R, Schäppi G, Schmid-Grendelmeier P. Clinical phenotypes and endophenotypes of atopic dermatitis: where are we, and where should we go? J Allergy Clin Immunol. 2017;139(4S):S58–64. https://doi.org/10.1016/j.jaci.2017.01.008.
6. Sroka-Tomaszewska J, Trzeciak M. Molecular mechanisms of atopic dermatitis pathogenesis. Int J Mol Sci. 2021;22(8):4130. https://doi.org/10.3390/ijms22084130. PMID: 33923629; PMCID: PMC8074061.
7. Suárez AL, Feramisco JD, Koo J, Steinhoff M. Psychoneuroimmunology of psychological stress and atopic dermatitis: pathophysiologic and therapeutic updates. Acta Derm Venereol. 2012;92(1):7–15. https://doi.org/10.2340/00015555-1188. PMID: 22101513; PMCID: PMC3704139.
8. Fabrazzo M, Cipolla S, Signoriello S, Camerlengo A, Calabrese G, Giordano GM, Argenziano G, Galderisi S. A systematic review on shared biological mechanisms of depression and anxiety in comorbidity with psoriasis, atopic dermatitis, and hidradenitis suppurativa. Eur Psychiatry. 2021;64(1):e71. https://doi.org/10.1192/j.eurpsy.2021.2249. PMID: 34819201; PMCID: PMC8668448.
9. Silverberg JI. Comorbidities and the impact of atopic dermatitis. Ann Allergy Asthma Immunol. 2019;123(2):144–51. https://doi.org/10.1016/j.anai.2019.04.020. Epub 2019 Apr 26.

10. Ali F, Vyas J, Finlay AY. Counting the burden: atopic dermatitis and health-related quality of life. Acta Derm Venereol. 2020;100(12):adv00161. https://doi.org/10.2340/00015555-3511. PMID: 32412644; PMCID: PMC9189752.
11. Stingeni L, Bianchi L, Antonelli E, Caroppo ES, Ferrucci SM, Ortoncelli M, Fabbrocini G, Nettis E, Schena D, Napolitano M, Gola M, Bonzano L, Rossi M, Belloni Fortina A, Balato A, Peris K, Foti C, Guarneri F, Romanelli M, Patruno C, Savoia P, Fargnoli MC, Russo F, Errichetti E, Bianchelli T, Bianchi L, Pellacani G, Feliciani C, Offidani A, Corazza M, Micali G, Milanesi N, Malara G, Chiricozzi A, Tramontana M, Hansel K, DADA - Dupilumab for Atopic Dermatitis of the Adolescence Study Group. Moderate-to-severe atopic dermatitis in adolescents treated with dupilumab: a multicentre Italian real-world experience. J Eur Acad Dermatol Venereol. 2022;36(8):1292–9. https://doi.org/10.1111/jdv.18141. Epub 2022 Apr 22. PMID: 35412683; PMCID: PMC9542087.
12. Stingeni L, Belloni Fortina A, Baiardini I, Hansel K, Moretti D, Cipriani F. Atopic dermatitis and patient perspectives: insights of bullying at school and career discrimination at work. J Asthma Allergy. 2021;21(14):919–28. https://doi.org/10.2147/JAA.S317009. PMID: 34321892; PMCID: PMC8312319.
13. Damiani G, Calzavara-Pinton P, Stingeni L, Hansel K, Cusano F, "Skin Allergy" Group of SIDeMaST; "ADOI" (Associazione Dermatologi Ospedalieri Italiani); "SIDAPA" (Società Italiana di Dermatologia Allergologica, Professionale e Ambientale); Pigatto PDM. Italian guidelines for therapy of atopic dermatitis-Adapted from consensus-based European guidelines for treatment of atopic eczema (atopic dermatitis). Dermatol Ther. 2019;32(6):e13121. https://doi.org/10.1111/dth.13121. Epub 2019 Nov 7. Erratum in: Dermatol Ther. 2021 Sep;34(5):e15091. PMID: 31625221.
14. Armstrong AW, Read C. Pathophysiology, clinical presentation, and treatment of psoriasis: a review. JAMA. 2020;323(19):1945–60. https://doi.org/10.1001/jama.2020.4006. PMID: 32427307.
15. Raharja A, Mahil SK, Barker JN. Psoriasis: a brief overview. Clin Med (Lond). 2021;21(3):170–3. https://doi.org/10.7861/clinmed.2021-0257. MID: 34001566; PMCID: PMC8140694.
16. Micali G, Verzì AE, Giuffrida G, Panebianco E, Musumeci ML, Lacarrubba F. Inverse psoriasis: from diagnosis to current treatment options. Clin Cosmet Investig Dermatol. 2019;12:953–9. https://doi.org/10.2147/CCID.S189000. PMID: 32099435; PMCID: PMC6997231.
17. Galili E, Levy SR, Tzanani I, Segal O, Lyakhovitsky A, Barzilai A, Baum S. New-onset guttate psoriasis: a long-term follow-up study. Dermatology. 2023;239(2):188–94. https://doi.org/10.1159/000527737. Epub 2022 Dec 8. PMID: 36481593; PMCID: PMC10015744.
18. Hoegler KM, John AM, Handler MZ, Schwartz RA. Generalized pustular psoriasis: a review and update on treatment. J Eur Acad Dermatol Venereol. 2018;32(10):1645–51. https://doi.org/10.1111/jdv.14949. Epub 2018 Apr 11. PMID: 29573491.
19. Trevisan G, Germi L, Naldi L. Erythrodermic psoriasis improved by Tildrakizumab. Dermatol Rep. 2022;14(4):9448. https://doi.org/10.4081/dr.2022.9448. PMID: 36483225; PMCID: PMC9724727.
20. Canal-García E, Bosch-Amate X, Belinchón I, Puig L. Nail psoriasis. Actas Dermosifiliogr. 2022;113(5):481–90. https://doi.org/10.1016/j.ad.2022.01.006. English, Spanish. Epub 2022 Feb 2. PMID: 35697407.
21. Fatahzadeh M, Schwartz RA. Oral psoriasis: an overlooked enigma. Dermatology. 2016;232(3):319–25. https://doi.org/10.1159/000444850. Epub 2016 Apr 2. PMID: 27035486.
22. Umezawa Y. Psoriatic arthritis. J Dermatol. 2021;48(6):741–9. https://doi.org/10.1111/1346-8138.15954. PMID: 34060132.
23. Mahé E. Childhood psoriasis. Eur J Dermatol. 2016;26(6):537–48. https://doi.org/10.1684/ejd.2016.2932. PMID: 27900946.
24. Rendon A, Schäkel K. Psoriasis pathogenesis and treatment. Int J Mol Sci. 2019;20(6):1475. https://doi.org/10.3390/ijms20061475. PMID: 30909615; PMCID: PMC6471628.
25. Yamazaki F. Psoriasis: comorbidities. J Dermatol. 2021;48(6):732–40. https://doi.org/10.1111/1346-8138.15840. Epub 2021 Mar 25. PMID: 33763899; PMCID: PMC8252780.

26. Marek-Jozefowicz L, Czajkowski R, Borkowska A, Nedoszytko B, Żmijewski MA, Cubała WJ, Slominski AT. The brain-skin axis in psoriasis-psychological, psychiatric, hormonal, and dermatological aspects. Int J Mol Sci. 2022;23(2):669. https://doi.org/10.3390/ijms23020669. PMID: 35054853; PMCID: PMC8776235.
27. Stewart TJ, Tong W, Whitfeld MJ. The associations between psychological stress and psoriasis: a systematic review. Int J Dermatol. 2018;57(11):1275–82. https://doi.org/10.1111/ijd.13956. Epub 2018 Mar 8. PMID: 29516474.
28. Balato N, Di Costanzo L, Balato A. Differential diagnosis of psoriasis. J Rheumatol Suppl. 2009;83:24–5. https://doi.org/10.3899/jrheum.090216. PMID: 19661533.
29. Adalsteinsson JA, Kaushik S, Muzumdar S, Guttman-Yassky E, Ungar J. An update on the microbiology, immunology and genetics of seborrheic dermatitis. Exp Dermatol. 2020;29(5):481–9. https://doi.org/10.1111/exd.14091. Epub 2020 Mar 16. PMID: 32125725.
30. Dessinioti C, Katsambas A. Seborrheic dermatitis: etiology, risk factors, and treatments: facts and controversies. Clin Dermatol. 2013;31(4):343–51. https://doi.org/10.1016/j.clindermatol.2013.01.001. PMID: 23806151.
31. Gupta AK, Bluhm R. Seborrheic dermatitis. J Eur Acad Dermatol Venereol. 2004;18(1):13–26. https://doi.org/10.1111/j.1468-3083.2004.00693.x; quiz 19–20. PMID: 14678527.
32. Saunte DML, Gaitanis G, Hay RJ. *Malassezia*-associated skin diseases, the use of diagnostics and treatment. Front Cell Infect Microbiol. 2020;20(10):112. https://doi.org/10.3389/fcimb.2020.00112. PMID: 32266163; PMCID: PMC7098993.
33. Misery L, Touboul S, Vinçot C, Dutray S, Rolland-Jacob G, Consoli SG, Farcet Y, Feton-Danou N, Cardinaud F, Callot V, De La Chapelle C, Pomey-Rey D, Consoli SM. Pour le Groupe Psychodermatologie. Stress et dermatite séborrhéique [Stress and seborrheic dermatitis]. Ann Dermatol Venereol. 2007;134(11):833–7. https://doi.org/10.1016/s0151-9638(07)92826-4. French. PMID: 18033062.
34. Borda LJ, Perper M, Keri JE. Treatment of seborrheic dermatitis: a comprehensive review. J Dermatolog Treat. 2019;30(2):158–69. https://doi.org/10.1080/09546634.2018.1473554. Epub 2018 May 24. PMID: 29737895.
35. Villasante Fricke AC, Miteva ṆM. Epidemiology and burden of alopecia areata: a systematic review. Clin Cosmet Investig Dermatol. 2015;24(8):397–403. https://doi.org/10.2147/CCID.S53985. PMID: 26244028; PMCID: PMC4521674.
36. Finner AM. Alopecia areata: clinical presentation, diagnosis, and unusual cases. Dermatol Ther. 2011;24(3):348–54. https://doi.org/10.1111/j.1529-8019.2011.01413.x. PMID: 21689244.
37. Chelidze K, Lipner SR. Nail changes in alopecia areata: an update and review. Int J Dermatol. 2018;57(7):776–83. https://doi.org/10.1111/ijd.13866. Epub 2018 Jan 10. PMID: 29318582.
38. Rajabi F, Drake LA, Senna MM, Rezaei N. Alopecia areata: a review of disease pathogenesis. Br J Dermatol. 2018;179(5):1033–48. https://doi.org/10.1111/bjd.16808. Epub 2018 Sep 9. PMID: 29791718.
39. Pratt CH, King LE Jr, Messenger AG, Christiano AM, Sundberg JP. Alopecia areata. Nat Rev Dis Primers. 2017;16(3):17011. https://doi.org/10.1038/nrdp.2017.11. PMID: 28300084; PMCID: PMC5573125.
40. Minokawa Y, Sawada Y, Nakamura M. Lifestyle factors involved in the pathogenesis of alopecia areata. Int J Mol Sci. 2022;23(3):1038. https://doi.org/10.3390/ijms23031038. PMID: 35162962; PMCID: PMC8835065.
41. Torales J, Castaldelli-Maia JM, Ventriglio A, Almirón-Santacruz J, Barrios I, O'Higgins M, García O, Navarro R, Melgarejo O, Jafferany M. Alopecia areata: a psychodermatological perspective. J Cosmet Dermatol. 2022;21(6):2318–23. https://doi.org/10.1111/jocd.14416. Epub 2021 Aug 27. PMID: 34449973.
42. Strazzulla LC, Wang EHC, Avila L, Lo Sicco K, Brinster N, Christiano AM, Shapiro J. Alopecia areata: disease characteristics, clinical evaluation, and new perspectives on pathogenesis. J Am Acad Dermatol. 2018;78(1):1–12. https://doi.org/10.1016/j.jaad.2017.04.1141. PMID: 29241771.

43. Manolache L, Benea V. Stress in patients with alopecia areata and vitiligo. J Eur Acad Dermatol Venereol. 2007;21(7):921–8. https://doi.org/10.1111/j.1468-3083.2006.02106.x. PMID: 17659001.
44. Rossi A, Muscianese M, Piraccini BM, Starace M, Carlesimo M, Mandel VD, Alessandrini A, Calvieri S, Caro G, D'arino A, Federico A, Magri F, Pigliacelli F, Amendolagine G, Annunziata MC, Arisi MC, Astorino S, Babino G, Bardazzi F, Barruscotti S, Belloni Fortina A, Borghi A, Bruni F, Caccavale S, Calzavara-Pinton P, Cameli N, Cardone M, Carugno A, Coppola R, Dattola A, De Felici Del Giudice MB, Di Cesare A, Dika E, Di Nunno D, D'ovidio R, Fabbrocini G, Feliciani C, Fulgione E, Galluzzo M, Garcovich S, Garelli V, Guerriero C, Hansel K, La Placa M, Lacarrubba F, Lora V, Marinello E, Megna M, Micali G, Misciali C, Monari P, Monfrecola G, Neri I, Offidani A, Orlando G, Papini M, Patrizi A, Piaserico S, Rivetti N, Simonetti O, Stan TR, Stingeni L, Talamonti M, Tassone F, Villa L, Vincenzi C, Fortuna MC. Italian Guidelines in diagnosis and treatment of alopecia areata. G Ital Dermatol Venereol. 2019;154(6):609–23. https://doi.org/10.23736/S0392-0488.19.06458-7. Epub 2019 Sep 26. PMID: 31578836.
45. Sadeghian A, Rouhana H, Oswald-Stumpf B, Boh E. Etiologies and management of cutaneous flushing: nonmalignant causes. J Am Acad Dermatol. 2017;77(3):391–402. https://doi.org/10.1016/j.jaad.2016.12.031. PMID: 28807107
46. Gallo RL, Granstein RD, Kang S, Mannis M, Steinhoff M, Tan J, Thiboutot D. Standard classification and pathophysiology of rosacea: the 2017 update by the National Rosacea Society Expert Committee. J Am Acad Dermatol. 2018;78(1):148–55. https://doi.org/10.1016/j.jaad.2017.08.037. Epub 2017 Oct 28. PMID: 29089180.
47. Anzengruber F, Czernielewski J, Conrad C, Feldmeyer L, Yawalkar N, Häusermann P, Cozzio A, Mainetti C, Goldblum D, Läuchli S, Imhof L, Brand C, Laffitte E, Navarini AA. Swiss S1 guideline for the treatment of rosacea. J Eur Acad Dermatol Venereol. 2017;31(11):1775–91. https://doi.org/10.1111/jdv.14349. Epub 2017 Aug 21. PMID: 28833645.
48. Vanstreels L, Megahed M. Lupoide Rosazea als Sonderform der Rosazea: Einblick in die Pathogenese und Therapieoptionen [Lupoid rosacea as a special form of rosacea: review of pathogenesis and therapeutic options]. Hautarzt. 2013;64(12):886–8. https://doi.org/10.1007/s00105-013-2685-z. German. PMID: 24173607.
49. Two AM, Wu W, Gallo RL, Hata TR. Rosacea: part I. Introduction, categorization, histology, pathogenesis, and risk factors. J Am Acad Dermatol. 2015;72(5):749–58. https://doi.org/10.1016/j.jaad.2014.08.028; quiz 759–60. PMID: 25890455.
50. Angileri L, Veraldi S, Barbareschi M. Rosacea fulminans: two case reports and review of the literature. J Dermatolog Treat. 2021;32(1):110–3. https://doi.org/10.1080/09546634.2019.1628175. Epub 2019 Jul 10. PMID: 31169436.
51. Buddenkotte J, Steinhoff M. Recent advances in understanding and managing rosacea. F1000Res. 2018;7:F1000 Faculty Rev-1885. https://doi.org/10.12688/f1000research.16537.1. PMID: 30631431; PMCID: PMC6281021.
52. Aktaş Karabay E, Aksu ÇA. Demodex folliculorum infestations in common facial dermatoses: acne vulgaris, rosacea, seborrheic dermatitis. An Bras Dermatol. 2020;95(2):187–93. https://doi.org/10.1016/j.abd.2019.08.023. Epub 2020 Feb 12. PMID: 32113677; PMCID: PMC7175027.
53. Haber R, El Gemayel M. Comorbidities in rosacea: a systematic review and update. J Am Acad Dermatol. 2018;78(4):786–792.e8. https://doi.org/10.1016/j.jaad.2017.09.016. Epub 2017 Oct 26. PMID: 29107339.
54. van Zuuren EJ, Arents BWM, van der Linden MMD, Vermeulen S, Fedorowicz Z, Rosacea TJ. New concepts in classification and treatment. Am J Clin Dermatol. 2021;22(4):457–65. https://doi.org/10.1007/s40257-021-00595-7. Epub 2021 Mar 23. PMID: 33759078; PMCID: PMC8200341.
55. Thiboutot D, Anderson R, Cook-Bolden F, Draelos Z, Gallo RL, Granstein RD, Kang S, Macsai M, Gold LS, Tan J. Standard management options for rosacea: The 2019 update by

the National Rosacea Society Expert Committee. J Am Acad Dermatol. 2020;82(6):1501–10. https://doi.org/10.1016/j.jaad.2020.01.077. Epub 2020 Feb 7. PMID: 32035944.
56. Semkova K, Gergovska M, Kazandjieva J, Tsankov N. Hyperhidrosis, bromhidrosis, and chromhidrosis: Fold (intertriginous) dermatoses. Clin Dermatol. 2015;33(4):483–91. https://doi.org/10.1016/j.clindermatol.2015.04.013. Epub 2015 Apr 8. PMID: 26051066.
57. Moraites E, Vaughn OA, Hill S. Incidence and prevalence of hyperhidrosis. Dermatol Clin. 2014;32(4):457–65. https://doi.org/10.1016/j.det.2014.06.006. Epub 2014 Jul 19. PMID: 25152338.
58. Ro KM, Cantor RM, Lange KL, Ahn SS. Palmar hyperhidrosis: evidence of genetic transmission. J Vasc Surg. 2002;35(2):382–6. https://doi.org/10.1067/mva.2002.119507. PMID: 11854739.
59. Nawrocki S, Cha J. The etiology, diagnosis, and management of hyperhidrosis: a comprehensive review: etiology and clinical work-up. J Am Acad Dermatol. 2019;81(3):657–66. https://doi.org/10.1016/j.jaad.2018.12.071. Epub 2019 Jan 31. PMID: 30710604.
60. Schote AB, Dietrich K, Linden AE, Dzionsko I, Molano Moreno LLA, Winnikes U, Zimmer P, Domes G, Meyer J. Real sweating in a virtual stress environment: investigation of the stress reactivity in people with primary focal hyperhidrosis. PLoS One. 2022;17(8):e0272247. https://doi.org/10.1371/journal.pone.0272247. PMID: 35917298; PMCID: PMC9345359.
61. Gross KM, Schote AB, Schneider KK, Schulz A, Meyer J. Elevated social stress levels and depressive symptoms in primary hyperhidrosis. PLoS One. 2014;9(3):e92412. https://doi.org/10.1371/journal.pone.0092412. PMID: 24647796; PMCID: PMC3960246.
62. Walling HW. Primary hyperhidrosis increases the risk of cutaneous infection: a case-control study of 387 patients. J Am Acad Dermatol. 2009;61(2):242–6. https://doi.org/10.1016/j.jaad.2009.02.038. Epub 2009 Apr 23. PMID: 19395123.
63. Arora G, Kassir M, Patil A, Sadeghi P, Gold MH, Adatto M, Grabbe S, Goldust M. Treatment of axillary hyperhidrosis. J Cosmet Dermatol. 2022;21(1):62–70. https://doi.org/10.1111/jocd.14378. Epub 2021 Aug 20. PMID: 34416078.
64. Saini S, Shams M, Bernstein JA, Maurer M. Urticaria and angioedema across the ages. J Allergy Clin Immunol Pract. 2020;8(6):1866–74. https://doi.org/10.1016/j.jaip.2020.03.030. Epub 2020 Apr 13. PMID: 32298850.
65. Radonjic-Hoesli S, Hofmeier KS, Micaletto S, Schmid-Grendelmeier P, Bircher A, Simon D. Urticaria and angioedema: an update on classification and pathogenesis. Clin Rev Allergy Immunol. 2018;54(1):88–101. https://doi.org/10.1007/s12016-017-8628-1. PMID: 28748365.
66. Zuberbier T, Abdul Latiff AH, Abuzakouk M, Aquilina S, Asero R, Baker D, Ballmer-Weber B, Bangert C, Ben-Shoshan M, Bernstein JA, Bindslev-Jensen C, Brockow K, Brzoza Z, Chong Neto HJ, Church MK, Criado PR, Danilycheva IV, Dressler C, Ensina LF, Fonacier L, Gaskins M, Gáspár K, Gelincik A, Giménez-Arnau A, Godse K, Gonçalo M, Grattan C, Grosber M, Hamelmann E, Hébert J, Hide M, Kaplan A, Kapp A, Kessel A, Kocatürk E, Kulthanan K, Larenas-Linnemann D, Lauerma A, Leslie TA, Magerl M, Makris M, Meshkova RY, Metz M, Micallef D, Mortz CG, Nast A, Oude-Elberink H, Pawankar R, Pigatto PD, Ratti Sisa H, Rojo Gutiérrez MI, Saini SS, Schmid-Grendelmeier P, Sekerel BE, Siebenhaar F, Siiskonen H, Soria A, Staubach-Renz P, Stingeni L, Sussman G, Szegedi A, Thomsen SF, Vadasz Z, Vestergaard C, Wedi B, Zhao Z, Maurer M. The international EAACI/GA²LEN/EuroGuiDerm/APAAACI guideline for the definition, classification, diagnosis, and management of urticaria. Allergy. 2022;77(3):734–66. https://doi.org/10.1111/all.15090. Epub 2021 Oct 20. PMID: 34536239.
67. Stingeni L, Bianchi L, Tramontana M, Pigatto PD, Patruno C, Corazza M, Foti C, Fabbrocini G, Micali G, Romita P, Napolitano M, Hansel K. Skin tests in the diagnosis of adverse drug reactions. G Ital Dermatol Venereol. 2020;155(5):602–21. https://doi.org/10.23736/S0392-0488.20.06698-5. Epub 2020 Sep 17. PMID: 32938165.
68. De Martinis M, Sirufo MM, Suppa M, Ginaldi L. New Perspectives in Food Allergy. Int J Mol Sci. 2020;21(4):1474. https://doi.org/10.3390/ijms21041474. PMID: 32098244; PMCID: PMC7073187.
69. Bansal CJ, Bansal AS. Stress, pseudoallergens, autoimmunity, infection and inflammation in chronic spontaneous urticaria. Allergy Asthma Clin Immunol. 2019;11(15):56. https://doi.org/10.1186/s13223-019-0372-z. PMID: 31528163; PMCID: PMC6737621.

70. Konstantinou GN, Konstantinou GN. Psychological stress and chronic urticaria: a neuro-immuno-cutaneous crosstalk. a systematic review of the existing evidence. Clin Ther. 2020;42(5):771–82. https://doi.org/10.1016/j.clinthera.2020.03.010. Epub 2020 Apr 29. PMID: 32360096
71. Peter J, Krause K, Staubach P, Wu MA, Davis M. Chronic urticaria and recurrent angio-edema: clues to the mimics. J Allergy Clin Immunol Pract. 2021;9(6):2220–8. https://doi.org/10.1016/j.jaip.2021.03.043. Epub 2021 Apr 24. PMID: 33906826.
72. Lofgren SM, Warshaw EM. Dyshidrosis: epidemiology, clinical characteristics, and therapy. Dermatitis. 2006;17(4):165–81. https://doi.org/10.2310/6620.2006.05021. PMID: 17150166.
73. Veien NK. Acute and recurrent vesicular hand dermatitis. Dermatol Clin. 2009;27(3):337–53, vii. https://doi.org/10.1016/j.det.2009.05.013. PMID: 19580928.
74. Guillet MH, Wierzbicka E, Guillet S, Dagregorio G, Guillet G. A 3-year causative study of pompholyx in 120 patients. Arch Dermatol. 2007;143(12):1504–8. https://doi.org/10.1001/archderm.143.12.1504. PMID: 18086998.
75. Nalluri R, Rhodes LE. Photoaggravated pompholyx. Photodermatol Photoimmunol Photomed. 2016;32(3):168–70. https://doi.org/10.1111/phpp.12237. Epub 2016 Mar 2. PMID: 26868937.
76. Gerstenblith MR, Antony AK, Junkins-Hopkins JM, Abuav R. Pompholyx and eczematous reactions associated with intravenous immunoglobulin therapy. J Am Acad Dermatol. 2012;66(2):312–6. https://doi.org/10.1016/j.jaad.2010.12.034. Epub 2011 May 20. PMID: 21601310.
77. Peera M, Smith A. Palmoplantar pompholyx secondary to interleukin 17A inhibitor therapy for psoriasis: a case series. JAAD Case Rep. 2021;13:46–8. https://doi.org/10.1016/j.jdcr.2021.03.052. PMID: 34141846; PMCID: PMC8188176.
78. Wollina U. Pompholyx: a review of clinical features, differential diagnosis, and management. Am J Clin Dermatol. 2010;11(5):305–14. https://doi.org/10.2165/11533250-000000000-00000.
79. Waldman RA, DeWane ME, Sloan B, Grant-Kels JM, Lu J. Dupilumab for the treatment of dyshidrotic eczema in 15 consecutive patients. J Am Acad Dermatol. 2020;82(5):1251–2. https://doi.org/10.1016/j.jaad.2019.12.053. Epub 2020 Jan 8. PMID: 31926220.
80. Gasmi Benahmed A, Noor S, Menzel A, Gasmi A. Oral aphthous: pathophysiology, clinical aspects and medical treatment. Arch Razi Inst. 2021;76(5):1155–63. https://doi.org/10.22092/ari.2021.356055.1767. PMID: 35355774; PMCID: PMC8934078.
81. Vaillant L, Samimi M. Aphtes et ulcérations buccales [Aphthous ulcers and oral ulcerations]. Presse Med. 2016;45(2):215–26. https://doi.org/10.1016/j.lpm.2016.01.005. French. Epub 2016 Feb 12. PMID: 26880080.
82. Femiano F, Lanza A, Buonaiuto C, Gombos F, Nunziata M, Piccolo S, Cirillo N. Guidelines for diagnosis and management of aphthous stomatitis. Pediatr Infect Dis J. 2007;26(8):728–32. https://doi.org/10.1097/INF.0b013e31806215f9. PMID: 17848886.
83. Huling LB, Baccaglini L, Choquette L, Feinn RS, Lalla RV. Effect of stressful life events on the onset and duration of recurrent aphthous stomatitis. J Oral Pathol Med. 2012;41(2):149–52. https://doi.org/10.1111/j.1600-0714.2011.01102.x. Epub 2011 Nov 12. PMID: 22077475; PMCID: PMC3323121.
84. Soto Araya M, Rojas Alcayaga G, Esguep A. Association between psychological disorders and the presence of Oral lichen planus, Burning mouth syndrome and Recurrent aphthous stomatitis. Med Oral. 2004;9(1):1–7. English, Spanish. PMID: 14704611.
85. Sánchez-Bernal J, Conejero C, Conejero R. Recurrent Aphthous Stomatitis. Actas Dermosifiliogr (Engl Ed). 2020;111(6):471–80. https://doi.org/10.1016/j.ad.2019.09.004. English, Spanish. Epub 2020 May 22. PMID: 32451064.
86. Jurge S, Kuffer R, Scully C, Porter SR. Mucosal disease series. Number VI. Recurrent aphthous stomatitis. Oral Dis. 2006;12(1):1–21. https://doi.org/10.1111/j.1601-0825.2005.01143.x. PMID: 16390463.
87. Giannetti L, Murri Dello Diago A, Lo Muzio L. Recurrent aphtous stomatitis. Minerva Stomatol. 2018;67(3):125–8. https://doi.org/10.23736/S0026-4970.18.04137-7. Epub 2018 Jan 11. PMID: 29332375.

Chapter 9
Group and Mass Population Disorders

Luca Stingeni, Katharina Hansel, and Elisa Cecchini

9.1 Sick Building Syndrome

The sick building syndrome (SBS) consists of a group of mucosal, skin, and general symptoms that arise during the stay in the workplace building and resolve shortly after leaving the site. These symptoms are of unclear etiology, unlike building-related illnesses. The latter may be caused by infectious diseases that spread from worker to worker or from the building itself, as in the case of mold, chemicals or toxins present or used in the workplace. Office workers are the most studied group but school, hospitals, and care homes employees can present similar problems [1].

First reported outbreaks of SBS go back to 1970–1980 when the first buildings with mechanical ventilation systems, humidity, and temperature control began to develop [2].

A general feeling of tiredness and non-migranous headache are the most common symptoms sometimes accompanied by lethargy and lack of concentration. Mucosal involvement is typical with stuffy nose, dryness of throat and eyes and can be associated with respiratory symptoms such as cough and shortness of breath. Sneezing, wheezing, and runny nose are more suggestive of an allergic condition due to sensitization to an allergen that may or may not be workplace specific but can also be reported in SBS. Skin rashes, itching, and dryness are the main dermatological complaints related to SBS and contrarily to other symptoms discussed above, they tend to persist for several days after leaving the suspected building [1]. Abnormal odor perception and visual disturbances are less frequent. Host factors and microenvironment interaction are major determinants for developing

L. Stingeni · K. Hansel · E. Cecchini (✉)
Department of Medicine and Surgery, Dermatology Section, University of Perugia, Perugia, Italy
e-mail: luca.stingeni@unipg.it; katharina.hansel@unipg.it; elisa.cecchini@specializzandi.unipg.it

G. Angelini et al. (eds.), *Psychocutaneous Diseases*,
https://doi.org/10.1007/978-3-031-70296-9_9

SBS. In fact, in the same building some individuals may be totally asymptomatic while those who are "sick" may report different types of symptoms. Also severity of symptoms can vary greatly among these patients thus determine different degrees of distress, reduced productivity, and loss of working days [3].

As previously said, none of the symptoms of SBS can be addressed to a specific organic cause. Indoor parameters of temperature, humidity, ventilation rate, CO_2 levels, microbial contamination (molds, viruses, bacteria), presence of dust and chemical compounds are the most studied factors. High indoor temperature over 23 °C, especially in overcrowded places, dust and poor cleaning are associated with SBS symptoms. Regarding ventilation, some studies show a relation between ventilation rates less than 10 L/s/person an increased symptoms. In fact, higher ventilation rates can help dilute pollutants of the office which are generated by occupants, machinery, or that come from the outside through windows or ventilation systems. On the other hand, augmented ventilation can also increase exposure to pollutants generated by ventilation systems themselves making the relationship between ventilation and SBS not of unique interpretation. Actually, patients show improvement of symptoms when given individual ventilation control regardless of rates, temperature, and dust presence. In fact, respect of the standard levels of air humidification have not been shown to reduce SBS symptoms but it is still important to respect them to avoid water stagnation, bacterial growth and the need to add bioceds:some of them, like isothiazolinones, glutaraldehyde, chloramine, chlorhexidine, and benzalkonium chloride, have a known irritant or allergenic potential. The role of microbial contamination is not clear in SBS etiology while it is more acknowledged in the genesis of alveolitis, humidifier fever, and asthma. Paper and presence of printers, cigarettes smoke, air conditioner, and prolonged use of computer are all factors related to increased prevalence of sick building syndrome [1]. Indoor CO_2 levels are mainly influenced by the number of people present and ventilation: a higher difference between indoor and outdoor CO_2 levels is related to symptoms such as fatigue and dizziness. This may have a biological explanation: an increase in blood CO_2 resulting in oxygen desaturation can lead to central nervous system symptoms. In addition, a slight association between VOC (volatile orgnanic compounds) levels and symptoms such as eye, nose, throat, and skin dryness irritation has been observed [4]. Moreover also the concentration of nanoparticles has been studied in work environments to assess its relationship with BSS and, interestingly, when results were adjusted for perception of air quality and its associated risk, no correlation was found [5]. What seems to influence the most the appearance of SBS symptoms is in fact the perception of air quality, regardless of respect of the indoor air quality standards. In fact, SBS is more common in buildings with mechanical ventilation or air conditioning than in those with natural ventilation, despite the fact that even in the latter sometimes environmental parameters are outside recommended values [6]. The perception of working in an unhealthy environment with poor air quality and thus the idea of being exposed to real health risks are the most frequently factors associated with the presence of symptoms of sick building syndrome. Path analytic models try to explain how risk perception, regardless of the cause, can increase stress which can exacerbate pre-existing diseases or SBS eliciting physiological responses of avoidance or adaptation [5]. Low social and supervisor support and thus a poor psychosocial working environment has also shown to be associated with a higher risk of developing SBS. Other patient factors associated with SBS are female gender, atopy, history of allergic disorders, self-reported work-stress, and personality traits such as anxiety and aggression [7]. Poor and inappropriate lighting with absence of sunlight, bad acoustics, poor ergonomics and humidity may also contribute to SBS [8].

Average number of work-related symptoms per occupant is known as the building symptom index and can be measured reproducibly by several questionnaire surveys. Most frequent and significant questions are shown in box 1 [1]. Diagnosis is made through an exclusion process: all other conditions that can cause the complaints symptoms by the workers needs to be ruled out as for example, allergic problems or underlying diseases associated or not with the working activity. Evaluating IAQ (indoor air quality) by air samples and establishing a relationship between certain air parameters and symptoms is essential to study SBS, and also a "walk-through" inspection of the suspected areas is recommended to collect information from occupants, to detect possible sources of contamination or to assess general conditions of workers. Timing of symptoms, as said, is specific: symptoms appear during the permanence in the building and spontaneously disappear after leaving it within a short time.

Reduced productivity and loss of work days due to the disorders are not the only costs and consequences of the syndrome since, especially if a substantial number of workers are involved, it makes a series of investigations aimed at highlighting environmental triggers necessary. Cause is often not found, and sometimes changing certain parameters of indoor air can reduce the symptoms of some and worsen those of others, effectively making it difficult to find a proper solution. Creating a good work environment from a psycho-emotional point of view is certainly necessary to reduce this issue, as is ensuring regular cleaning, maintenance, achievement of good air standard parameters, and avoiding the use of possibly irritating products [8].

9.2 Epidemic Hysteria

Epidemic hysteria, also known as mass psychogenic illness (MPI) or mass hysteria, is a phenomenon characterized by outbreaks of psychogenic signs and symptoms suggesting the presence of organic illness but with no clinical and laboratory evidence of disease. The spread of symptoms is usually rapid and affects members of a cohesive group or people who spend a lot of time together. However, today mass media and technology can result in a greater spread of epidemic hysteria because of their ability to reach a wide audience [9]. Mass hysteria is classified as conversion disorder which is a psychiatric disease characterized by signs and symptoms affecting sensory or motor function inconsistent with any medical conditions. Symptoms are not under voluntary control of patients [10].

First episodes of epidemic hysteria have been described since the fourteenth century in various cultural groups with similar presentations despite differences in sociocultural setting, religion, or age. Adolescents and females are the most affected, and almost 60% of literature reports outbreaks in schools. Mass hysteria has been also common among developing nations with cases associated with mass deworming of children or school feeding program [11]. Interestingly, the main triggers in western setting are chemical toxins, environmental pollution, and infectious diseases while in Africa, for example, evil spirits or religious topic have a major role [9].

Clinical manifestations of epidemic hysteria are subdivided into two main forms: anxiety and motor. The former is typical of children in a school setting and spreads rapidly through a group via sight and physical contact with affected individuals: headache, dizziness, hyperventilation, and fainting are the main manifestations. Mass anxiety hysteria has a good prognosis, separating the group generally helps to stop outbreaks and reduce their duration. Mass motor hysteria is less common and may affect different age groups, with a more gradual spread and a prolonged outbreak. The most common symptoms are twitching, difficulty walking, and inappropriate laughter. In this form, removal of the stressor is essential for treatment [12].

The outbreak tends to begin with and index case in the community (schools, factories, villages, or other institutions) which can have an organic illness or not. The presence of symptoms with no organic basis in a segregated group is a major feature of epidemic hysteria. However, when concerning diagnosis, the presence of organic causes like infections or poisoning needs to be investigated. MPI and organic outbreak can also coexist and overlap.

Epidemic hysteria outbreaks can be difficult to manage, especially for emergency departments. Moreover, site of outbreaks as schools are often closed during epidemic which implies loss of days of work, both for teachers and sometimes parents, postponement of examinations and compromised teaching programs. A prompt recognition of the phenomena is essential for its management, early intervention can significantly reduce the duration of event and the number of subjects involved. Coordinated investigations, proper communication strategy, and environmental modifications are fundamental to manage the outbreaks [13].

References

1. Burge PS. Sick building syndrome. Occup Environ Med. 2004;61(2):185–90.
2. Grant IWB. The sick building syndrome. Br Med J (Clin Res Ed). 1985;290(6464):321–2.
3. Redlich CA, Sparer J, Cullen MR. Sick-building syndrome. Lancet. 1997;349(9057):1013–6.
4. Lu CY, Lin JM, Chen YY, Chen YC. Building-related symptoms among office employees associated with indoor carbon dioxide and total volatile organic compounds. Int J Environ Res Public Health. 2015;12:5833–45.
5. Orru H, Olstrup H, Hagenbjörk A, Nordin S, Orru K. Exposures, symptoms and risk perception among office workers in relation to nanoparticles in the work environment. Int J Environ Res Public Health. 2022;19(10):5789.

6. Burge PS, Hedge A, Wilson S, et al. Sick building syndrome; a study of 4373 office workers. Ann Occup Hyg. 1987;31:493–504.
7. Runeson-Broberg R, Norbäck D. Sick building syndrome (SBS) and sick house syndrome (SHS) in relation to psychosocial stress at work in the Swedish workforce. Int Arch Occup Environ Health. 2013;86(8):915–22.
8. Joshi SM. The sick building syndrome. Indian J Occup Environ Med. 2008;12(2):61–4.
9. Ayehu M, Endriyas M, Mekonnen E, Shiferaw M, Misganaw T. Chronic mass psychogenic illness among women in Derashe Woreda, Segen Area People Zone, southern Ethiopia: a community based cross-sectional study. Int J Ment Health Syst. 2018;7(12):31.
10. Balaratnasingam S, Janca A. Mass hysteria revisited. Curr Opin Psychiatry. 2006;19(2):171–4.
11. Jebessa S, Deksiso H, Tefera M, Bahretibeb Y. Mass Hysteria among Beneficiary Students of the School-Feeding Program in Addis Ababa. Ethiopia. Ethiop J Health Sci. 2022;32(3):563–8.
12. Siamisang K, Phologolo T, Mukuhwa T, Schafrick N, Mhaladi B, Phuthego B, Mmati M, Masupe T. Predictors of mass psychogenic illness in a junior secondary school in rural Botswana: a case control study. S Afr J Psychiatr. 2022;30(28):1671.
13. Tarafder BK, Khan MA, Islam MT, Mahmud SA, Sarker MH, Faruq I, Miah MT, Arafat SM. Mass psychogenic illness: demography and symptom profile of an episode. Psychiatry J. 2016;2016:2810143.

Chapter 10
Medico-Legal Implications in the Management of Psychocutaneous Diseases

Biagio Solarino, Davide Ferorelli, Luigi Buongiorno, Marcello Benevento, and Gabriele Mandarelli

10.1 Introduction

From the medico-legal standpoint, diagnosing and managing psychocutaneous diseases might be challenging. The pathologic interaction of mind and skin may be classified as follows: (a) psychophysiological disorders (i.e., the skin disease is not caused by psychiatric disorders, but it may be triggered by emotional stress), (b) psychiatric disorders with dermatological symptoms, (c) dermatological disorders with psychiatric symptoms [1, 2]. Hence, patients with psychocutaneous conditions may show skin lesions arising from the dermatological disease, or skin artifacts due to pathomimesis. Some patients may cause self-skin lesions with illicit intent (malingering) or be subjected to skin injuries due to abuse or other violent crime.

Hence, one of the aims of medico-legal consultation is to evaluate characteristics of skin lesions to recognize suspected traumatic lesions and distinguish self-inflicted from injuries inflicted by others. The traumatic skin lesions (bruises, burns and scalds, abrasions, cuts, lacerations, etc.) are indeed associated with abuse, neglect, or self-harm behaviors.

Pathomimesis and malingering may increase the odds of diagnostic and therapeutic errors and conduce to medical claims.

B. Solarino · D. Ferorelli · L. Buongiorno · M. Benevento (✉) · G. Mandarelli
Department of Interdisciplinary Medicine, University of Bari "Aldo Moro", Bari, Italy
e-mail: Biagio.solarino@uniba.it; davide.ferorelli@uniba.it; luigi.buongiorno@uniba.it; marcello.benevento@uniba.it; gabriele.mandarelli@uniba.it

G. Angelini et al. (eds.), *Psychocutaneous Diseases*,
https://doi.org/10.1007/978-3-031-70296-9_10

10.2 Medico-Legal Examination of Skin Injuries

10.2.1 Forensic Assessment

Inadequate or incorrect diagnosis of an external wound may influence the clinical management of the patient, but also any subsequent criminal investigation or court proceedings. A proper forensic assessment of external injuries should allow differentiating wounds from any other pathological skin signs but also define the cause and the manner of the wounds. This paragraph will give a compendium of the basis of forensic examination of external injuries.

10.2.1.1 Informed Consent

All medical procedures require adequate patient informed consent. The fundamental underpinnings of a valid informed consent are complete information disclosure, voluntariness of consent, and patient's mental capacity to decide.

Informed consent for treatment or diagnostic procedures usually includes information disclosure about (1) the procedure characteristics; (2) risks, benefits, and possible alternatives; (3) consequences of procedures refusing [3]. Medical examination of wounds may involve the collection of samples and pictures, and the practitioner should obtain patient informed consent for such procedures. The exemption from the requirement to obtain consent covers a limited number of cases, where there is a warrant and a subsequent obligation, by the judicial authority.

Vulnerable patients, including those suffering from severe psychiatric disorders or cognitive impairment, could deserve a second-line assessment of their mental capacity to give informed consent [4, 5]. An easy way to assess patients' capacity to consent to diagnostic procedures is to evaluate patients' understanding and appreciation by asking them to repeat the information disclosed, to encourage questions and reasoning. States regulations normally required patients or guardians to give consent on behalf of minors or incapable patients.

10.2.1.2 Case History

The medical history is a set of information that the doctor collects from the patients or their informants (parents, etc.). The practitioner should elicit information about the skin lesions' symptoms and characteristics (appearance, timing, evolution, precipitating and healing factors, etc.).

Sometimes, information regarding suspected injuries may be distorted or incomplete. It happens because the patients may forgive something in good faith, but also wittingly lie.

10.2.1.3 Collecting Pictures

Pictures taken for forensic aims should have a good quality color and good resolution. It is important to take two pictures of each lesion: a wide-angle picture to well localize the injury; a macro picture to enhance its morphologic characteristics. The macro picture should be near enough to frame the whole required object. To take a reliable picture, the camera should be perpendicular to the surface of the skin both in frontal and sagittal planes. It's advisable to frame a measuring tape to give a reference.

Nowadays, many smartphones have high-quality cameras, with electronic flashes and automatic focusing. However, Knight et al. suggested using a 35-mm single-lens reflex [6].

10.2.1.4 Clothes Examination

From a forensic perspective, clothing is like a "crime scene" as garments retain multiple traces of both the victim and the aggressor during a crime [7, 8].

A simple observation of the clothing style, items, and hygiene should inform about psychiatric conditions such as schizophrenia or compulsive disorders [9, 10].

First, the examinator should describe the clothing: type, color, hygiene, and the number of items; color, position, and shape of the stains; type and shape of the lacerations. The examinator should take pictures of the clothes, especially any biological or non-biological traces, ruptures, and tears. Then, every biological or non-biological trace should be carefully collected trying to avoid any contamination.

The patients should undress themselves standing on a white cloth to collect the falling trace (hair, soil remains, glass or metallic fragments, etc.).

10.2.2 Wounds Examination

Bernard Knight defines a wound as "damage to any part of the body due to the application of mechanical force" [6]. The intensity of a mechanical force varies directly with the mass of the hitting item and directly with the square of impact velocity (kinetic energy= ½ mass × velocity^2). The effects on the tissue can result in compression, traction, torsion, and tangential stresses.

Soft tissue's resilience and elasticity entail a certain capacity to absorb mechanical forces. However, tissue resistance also depends on the surface on which face the force: blunt objects need more energy to break the skin compared to edged or pointed items [6]. For this reason, it is possible to distinguish wounds resulting from blunt injuries (abrasions, bruises, and lacerations) and incised wounds caused by sharped or pointed objects (cuts, chops, and stabs).

10.2.2.1 Abrasions

Also known as "scratches," abrasions are the most superficial skin injuries as they resulted from the traumatic removal of some keratinized layers of the epidermis. However, abrasions commonly involve some dermis vessels causing little bleeding (Fig. 10.1). Abrasions are caused by tangential stresses of the skin. A wide impact causes a "brush" abrasion (typically resulting from the contact of a moving body with a rough surface), while irregular surfaces or small objects may cause multiple linear marks [6].

In forensics, patterned wounds should be carefully examined as the shape and the localization of the abrasion may inform about the cause and the manner of the wound [11]. Multiple small linear scratches or short curved marks may be caused by the nails (fingernail marks). The localization of such marks should help distinguish their origin, as fingernail marks are frequent in assaults and smothering. strangulation, sexual attacks, and abuse.

Circumferential abrasions of the wrist, ankle, or neck should originate from ligature marks, which result from the skin's pressure and transversal stress due to a rope or other ligature. A ligature mark on the neck may indicate hanging or strangulation. Hanging is one of the commonest means of suicide. The hanging mark is usually a single circumferential wrap. The mark proceeds obliquely from the neck anteriorly, passes round beneath the jawbones, and rises at the sides or back of the neck to the usual gap under the knot [12]. On the other hand, the strangulation mark is a multiple circumferential wrap; it proceeds transversally to the neck's axis without gaps. Finally, ligature marks on wrists or ankles should be referred to as immobilization attempts.

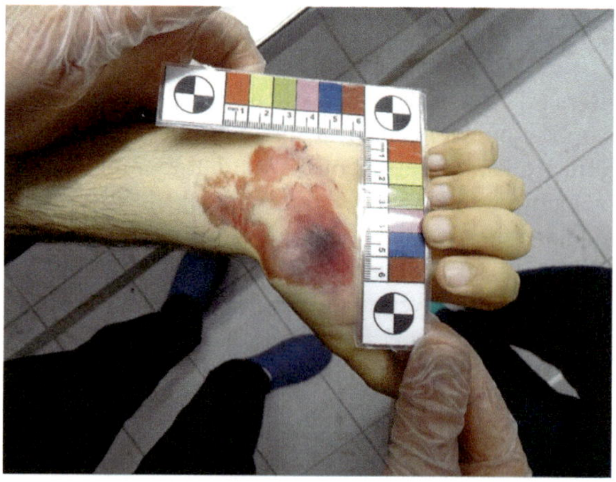

Fig. 10.1 Reddish abrasion due to contact with asphalt

10.2.2.2 Bruises

A bruise (or contusion) consists of an extravascular collection of blood due to the mechanical damage of vessels. The word "contusion" is often used to indicate internal blood spreading, such as in the spleen or muscles. The term "ecchymosis" usually refers to a small bruise and is little used nowadays.

The bruise may be caused by compression, traction, and torsion of the soft tissues. Even though the pure bruise lies beneath the intact epidermis, it is common to find it in combination with abrasions or lacerations. The intradermal bruises are usually visible through the overlying epidermic layers and appear as colored, slightly swollen, painful areas. Sometimes, deeper collections of blood due to hemorrhage may be visible through the skin surface and may be confused with a proper intradermal bruise (e.g., "black eye" due to cranial fractures).

The color of the bruise changes with time: fresh extravasations of blood appear purple or dark purple; while due to the enzymatic progressive degradation of blood pigments, the bruise turned into bluish-brown, greenish-brown, and yellowish, before completely fading [13]. The duration of the whole process depends on the dimension and deepness of the bruise and the characteristics of the victim: it takes a few days for a "love bite," up to 15–20 days in old patients with bigger bruises [14]. Therefore, accurately pinpointing the precise time an injury occurred becomes challenging due to the influence of subjective factors. Nevertheless, distinguishing lesions from different periods within the same individual can still offer valuable information and aid analysis.

Patterned bruises are caused by the impact of patterned objects (kicks with the shod foot, hits with a patterned floor). The impact with a rod or similar objects usually gives the "tram line" bruise, as the edges of the impact surface suffer powerful traction and compression.

Due to their pattern or site, certain types of bruises have special significance: clusters of small discoid bruises may indicate fingertip pressure (gripping lesions). Such gripping lesions are commonly seen on the arm or forearm in child abuse.

10.2.2.3 Lacerations

A blunt trauma penetrating the whole thickness of the skin produces a laceration. The skin is lacerated by tearing so that the margins of the wounds are irregular. As the different components of soft tissues have different resistance to blunt force tearing, lacerations show an incomplete separation of vessels, nerves, or fibrous tissues which causes "bridges" of tissue running from side to side of the wound. Due to the blunt force of a crushing component, lacerations show often abrasions and bruises on the margins [15].

The tearing effect is more evident in over-bony prominences (head, thorax) where the soft tissues are thinner and pinned against the bones. Whereas soft areas like the buttock or abdomen require more energy to be lacerated (Fig. 10.2).

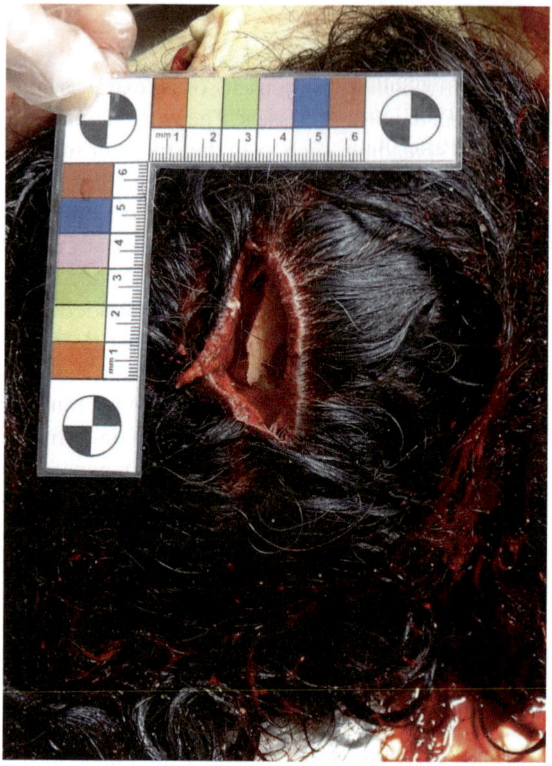

Fig. 10.2 Head laceration due to a high-energy impact

Due to the mechanisms of injury, the laceration shape does not reproduce the shape of the injuring agent.

10.2.2.4 Cuts

Cuts are incised wounds due to the slicing action of a blade, but also any other sharp object (e.g., a broken glass). Due to the sharpness of the blade, weak energy is sufficient to cut soft tissues and the cut's margins do not show any abrasions or bruises. The wound is longer than deeper; the margins are clean, regular, and straight. The wound may be deeper near the entrance point and shallower through the exit point of the blade.

The dimensions or shape of the injury agents do not determine any effects on wound appearance. However, the localization of cuts may be linked to the manner of the injury in some cases (self-inflicted or third-part inflicted, see the next paragraphs) [16].

10.2.2.5 Chops

Chops are deep incised mutilating wounds caused by a sharp-edged object that perpendicularly strikes the skin with a certain kinetic energy. The chop is caused by the impact with a sharp component, while cuts result from the tangential slice of the blade. So, chops are deeper than longer and cause internal organ injuries, bone injuries, or mutilations (fingers, extremities, head) [17, 18]. The chops are commonly caused by heavy sharp objects (e.g., axes or machetes) which may transmit sufficient kinetic energy easily [19].

10.2.2.6 Stabs

Stab wounds are produced by pointed instruments penetrating the skin and the soft tissues. The shape of the injuring component determines the force needed to perforate the skin: sharp-pointed objects or pointed weapons with or without blades penetrate more easily than smooth pointed objects (e.g., umbrellas) [20].

The wound is deeper than wider and may cause serious damage to the internal organs. The characteristics of the weapon may determine the shape of the wound. The external wound appears circular when the weapon has no sharp edges, triangular or buttonhole-shaped whether the weapon is single- or double-edged (Fig. 10.3).

Normally, stab wound margins are clean and regular. However, in the victim is struck with sufficient energy, the hilt guard may hit the skin surface producing a patterned bruise. In this case, it is also possible to estimate the length of the blade by measuring the deepness of the wound [21]. The width of the blade is difficult to estimate because of the modification of wounds' dimensions and the movement of injuring objects into the wound [22].

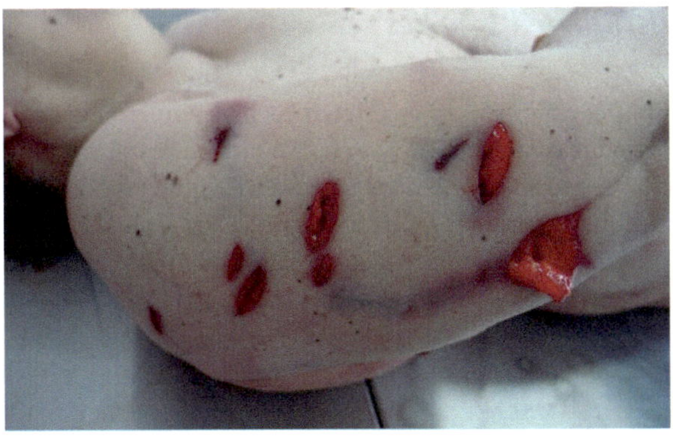

Fig. 10.3 Multiple stabs on the right arm

10.2.2.7 Burns and Scalds

Burns are injuries arising from the application of heat to the body; scalds are caused by hot liquids. The forensic evaluation of heat injuries is challenging. This type of injury is common in accidents and cases of maltreatment or as a means to cover up homicide [23–25].

A steaming object may produce patterned burns, while flames, explosions, or liquids produce wider lesions. The clothes and skin appendages may be wet (hot liquids) or may be burned (flames or explosions).

10.2.2.8 Electrocution

The passage through the body of electrical current (electrocution) may cause different kinds of injury. Due to some physical factors (current, voltage, resistance), a substantial electrical current may cause death, severe organ damage, or mutilations. In some cases, it can cause different degrees of skin lesions [6, 26].

The point of contact between the body and the electrical conductor shows the "targetoid" lesion, also known as the "electrical" burn or "electrical" mark. The skin lesion is a thermal burn: if there is firm contact with the skin the current causes skin blisters, if the contact is less firm, the keratin layer melts forming the "spark lesion" entailing a fused node of keratin surrounded by a pale areola [27].

10.3 Manner of Injury

The next paragraphs will examine some injury patterns whose manner can be recognized after a proper forensic assessment.

10.3.1 Self-Inflicted Injuries

Self-inflicted injuries include suicide, attempted suicide, suicidal acts, and self-inflicted non-suicidal trauma [28]. Self-inflicted injuries are generally associated with psychiatric disorders, particularly personality, eating, mood, and psychotic disorders [29]. Still, they are often motivated by pursuing secondary gains especially in insurance, military, or prison settings [28, 30]. Although data on the phenomenon's prevalence are not exhaustive due to underreporting and undetecting, the standardized incidence rate of self-harm is reported to be 62.5 per 100,000 individuals. Notably, there are gender disparities with a higher incidence of self-inflicted injuries in women (74.0 per 100,000; 95% CI 62.6–87.6) than in men (51.0 per 100,000; 95% CI 43.6–60.0) [31, 32].

Clinical examination of self-inflicted injuries poses a difficult challenge for physicians to distinguish accurately between pathologies, aggression-related injuries, and other types of self-harm. Failure to do so may lead to the start or end of a forensic investigation [32].

Conducting a thorough assessment of topographical arrangement is advisable. In particular, the anatomical region's self-attackability and how it correlates with the subject's handedness—left or right—should be carefully considered. For example, in right-handed individuals, usually, most lesions are observed on the left side [28, 33]. Moreover, generally, self-inflicted injuries tend to save more vulnerable areas, such as the ocular, aural, nasal, and labial regions, in favor of targeting sites such as the mandibular area, temporal region, frontal region, cervical region, pectoral region, deltoid region, brachial region, dorsum of the hand, and femoral region [28, 34, 35].

In the self-inflicted injuries examination, particularly those inflicted by a bladed weapon, it is essential to recognize the consistent nature of the pattern in which wounds manifest [28, 32].

These models typically involve multiple lesions arranged parallel to each other [28, 36, 37]. Such agreements strongly suggest that an external aggressor did not cause the injuries, as a victim is unlikely to remain stationary and allow the precise execution of several lights and evenly aligned wounds; in such circumstances, defensive injuries are highly likely to occur [28, 32].

Usually, self-inflicted injuries exhibit regularity of the margins of the wounds, a tendency to be superficial, and rarely pose a fatality risk and exhibit consistent depth. This contrasts with other bladed wounds, which progressively deepen from the surface toward the body's interior [28, 32, 33].

Moreover, in self-inflicted injuries, when incisions are made on coated areas, the corresponding clothes may not show cuts or cuts not aligned with the lesions in position or direction. Notably, in these instances, the integrity of the affected tissue is often preserved, suggesting a deliberate intent to minimize structural damage [28, 38].

10.3.1.1 Diagnosis and Assessment of Self-Harm

The evaluation of the characteristics of the injurious model constitutes an initial and essential step in establishing an appropriate differential diagnosis. This assessment examines the consistency between the narration of the victim and the number of lesions, their spatial arrangement, and their temporal and morphological manifestations (Table 10.1).

To accurately diagnose the cause of a patient's injuries, it is important to evaluate the injury, review the patient's medical history, and thoroughly investigate the circumstances surrounding the injury. This will help distinguish between potential causes of the observed injuries.

By carefully considering all these aspects, healthcare professionals can gather valuable insights that aid in distinguishing between potential causes and

Table 10.1 Common characteristics of self-inflicted injuries compared with injuries inflicted by others

	Injury inflicted by others	Self-inflicted injury
Type	Stab wounds, abrasions, or bruises; occasionally cuts	Cuts or abrasions; occasionally lacerations or blunt trauma
Location	Anywhere on the body	Easily accessible body areas not covered by clothing, avoiding sensitive areas, usually on the side opposite the dominant hand
Arrangement	Random	In groups of lesions arranged neatly, often in symmetrical and parallel rows
Form	Usually short and variable shape	Often long and constant in shape and may form geometric shapes, symbols, letters, or words
Intensity	Highly variable, often deep	Generally superficial
Severity	Highly variable, usually severe or very severe	Usually mild or very mild
Self-defense injuries	Common	Absent or atypical
Clothing	Tears and stains associated with the injury	Usually not included in the injury or harmed congruently with the presumed dynamic of the struggle
Repeated	Rare	Often, linear scars of varying ages (old scars)

contributing factors for the observed injuries. This systematic approach helps ensure a comprehensive analysis of the injurious model, facilitating a more accurate differential diagnosis.

In general, suicide and self-harm represent multifaceted phenomena that arise from a confluence of factors and are rarely attributable to a single cause. Various nonspecific risk factors contribute to developing suicidal tendencies, self-harm behaviors, and psychological distress. Therefore, comprehensive assessments that delve into individuals' contextual, mental, and treatment-related aspects are crucial. These assessments, often called psychosocial or biopsychosocial assessments, have demonstrated an association with decreased rates of repeated self-harm among patients seeking help in emergency departments [36].

Consequently, it is imperative to ensure the availability of such assessments for all individuals presenting with these concerns. By conducting in-depth evaluations that consider the multidimensional nature of these issues, healthcare professionals can better understand the underlying factors, tailor interventions to address specific needs, and ultimately reduce the risk of future self-harm incidents.

10.3.1.2 Skin Lesions from Recreative Drug Abuse

Many recreative drugs may cause skin damage directly or indirectly. Desomorphine is an injectable opioid whose recreative use is rapidly spreading across Europe. Desomorphine is a good substitute for the heroine, as they have similar effects. It is also commonly known as "krokodil" (the Russian word for crocodile) because of the skin lesions that causes in users [39].

The skin lesions from krokodil abuse refer to large eschars or ulcers of necrotized skin due to the thrombosis of skin vessels and infections of soft tissues [40, 41].

10.3.2 Defense Wounds

Another valuable element in the differential diagnosis is the detection of common defensive injuries, indications of self-protective actions undertaken by individuals when subjected to an assault. These injuries manifest in various forms, such as bruises, abrasions, lacerations, or fractures, and they are typically found in body regions susceptible to defensive actions, such as the hands, forearms, and head [42].

Evaluating the characteristics of defensive injuries involves comprehensively analyzing their location, distribution, and morphological attributes. The location of these injuries can provide valuable insights into the type and direction of the threat encountered, the defensive actions employed by the victim, and the dispute's duration and intensity. Morphologically, defensive injuries often exhibit features consistent with impact or contact with external objects, such as linear or curvilinear patterns, imprints, or patterns corresponding to the nature of the assailant's weapon or mode of attack [43] (Fig. 10.4).

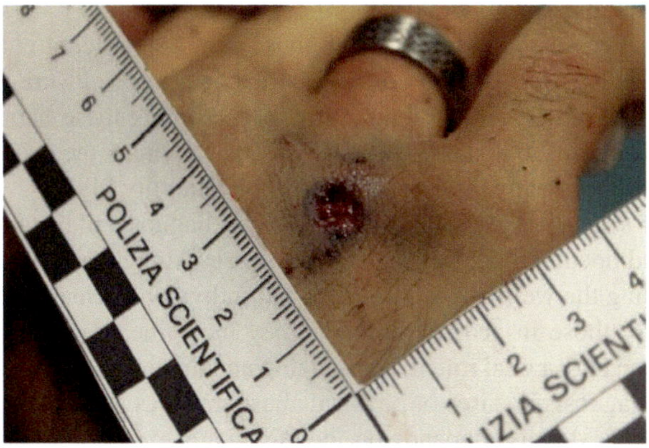

Fig. 10.4 Defensive injury from a gunshot wound. The location of the wound allows partial dynamics reconstruction

These features can help reconstruct the sequence of events and corroborate the victim's narrative regarding the dynamics of the incident. Meticulously examining and documenting the presence and characteristics of defensive injuries can derive crucial information to help determine the plausibility and veracity of the victim's account, further enhancing the overall understanding of the events under investigation.

10.3.3 Suspected Child Abuse

Child abuse is defined as all forms of physical, emotional, or sexual abuse resulting in harm to the child's health or dignity [44]. Also, neglect may represent a form of child abuse. Despite advances in human rights advocacy and increasing awareness surrounding abuse, physical abuse remains pervasive in familial and institutional settings [45, 46]. Moreover, it is often veiled in secrecy, perpetuating a cycle of silence that hinders the identification and intervention necessary to protect victims [47].

Often prominently visible, bruises are tangible evidence of the harm inflicted, reflecting the devastating physical toll, which can result in both short-term and long-term physical, psychological, and social impacts [45, 47].

Understanding the prevalence and scope of physical abuse is crucial for developing effective prevention and intervention strategies. Globally, physical abuse varies across regions, influenced by cultural, social, and economic factors [48]. Both children and adults can fall victim to physical abuse; fragile individuals, especially children, are at a higher risk of experiencing physical abuse [49].

The consequences of physical abuse extend far beyond immediate physical injuries. Survivors often experience long-lasting psychological and emotional effects, including anxiety, depression, post-traumatic stress disorder, and low self-esteem. The societal costs of physical abuse are profound, impacting healthcare systems, productivity, and the overall well-being of communities [50].

Yet, the silence surrounding physical abuse poses significant challenges to its detection and prevention. Victims often face barriers to disclosure rooted in fear, shame, power dynamics, and societal norms. Overcoming these barriers requires a comprehensive approach that empowers individuals to break the cycle of abuse and promotes a culture of empathy, support, and accountability [48].

In cases of suspected physical abuse, medical diagnosis plays a crucial role in identifying and documenting the signs of abuse, ensuring appropriate intervention, and safeguarding the well-being of the affected individuals. Healthcare professionals, particularly those in pediatrics, emergency medicine, forensic medicine, and family medicine play a vital role in recognizing and diagnosing physical abuse [51]. The medical diagnosis in cases of physical abuse involves several key components. Identifying physical abuse depends on the clinician's expertise in detecting suspicious injuries, performing a comprehensive physical exam with suitable supplementary tests, and evaluating whether the explanation for the physical evidence aligns with the patient's history. A detailed medical history should include previous trauma, admissions to the hospital, chronic illness, and treatment adherence. To comprehend a family's situation, asking about past experiences with substance abuse, mental health, domestic violence, disciplinary actions, stress levels, and any prior involvement with child protection services is essential. Inconsistent or unclear explanations for a child's injury and delayed medical care may indicate abuse, but it is crucial to approach these situations with sensitivity and consider potential factors contributing to inconsistencies, such as fear, coercion, or the victim's developmental stage [51]. Ideally, careful documentation with photographs and an interdisciplinary approach is necessary.

10.3.3.1 Bruises in Suspected Abuse

In general, bruises are the most common manifestation of physical abuse, although some bruises' frequency, number, and location are linked to motor development [52]. Accidental bruises are characteristically anterior and over-bony prominences, such as shins and forehead, usually due to falls [53, 54]. Bruises in infants younger than 9 months who have not started walking should lead the physician to consider abuse or illness as likely causes. Well-padded areas are unlikely to be bruised during most childhood activities. Thus, bruises on the buttocks, cheeks, and thighs suggest abuse [54, 55]. The bruise color depends on several factors, particularly the depth of the lesion, the force of impact, location, and vascularity of tissues, time since injury, skin color, and ambient lighting. If an implement was used, bruises can carry an imprint [56]. Sometimes ecchymosis in a child with a medical explanation (such as idiopathic thrombocytopenic purpura, leukemia, *Henoch Schönlein* purpura, coagulation disorders, connective tissue disorders like *Ehlers-Danlos* syndrome, or osteogenesis imperfecta) may mimic bruises. Moreover, birthmarks and Mongolian spots can be confused with bruises, but these marks are not tender and do not rapidly change color or size [57].

10.3.3.2 Bite Marks

Other possible evidence of abuse during a physical examination is bite marks associated with an adult, another child, an animal, or the patient depending on the characteristics. Animal bites vary, but they usually have narrower arches than human bites and are often profound. Self-inflicted bites are limited to accessible areas, especially the hands. Adult bites generally have more than an inch between the canines and often cause the most critical bruises. Many bites of another child suggest inadequate supervision and neglect [51].

Additionally, while abuse is often the cause of childhood burns, negligence or insufficient supervision are also major contributing factors; children may draw hot substances onto themselves while investigating their surroundings. The likely mechanism can be inferred from the pattern or distribution of the burn; burns from hot items have geometries that are similar to those of other burns. Symmetrical burns, like those of the buttocks and perineum, are especially suspicious. Also, in these cases, several circumstances could mimic abusive burns, such as brushing against car seat burns, enuresis blanket marks, and impetigo [51, 58–61]. Impetigo can resemble cigarette burns, but cigarette burns are usually 7–10 mm across; impetigo has lesions of varying sizes [61].

10.3.3.3 Fractures in Suspected Abuse

The American Academy of Pediatrics recommends a mandatory skeletal survey of all suspected physical abuse cases in children under 2 years. Bone fractures are the second most common presentation of physical abuse after bruises [52]. No lesion is pathognomonic of abuse; however, some strongly suggest abuse, like metaphyseal lesions, rib (especially posterior), scapula, spinous process, and sternum [51]. The metaphyseal lesion usually suggests abuse although it has been identified after a difficult cesarean section [62]. Rib fractures are unusual in children without mineral deficiencies also after cardiopulmonary resuscitation [63].

Skull fractures happen in only 1–3% of children after falls from heights and are usually linear, narrow, and uncomplicated. Many complex fractures on both sides of the skull and depressed or growing fractures (leptomeningeal cysts) are typical of abuse. Skull fractures with intracranial injury in infants are usually due to abuse although simple skull fractures could have a thin adjacent subdural hematoma [64].

10.3.3.4 Internal Organs Damage in Suspected Abuse

Abusive head injuries result from mechanisms including shaking, direct impact, penetration, and asphyxiation or hypoxia, alone or in combination. Results of studies strongly accord with the contention that adults do shake infants and that shaking alone can cause widespread brain injury. Abusive head trauma can result from frustration associated with a baby's crying or irritability. In these cases, in the child occurs shaken baby syndrome because of the impact of the brain against the skull linked to the severe forces of acceleration-deceleration [65].

In abused children, abdominal trauma is a leading cause of morbidity and mortality. An impact or forceful blow can cause bleeding or rupturing of hollow organs, and solid organs can also be injured. The signs of abdominal trauma may not be immediately apparent, and even severe injuries may not result in visible bruising of the abdominal wall. Abdominal injuries can occur slowly, making it essential to be vigilant for subtle symptoms and signs of physical abuse. If a young child presents with bilious vomiting but no fever or peritoneal irritation, it may indicate a duodenal hematoma often linked to abuse [51, 66].

Physicians should conduct tests on urine and stool samples to check for any blood and examine liver and pancreatic enzymes.

10.3.4 Neglect

Neglect is a severe form of maltreatment characterized by a caregiver's failure to provide the necessary care, support, and protection to meet the individual's basic needs. Neglect can take on different forms, such as physical neglect, medical neglect, emotional neglect, educational neglect, and supervisory neglect [67, 68]. Neglected individuals face various physical health problems, including malnutrition, dehydration, poor hygiene, untreated medical conditions, and developmental delays. Neglect affects physical health and can have severe emotional and psychological consequences such as low self-esteem, depression, anxiety, and difficulty forming and maintaining relationships.

10.3.4.1 Neglect and Malnutrition

In individuals who experience neglect and are unable to independently nutrition, a notable and pronounced consequence is the development of severe malnutrition due to inadequate dietary intake. Individual daily calorie needs vary by age, sex, and physical activity level, but active adults generally need at least 1500–2500 calories/day to maintain body weight [69]. Life-threatening conditions arise when an individual loses more than 40% of the original body weight although the speed of weight loss is also relevant. Without food, death can occur in about 50–60 days if adequate water is available, but this time frame depends on the individual's initial time, temperature, fitness, and fat. Water deprivation can lead to death in about 10 days or less at higher ambient temperatures [28, 70].

In fatal and nonfatal starvation cases, two main types are described: "dry" and "wet." The "dry" type is characterized by emaciation with only edema of the legs, with body weight up to half the average. Individuals with this type typically exhibit marked hypotension, weak pulse, and cyanosis. The "wet" type, on the other hand, involves marked edema of the face, trunk, and limbs, with ascites and pleural effusions [71].

Hunger can lead to various issues, including skin problems, infections, vitamin deficiencies, and swelling caused by a lack of proper nutrition. However, the most severe consequences that can result in death are dehydration, hypothermia, and necrosis in the extremities. Dehydration is especially common in infants and can significantly affect their mortality. Dehydrated skin can become dry and wrinkled, and when pinched, it retains its ridges due to the loss of subcutaneous fat and fluids. Malnutrition can be visible in the face, which may appear elongated through the cheekbones, with sunken cheeks, prominent maxillary lines, and sunken eyes due to fat loss and dehydration. The chest may show prominent ribs, concavity in the intercostal spaces, and a sunken supraclavicular fossa. The abdomen may appear concave, with the rib margin at the iliac ridges concave and the iliac ridges protruding like wings. The limbs may appear skeletal due to the loss of fat and muscles, while the head may appear disproportionately large compared to the narrow neck [28, 70, 71].

In general, the appearance of the skin can vary depending on the duration of nutritional loss and specific dietary deficiencies, especially of vitamins. The skin may appear pale, shiny, and semi-translucent, with a bluish tinge in newborns, partly due to subcutaneous fat loss. Alternatively, it may be coarse, rough, and present with flaking hyperkeratosis, commonly seen in older individuals due to senile changes [28]. In infants, fontanelles may be depressed due to loss of cerebrospinal fluid pressure and avitaminosis.

Skin infections are frequently occurring, often caused by altered immunity caused by malnutrition and also by inadequate attention to hygiene and care, especially in babies [28, 70, 72, 73].

When infants or older individuals remain immobile for extended periods due to weakness, they may develop pressure sores on their gluteal region, heels, and spine. These sores can worsen in infants due to urinary dermatitis and lack of proper skin care after defecation. Sores can also appear on areas of the body that experience pressure or friction, such as the elbows, knees, shoulders, and back of the head. Other signs of malnutrition include sores on the lips, blepharitis, conjunctivitis, dry and brittle hair, and loss of skin pigmentation.

It can be difficult to determine the relationship between neglect and cachexia, especially when other medical conditions can also cause cachexia, such as neoplastic diseases [28, 74]

10.3.4.2 Diagnosis and Assessment of Neglect

Healthcare workers should examine various medical records and relevant documents to accurately assess neglected individuals, including growth charts, vaccination records, and other health history information. This comprehensive approach might allow physicians to fully understand the neglected person's medical background, evaluate chronic illnesses, and address malnutrition. When dealing with children, it is essential to consider familial metabolic disorders [75–77].

Identifying neglect in older victims is crucial, especially as they often lack social interactions. Physicians play a critical role in identifying and intervening in such cases. The emergency department provides a valuable opportunity to spot victims and initiate intervention, which can significantly enhance their quality of life.

Obtaining a thorough and precise medical history is vital to assess potential abuse or neglect. It is also essential to perform thorough physical exams, laboratory tests, and radiological assessments to evaluate and record the individual's physical and mental health status that has been neglected. In elder abuse cases, healthcare workers should carefully observe the patient–caregiver interaction for any signs of a strained relationship if a caregiver is present at the patient's bedside [78–81].

In child-neglected cases, precise measurements of body weight and standard anatomical lengths are crucial for comparison with age-specific pediatric growth charts, considering factors such as birth weight, gender, and ethnicity [71, 72, 78].

Comprehensive documentation of test results, laboratory reports, and photographic tests is essential for providing evidence in forensic evaluations. Depending on local laws and regulations, this evidence may be used to report suspected negligence to child protection services or other competent authorities, such as adult protection services and law enforcement.

10.4 Pathomimesis and Malingering

10.4.1 Pathomimesis

Pathomimesis refers to artificial dermatological disorders associated with psychological and psychosomatic conditions [82]. From a medico-legal point of view, managing pathomimesis or other psychocutaneous disorders may increase the odds of diagnostic or therapeutic errors [83].

One strategy that can potentially enhance the detection of pathomimesis in clinical settings is the increased implementation of comprehensive screening measures for psychosocial correlates in primary care facilities. Established assessment instruments, such as the Personality Assessment Inventory (PAI) and the Minnesota Multiphasic Personality Inventory-2 (MMPI-2), incorporate scales designed to capture false or exaggerated reporting [84, 85]. However, it is noteworthy that these scales are infrequently utilized for identifying factitious symptom presentations within healthcare settings.

The proliferation of online resources poses additional challenges in diagnosing pathomimesis. Individuals engaging in deceptive behaviors often exploit the internet to facilitate their actions, thus augmenting the complexity of identifying and diagnosing pathomimesis in a clinical context. Accurately diagnosing pathomimesis necessitates a meticulous evaluation of presenting symptoms, which can prove arduous within high-volume medical facilities with limited time for comprehensive patient–physician interactions. Nonetheless, the increasing adoption of electronic medical records (EMRs) represents a potential avenue for mitigating logistical barriers to diagnosis within the healthcare system. Electronic medical records offer healthcare providers access to patients' longitudinal health information from diverse clinical settings. Leveraging this information can be valuable in identifying patterns of excessive and unnecessary treatment-seeking behaviors, ultimately supporting the diagnosis of pathomimesis. Furthermore, using EMRs undermines the patient's ability to evade suspicion by transitioning between facilities, as their comprehensive health records remain accessible to providers [86].

10.4.2 *Malingering*

Malingering is defined as deliberate deception regarding the exaggeration or simulation of signs and symptoms. When associated with litigation or compensation, the rate of malingering is reported to affect about 30% of cases [87].

Many countries adopted special laws to protect occupational health or compensate the workers. Given such context, it is essential to identify possible malingering [88]. The skin is one of the organs most affected by occupational diseases. Contact dermatitis is the most common manifestation of occupational skin disease; the lesions are often localized on the hands. The construction industry, hairdressing, metal manufacturing, and food industry are some of the fields most affected [89].

The recent position paper of the European Society for Dermatology and Psychiatry suggests that a deep examination of medical history is the best approach to recognizing a factitious skin disorder, with special attention to the frequency of symptoms presentation (isolated, episodic, or repeated), the presence of psychiatric symptoms, and any external incentive related to the skin disorder [90].

10.5 Practical Tips

Properly managing dermatological injuries considered suspect or unusual requires a multidisciplinary team. When a healthcare professional in a medical setting suspects an unusual or suspect dermatological condition during the clinical evaluation, it is essential to involve a branch specialist who may vary according to the specific characteristics of the lesion. The objective is to determine whether the injury is traumatic or non-traumatic.

In cases of traumatic injuries, a forensic approach may be necessary. Comparison with a specialist in the field can help to identify the dynamics that caused the injury and proceed in the protection of the psycho-physical health of the patient. Therefore, it is essential to have a multidisciplinary team, including medical professionals, forensic experts, and other specialists, to effectively manage dermatological injuries considered suspect or unusual (Fig. 10.5).

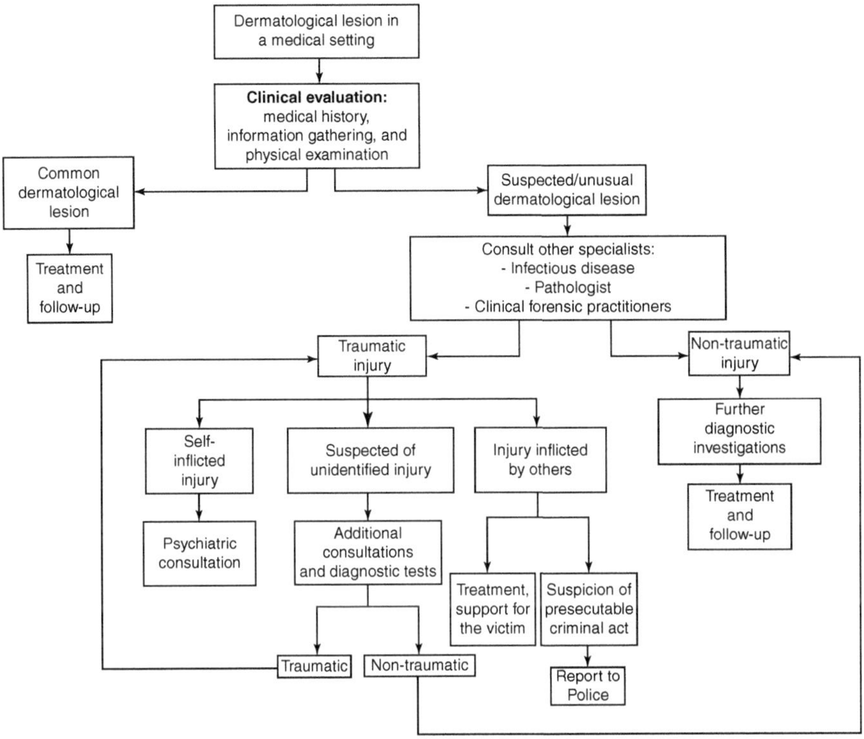

Fig. 10.5 A suggested flowchart for medico-legal management. Starting at the location of the "dermatological lesion in a medical setting" and working your way down the branches according to the findings' existence or absence will allow you to manage suspected dermatological lesions effectively

Competing Interest The authors have no competing interest to declare.

Ethical Approval Ethical approval was not needed as the present manuscript involves information freely available in the public domain, no personal information was needed.

References

1. Jafferany M. Psychodermatology: a guide to understanding common psychocutaneous disorders. Prim Care Companion J Clin Psychiatry. United States. 2007;9(3):203–13.
2. Koo JYM, Lee CS. General approach to evaluating psychodermatological disorders. Basic Clin Dermatol. 2003;25:1–12.
3. Cocanour CS. Informed consent-It's more than a signature on a piece of paper. Am J Surg. United States. 2017;214(6):993–7.

4. Fields LM, Calvert JD. Informed consent procedures with cognitively impaired patients: a review of ethics and best practices. Psychiatry Clin Neurosci. Australia. 2015;69(8):462–71.
5. Parmigiani G, Mandarelli G, Dacquino C, Pompili P, Lelli Chiesa G, Ferracuti S. Decisional capacity to consent to clinical research involving placebo in psychiatric Patients. J Forensic Sci. United States. 2016;61(2):388–93.
6. Saukko P, Knight B. Knight's forensic pathology. 3rd ed; 2004.
7. Blackie R, Taylor D, Linacre A. DNA profiles from clothing fibers using direct PCR. Springer; 2016.
8. Ueland M, Forbes SL, Stuart BH. Understanding clothed buried remains: the analysis of decomposition fluids and their influence on clothing in model burial environments. Forensic Sci Med Pathol. Springer. 2019;15:3–12.
9. Arnold VK, Rosenthal TL, Dupont RT, Hilliard D. Redundant clothing: a readily observable marker for schizophrenia in the psychiatric emergency room population. J Behav Ther Exp Psychiatry. Elsevier. 1993;24(1):45–7.
10. Trottier DG, Hilt L. I don't feel naked: the use of embodied supervision to examine the impact of patient clothing on clinical countertransference on an inpatient psychiatry unit. Drama Ther Rev. Intellect. 2017;3(2):261–83.
11. Langlois NEI. A patterned abrasion on the neck of an infant: inflicted injury or not. Forensic Sci Med Pathol [Internet]. 2009;5(4):324–5. Available from: https://doi.org/10.1007/s12024-009-9111-y
12. Suárez-Peñaranda JM, Alvarez T, Miguéns X, Rodríguez-Calvo MS, De Abajo BL, Cortesão M, et al. Characterization of lesions in hanging deaths. J Forensic Sci. Wiley Online Library. 2008;53(3):720–3.
13. Scafide KRN, Sheridan DJ, Campbell J, DeLeon VB, Hayat MJ. Evaluating change in bruise colorimetry and the effect of subject characteristics over time. Forensic Sci Med Pathol [Internet]. 2013;9(3):367–76. Available from: https://doi.org/10.1007/s12024-013-9452-4
14. Langlois NE, Gresham GA. The ageing of bruises: a review and study of the colour changes with time. Forensic Sci Int. Ireland. 1991;50(2):227–38.
15. Hamilton JR, Sunter JP, Cooper PN. Fatal hemorrhage from simple lacerations of the scalp. Forensic Sci Med Pathol [Internet]. 2005;1(4):267–71. Available from: https://doi.org/10.1385/FSMP:1:4:267
16. Schmidt U, Pollak S. Sharp force injuries in clinical forensic medicine—findings in victims and perpetrators. Forensic Sci Int. 2006;159(2):113–8.
17. DiMaio D, DiMaio VJ. Forensic pathology. CRC Press; 2001.
18. Wittschieber D, Beck L, Vieth V, Hahnemann ML. The role of 3DCT for the evaluation of chop injuries in clinical forensic medicine. Forensic Sci Int. Ireland. 2016;266:e59–63.
19. Nikolić S, Živković V. Attempted suicide with an axe: a hanged waiter with multiple healed chop wounds to the crown of the head. Forensic Sci Med Pathol [Internet]. 2013;9(1):117–21. Available from: https://doi.org/10.1007/s12024-012-9330-5
20. Rouse DA. Patterns of stab wounds: a six year study. Med Sci Law. SAGE Publications London, England; 1994;34(1):67–71.
21. Swann IJ, MacMillan R, Watson AA. A study of stab wounds. Emer Med J. British Association for Accident and Emergency Medicine. 1985;2(1):31–6.
22. Burke MP, Baber Y, Cheung Z, Fitzgerald M. Single stab injuries. Forensic Sci Med Pathol. Springer. 2018;14:295–300.
23. Fanton L, Jdeed K, Tilhet-Coartet S, Malicier D. Criminal burning. Forensic Sci Int. Ireland. 2006;158(2–3):87–93.
24. Kemp AM, Hollén L, Emond AM, Nuttall D, Rea D, Maguire S. Raising suspicion of maltreatment from burns: derivation and validation of the BuRN-Tool. Burns. Elsevier. 2018;44(2):335–43.
25. Maguire S, Okolie C, Kemp AM. Burns as a consequence of child maltreatment. Paediatr Child Health. Elsevier. 2014;24(12):557–61.

26. Mittal P, Bohnert M. Intramuscular hemorrhages in the pathway of an electric current through the body—two case reports. Forensic Sci Med Pathol [Internet]. 2023;19(1):72–7. Available from: https://doi.org/10.1007/s12024-022-00558-2
27. Byard RW. Electrocution—post-mortem presentations, problems and pitfalls. Forensic Sci Med Pathol [Internet]. 2023;19(1):91–3. Available from: https://doi.org/10.1007/s12024-022-00544-8
28. Saukko P, Knight B. Knight's forensic pathology. 4th ed. London: Taylor & Francis Ltd/CRC Press; 2015.
29. Ose SO, Tveit T, Mehlum L. Non-suicidal self-injury (NSSI) in adult psychiatric outpatients—a nationwide study. J Psychiatr Res. Pergamon. 2021;133:1–9.
30. Schnellbacher S, O'Mara H. Identifying and managing malingering and factitious disorder in the military. Curr Psychiatry Rep [Internet]. Current Medicine Group LLC 1. 2016;18(11):1–7. [cited 2023 Jul 11]. Available from: https://link.springer.com/article/10.1007/s11920-016-0740-z
31. Abbafati C, Abbas KM, Abbasi-Kangevari M, Abd-Allah F, Abdelalim A, Abdollahi M, et al. Global burden of 369 diseases and injuries in 204 countries and territories, 1990–2019: a systematic analysis for the Global Burden of Disease Study 2019. The Lancet [Internet]. Elsevier B.V. 2020;396(10258):1204–22. [cited 2023 Jul 6]. Available from: http://www.thelancet.com/article/S0140673620309259/fulltext
32. Knipe D, Padmanathan P, Newton-Howes G, Chan LF, Kapur N. Suicide and self-harm. Lancet [Internet]. Lancet. 2022;399(10338):1903–16. [cited 2023 Jul 6]. Available from: https://pubmed.ncbi.nlm.nih.gov/35512727/
33. Saukko P, Pollak S. Self-inflicted injury. encyclopedia of forensic sciences. 2nd ed. Academic Press; 2013. p. 110–5.
34. Nishimura T, Naito H, Nakao A, Nakayama S. Characteristics of self-inflicted injury among suicidal patients: analysis of nation-wide trauma registry. Trauma Surg Acute Care Open. BMJ Publishing Group. 2021;6(1)
35. Segal P, Mrzyglod S, Alichniewicz-Czaplicka H, Dunin-Horkawicz W, Zwyrzykowski E. Self-inflicted eye injuries. Am J Ophthalmol. Elsevier. 1963;55(2):349–62.
36. Guideline number NG225 N. Self-harm: assessment, management and preventing recurrence. Methods. 2022;
37. Nikolić S, Cvetković D, Ječmenica D, Živković V. Atypical longitudinal self-inflicted incised wounds as a cause of death in an ecstasy user. Forensic Sci Med Pathol [Internet]. 2022;18(2):197–200. Available from: https://doi.org/10.1007/s12024-021-00436-3
38. Venara A, Jousset N, Airagnes G, Arnaud JP, Rougé-Maillart C. Abdominal stab wounds: self-inflicted wounds versus assault wounds. J Forensic Leg Med [Internet]. J Forensic Leg Med. 2013;20(4):270–3. [cited 2023 Jul 10]. Available from: https://pubmed.ncbi.nlm.nih.gov/23622473/
39. Haskin A, Kim N, Aguh C. A new drug with a nasty bite: a case of krokodil-induced skin necrosis in an intravenous drug user. JAAD Case Rep [Internet]. 2016;2(2):174–6. Available from: https://www.sciencedirect.com/science/article/pii/S2352512616000230
40. Grund J-PC, Latypov A, Harris M. Breaking worse: the emergence of krokodil and excessive injuries among people who inject drugs in Eurasia. Int J Drug Policy [Internet]. 2013;24(4):265–74. Available from: https://www.sciencedirect.com/science/article/pii/S0955395913000510
41. Sorrentino A, Trotta S, Colucci AP, Aventaggiato L, Marzullo A, Solarino B. Lethal endomyocarditis caused by chronic "Krokodil" intoxication. Forensic Sci Med Pathol [Internet]. 2018;14(2):229–35. Available from: https://doi.org/10.1007/s12024-018-9967-9
42. Mohanty MK, Panigrahi MK, Mohanty S, Dash JK, Dash SK. Self-defense injuries in homicidal deaths. J Forensic Leg Med [Internet]. J Forensic Leg Med. 2007;14(4):213–5. [cited 2023 Jul 6]. Available from: https://pubmed.ncbi.nlm.nih.gov/16931102/

43. Katkici U, Ozkök MS, Orsal M. An autopsy evaluation of defence wounds in 195 homicidal deaths due to stabbing. J Forensic Sci Soc [Internet]. J Forensic Sci Soc. 1994;34(4):237–40. [cited 2023 Jul 6]. Available from: https://pubmed.ncbi.nlm.nih.gov/7844516/
44. Lupariello F. Child abuse and traditional medicine practices. Forensic Sci Med Pathol [Internet]. 2020;16(1):203. Available from: https://doi.org/10.1007/s12024-019-00160-z
45. Edwards VJ, Holden GW, Felitti VJ, Anda RF. Relationship between multiple forms of childhood maltreatment and adult mental health in community respondents: results from the adverse childhood experiences study. Am J Psychiatry [Internet]. Am J Psychiatry. 2003;160(8):1453–60. [cited 2023 Jul 11]. Available from: https://pubmed.ncbi.nlm.nih.gov/12900308/
46. Kilpatrick DG. Interpersonal violence and public policy: what about the victims? Journal of Law, Medicine and Ethics [Internet]. American Society of Law, Medicine and Ethics. 2004;32(1):73–81. [cited 2023 Jul 1. Available from: https://journals.sagepub.com/doi/10.1111/j.1748-720X.2004.tb00450.x
47. Vrolijk-Bosschaart TF, Brilleslijper-Kater SN, Benninga MA, Lindauer RJL, Teeuw AH. Clinical practice: recognizing child sexual abuse-what makes it so difficult? Eur J Pediatr [Internet]. Eur J Pediatr. 2018;177(9):1343–50. [cited 2023 Jul 11]. Available from: https://pubmed.ncbi.nlm.nih.gov/29938356/
48. Petersen AC, Joseph J, Feit M, Committee on Child Maltreatment Research P and P for the NDPI, Board on Children Y and F, Justice C on L and, et al. Describing the Problem. National Academies Press (US); 2014. [cited 2023 Jul 12]. Available from: https://www.ncbi.nlm.nih.gov/books/NBK195982/
49. Dubowitz H, Bennett S. Physical abuse and neglect of children. Lancet [Internet]. Elsevier B.V. 2007;369(9576):1891–9. [cited 2023 Jul 11]. Available from: http://www.thelancet.com/article/S0140673607608563/fulltext
50. Springer KW, Sheridan J, Kuo D, Carnes M. The long-term health outcomes of childhood abuse: an overview and a call to action. J Gen Intern Med [Internet]. Springer. 2003;18(10):864. [cited 2023 Jul 12]. Available from: /pmc/articles/PMC1494926/
51. Dubowitz H, Bennett S. Physical abuse and neglect of children. Lancet [Internet]. Elsevier B.V. 2007;369(9576):1891–9. [cited 2023 Jul 12]. Available from: http://www.thelancet.com/article/S0140673607608563/fulltext
52. McMahon P, Grossman W, Gaffney M, Stanitski C. Soft-tissue injury as an indication of child abuse. J Bone Joint Surg Am [Internet]. J Bone Joint Surg Am. 1995;77(8):1179–83. [cited 2023 Jul 12]. Available from: https://pubmed.ncbi.nlm.nih.gov/7642662/
53. Carpenter RF. The prevalence and distribution of bruising in babies. Arch Dis Child [Internet]. Arch Dis Child. 1999;80(4):363–6. [cited 2023 Jul 12]. Available from: https://pubmed.ncbi.nlm.nih.gov/10086945/
54. Labbé J, Caouette G. Recent skin injuries in normal children. Pediatrics [Internet]. Pediatrics. 2001;108(2):271–6. [cited 2023 Jul 12]. Available from: https://pubmed.ncbi.nlm.nih.gov/11483787/
55. Sugar NF, Taylor JA, Feldman KW. Bruises in infants and toddlers: those who don't cruise rarely bruise. Puget Sound Pediatric Research Network. Arch Pediatr Adolesc Med [Internet]. Arch Pediatr Adolesc Med. 1999;153(4):399–403. [cited 2023 Jul 12]. Available from: https://pubmed.ncbi.nlm.nih.gov/10201724/
56. Maguire S, Mann MK, Sibert J, Kemp A. Can you age bruises accurately in children? A systematic review. Arch Dis Child [Internet]. Arch Dis Child. 2005;90(2):187–9. [cited 2023 Jul 12]. Available from: https://pubmed.ncbi.nlm.nih.gov/15665179/
57. Wardinsky TD. Genetic and congenital defect conditions that mimic child abuse—PubMed. J Fam Pract [Internet]. 1995;41(4):377–83. Available from: https://pubmed.ncbi.nlm.nih.gov/7561712/
58. Andronicus M, Oates RK, Peat J, Spalding S, Martin H. Non-accidental burns in children. Burns [Internet]. Burns. 1998;24(6):552–8. [cited 2023 Jul 12]. Available from: https://pubmed.ncbi.nlm.nih.gov/9776094/

59. Angel C, Shu T, French D, Orihuela E, Lukefahr J, Herndon DN. Genital and perineal burns in children: 10 years of experience at a major burn center. J Pediatr Surg [Internet]. J Pediatr Surg. 2002;37(1):99–103. [cited 2023 Jul 12]. Available from: https://pubmed.ncbi.nlm.nih.gov/11781996/
60. Chester DL, Jose RM, Aldlyami E, King H, Moiemen NS. Non-accidental burns in children--are we neglecting neglect? Burns [Internet]. Burns. 2006;32(2):222–8. [cited 2023 Jul 12]. Available from: https://pubmed.ncbi.nlm.nih.gov/16448766/
61. Forjuoh SN. Pattern of intentional burns to children in Ghana. Child Abuse Negl [Internet]. Child Abuse Negl. 1995;19(7):837–41. [cited 2023]. Available from: https://pubmed.ncbi.nlm.nih.gov/7583740/
62. Grayev AM, Boal DKB, Wallach DM, Segal LS. Metaphyseal fractures mimicking abuse during treatment for clubfoot. Pediatr Radiol [Internet]. Pediatr Radiol. 2001;31(8):559–63. [cited 2023 Jul 12]. Available from: https://pubmed.ncbi.nlm.nih.gov/11550767/
63. Barsness KA, Cha ES, Bensard DD, Calkins CM, Partrick DA, Karrer FM, et al. The positive predictive value of rib fractures as an indicator of nonaccidental trauma in children. J Trauma [Internet]. J Trauma. 2003;54(6):1107–10. [cited 2023 Jul 12]. Available from: https://pubmed.ncbi.nlm.nih.gov/12813330/
64. Hobbs CJ. Skull fracture and the diagnosis of abuse. Arch Dis Child [Internet]. Arch Dis Child. 1984;59(3):246–52. [cited 2023 Jul 12]. Available from: https://pubmed.ncbi.nlm.nih.gov/6712273/
65. Mian M, Shah J, Dalpiaz A, Schwamb R, Miao Y, Warren K, et al. Shaken Baby Syndrome: a review. Fetal Pediatr Pathol [Internet]. Fetal Pediatr Pathol. 2015;34(3):169–75. [cited 2023 Jul 12]. Available from: https://pubmed.ncbi.nlm.nih.gov/25616019/
66. Barnes PM, Norton CM, Dunstan FD, Kemp AM, Yates DW, Sibert JR. Abdominal injury due to child abuse. Lancet [Internet]. Lancet. 2005;366(9481):234–5. [cited 2023 Jul 12]. Available from: https://pubmed.ncbi.nlm.nih.gov/16023514/
67. Ross AH, Juarez CA. A brief history of fatal child maltreatment and neglect. Forensic Sci Med Pathol [Internet]. 2014;10(3):413–22. Available from: https://doi.org/10.1007/s12024-014-9531-1
68. Sarkar R, Ozanne-Smith J, Bassed R. Mandatory reporting of child physical abuse and dental neglect by Australian dentists. Forensic Sci Med Pathol [Internet]. 2020;16(1):134–42. Available from: https://doi.org/10.1007/s12024-019-00180-9
69. McKinnon RA, Oladipo T, Ferguson MS, Jones OE, Maroto ME, Wolpert B. Reported knowledge of typical daily calorie requirements: relationship to demographic characteristics in US adults. J Acad Nutr Diet. Elsevier. 2019;119(11):1831–1841.e6.
70. Frølich J, Palm CVB, Støving RK. To the limit of extreme malnutrition. Nutrition [Internet]. Nutrition. 2016;32(1):146–8. [cited 2023 Jul 12]. Available from: https://pubmed.ncbi.nlm.nih.gov/26520917/
71. Solarino B, Tsokos M, Di Vella G, Tattoli L. Child starvation and neglect. Handbook of famine, starvation, and nutrient deprivation: from biology to policy [Internet]. Springer International Publishing; 2019. p. 961–79. [cited 2023 Jul 12]. Available from: https://link.springer.com/referenceworkentry/10.1007/978-3-319-55387-0_57
72. Bhutta ZA, Berkley JA, Bandsma RHJ, Kerac M, Trehan I, Briend A. Severe childhood malnutrition. Nat Rev Dis Primers [Internet]. Nat Rev Dis Primers. 2017;3(1) [cited 2023 Jul 12]. Available from: https://pubmed.ncbi.nlm.nih.gov/28933421/
73. Haffner D, Leifheit-Nestler M, Grund A, Schnabel D. Rickets guidance: part I-diagnostic workup. Pediatr Nephrol [Internet]. Pediatr Nephrol. 2022;37(9):2013–36. [cited 2023 Jul 12]. Available from: https://pubmed.ncbi.nlm.nih.gov/34910242/
74. Defloor T. The risk of pressure sores: a conceptual scheme. J Clin Nurs [Internet]. Blackwell Publishing Ltd. 1999;8(2):206–16. [cited 2023 Jul 12. Available from: https://europepmc.org/article/med/10401354
75. Glickman EA, Choi KW, Lussier AA, Smith BJ, Dunn EC. Childhood emotional neglect and adolescent depression: assessing the protective role of peer social support in a longitudinal

birth cohort. Front Psychiatry [Internet]. Frontiers Media S.A. 2021;12:681176. [cited 2023 Jul 12] Available from: /pmc/articles/PMC8381469/
76. Maguire SA, Williams B, Naughton AM, Cowley LE, Tempest V, Mann MK, et al. A systematic review of the emotional, behavioural and cognitive features exhibited by school-aged children experiencing neglect or emotional abuse. Child Care Health Dev [Internet]. Child Care Health Dev. 2015;41(5):641–53. [cited 2023 Jul 12]. Available from: https://pubmed.ncbi.nlm.nih.gov/25733080/
77. Young JC, Widom CS. Long-term effects of child abuse and neglect on emotion processing in adulthood. Child Abuse Negl [Internet]. Child Abuse Negl. 2014;38(8):1369–81. [cited 2023 Jul 12]. Available from: https://pubmed.ncbi.nlm.nih.gov/24747007/
78. Gonzalez D, Mirabal AB, McCall JD, Doerr C. Child abuse and neglect (Nursing). StatPearls [Internet]. StatPearls Publishing. 2022; [cited 2023 Jul 12]. Available from: https://www.ncbi.nlm.nih.gov/books/NBK568689/
79. Lachs MS, Pillemer K. Elder abuse. Lancet [Internet]. Elsevier B.V. 2004;364(9441):1263–72. [cited 2023 Jul 12]. Available from: https://pubmed.ncbi.nlm.nih.gov/15464188/
80. Lachs MS, Pillemer KA. Elder abuse. Campion EW, editor. N Engl J Med [Internet]. N Engl J Med; 2015. 373(20):1947–56. [cited 2023 Jul 12]. Available from: https://pubmed.ncbi.nlm.nih.gov/26559573/
81. Rosen T, Stern ME, Elman A, Mulcare MR. Identifying and initiating intervention for elder abuse and neglect in the emergency department. Clin Geriatr Med [Internet]. NIH Public Access. 2018;34(3):435. [cited 2023 Jul 12]. Available from: /pmc/articles/PMC6057151/
82. Milich MV, Suvorova KN, Shevarova VN. A case of pathomimesis. Vestn Dermatol Venerol. 1990;5:75–6.
83. Popescu MA, Diaconu D-J, Vicu R, Vasile S, Geantă M, Mîinea MM. Pathomimesis: psychiatric and medico-legal interference in dermatology. Rom J Leg Med. 2011;19:277–82.
84. Morey LC, Staff P. Personality Assessment Inventory™ Clinical Interpretive Report Client name: Sample Client. 1990.
85. Rogers R, Sewell KW, Martin MA, Vitacco MJ. Detection of feigned mental disorders. [Internet]. SAGE Publications. 2003;10(2):160–77. [cited 2023 Jul 18]. Available from: https://journals.sagepub.com/doi/abs/10.1177/1073191103010002007
86. Rogers R, Bender SD. Clinical assessment of malingering and deception [Internet]. [cited 2023 Jul 18]. Available from: https://www.routledge.com/Clinical-Assessment-of-Malingering-and-Deception/Rogers-Bender/p/book/9781462544189
87. Bass C, Wade DT. Malingering and factitious disorder. Pract Neurol. England. 2019;19(2):96–105.
88. Jakasa I, Thyssen JP, Kezic S. The role of skin barrier in occupational contact dermatitis. Exp Dermatol. Denmark. 2018;27(8):909–14.
89. Diepgen TL. Occupational skin diseases. JDDG: Journal der Deutschen Dermatologischen Gesellschaft [Internet]. Wiley Online Library. 2012;10(5):297–315. Available from: https://onlinelibrary.wiley.com/doi/10.1111/j.1610-0387.2012.07890.x
90. Gieler U, Consoli SG, Tomás-Aragones L, Linder DM, Jemec GBE, Poot F, et al. Self-inflicted lesions in dermatology: terminology and classification--a position paper from the European Society for Dermatology and Psychiatry (ESDaP). Acta Derm Venereol. Sweden. 2013;93(1):4–12.

Index

G. Angelini et al. (eds.), *Psychocutaneous Diseases*,
https://doi.org/10.1007/978-3-031-70296-9

GPSR Compliance

The European Union's (EU) General Product Safety Regulation (GPSR) is a set of rules that requires consumer products to be safe and our obligations to ensure this.

If you have any concerns about our products, you can contact us on ProductSafety@springernature.com

In case Publisher is established outside the EU, the EU authorized representative is:

Springer Nature Customer Service Center GmbH
Europaplatz 3
69115 Heidelberg, Germany

Batch number: 10732044

Printed by Printforce, the Netherlands